RENAL, METABOLIC AND UROLOGIC DISORDERS

MEDICINAL PLANTS FOR THE TREATMENT OF METABOLIC DISORDERS

PART 2

RENAL, METABOLIC AND UROLOGIC DISORDERS

Additional books and e-books in this series can be found on Nova's website under the Series tab.

RENAL, METABOLIC AND UROLOGIC DISORDERS

MEDICINAL PLANTS FOR THE TREATMENT OF METABOLIC DISORDERS

PART 2

ANABERTA CARDADOR MARTÍNEZ
VÍCTOR M. RODRÍGUEZ GARCÍA
PATRICIA MANZANO
AND
MARITZA ALONZO-MACÍAS
EDITORS

nova
Medicine & Health
New York

NOTICE TO THE READER

Library of Congress Cataloging-in-Publication Data

ISBN: 978-1-53618-061-9

Published by Nova Science Publishers, Inc. † New York

CONTENTS

PREFACE

This book provides a complete review of multiple metabolic disorders and the use of phytochemicals for their prevention and treatment. When describing each metabolic disorder, all authors describe the main health alterations, providing the most current figures and statistics worldwide; medicinal plants used in traditional medicine for its treatment and scientific information related to their potential to prevent or treat each condition. Authors also include a complete scientific background check, complete analysis of all phytochemicals recommended for each disorder, a description of the mechanism(s) of action and *in vivo* and/or *in vitro* studies. Within this volume, a series of 3 plant species, recommended to treat or prevent the previously described disorders, are presented with their botanical information, traditional use in different cultures and countries, and the available scientific information validating their health benefits. Besides, six main metabolic disorders are described, providing a full scientific background for its general understanding, and three study cases are presented, where metabolic disorders are analyzed and approached from different medical and pharmaceutical angles.

Chapter 1 – Obesity is a disease of multifactorial origin, but its well known that a sedentary lifestyle and consumption of high energy density food increase the probability of presenting this disease. Besides, obesity represents a risk factor for diabetes mellitus, hypertension, dyslipidemias, insulin resistance, cancer, and others. Its increased prevalence in both, developed and underdeveloped countries is recently related not only to lifestyle and food but also to genetic elements that can cause this metabolic disorder.

Chapter 2 – Hypertension or high blood pressure is a prevalent condition in the world. According to the World Health Organization, one out of five people is hypertensive. There are several drugs to treat hypertension, among them, vasorelaxants, diuretics, calcium modulators, and inhibitors of the angiotensin-converting enzyme are commonly used. This book chapters focused on the description of medicinal plants with inhibitory activity of the angiotensin-converting enzyme. The potential of plant extracts for the treatment of hypertension is continuously studied, and the possibility of finding new hypertensive drugs is constantly increasing.

Chapter 3 – From the point of view of public health, cancer is considered as a group of diseases whose primary feature is disorderly growth and dysfunction of the affected tissue. Still, these physiological and anatomical characteristics are regulated by the metabolism, which is adapted to allow cell survival. Throughout this review, the main metabolic alterations in the main types of cancer will be analyzed from the epidemiological point of view, focusing on specific metabolic or molecular markers of each, as well as the differences and/or similarities that characterize them. Also, the main compounds of plant extracts are also addressed, as well as promising natural therapies that are currently in clinical or pre-clinical evaluations that could add to current cancer therapies.

Chapter 4 – The study of medicinal plants today offers possible pharmacological agents for treatments of chronic degenerative diseases such as Alzheimer's with a more significant therapeutic effect and lower toxic effects than conventional therapies in force. However, the most significant limitation that still exists is to replicate the results obtained in the pre-clinical phase into the clinical phase, which implies time and money. It also concluded that natural compounds that have amphipathic characteristics and small molecular weight are the most viable candidates, for example, modified alkaloids and flavonoids, which exert a therapeutic multi-effect at various levels of Alzheimer's disease, mainly in the inhibition of key enzymes like acetyl and butyrylcholine esterase.

Chapter 5 – Authors of this chapter performed a literature review of PubMed®/ScienceDirect on March 15, 2019, using the following search items "Infectious diseases and cancer", "cancer of infectious origin." The authors (AOM, DM) screened titles and abstracts for relevance. Articles that did not include an abstract or full-text available in English or Spanish and original articles were excluded. The remaining publications that included information on infectious diseases and cancer were analyzed in-depth. After this literature research, sixteen scientific studies were selected and compared according to the WHO statistics in cancer.

Chapter 6 – The most studied parts of *Moringa oleifera* tree are leaves and seeds, either as extracts or as flours. These have shown to be effective against several conditions, including cancer, obesity, diabetes, hypercholesterolemia,

Parkinson, and Alzheimer's disease, among others. Phytochemicals are responsible for the observed effects with nutraceutical properties, such as polyphenols, carotenoids, glucosinolates, alkaloids, and phytosterols. This chapter describes the phytochemical profile found in all parts of the *Moringa oleifera* tree and the role they play as preventive and curative agents in high prevalence diseases.

Chapter 7 – Rue is used in cases of dysmenorrhoea (only in high doses is abortive), as a uterine stimulant, in gargles, in cases of angina, heart palpitations, pleurisy, respiratory complications, and cramps. Phytochemicals present in *Ruta* include furanocoumarins (bergapten, psoralen), flavonoids (rutin, quercetin), and alkaloids (skimmianine, isotaifine, taifine). These compounds have been studied for anticancer, antidiabetic, antioxidant, and anti-inflammatory activities. Moreover, because of the phototoxic activity of *Ruta* furanocoumarins, its extract has been used to treat psoriasis.

Chapter 8 – Ginger contains chemical constituents such as gingerol and shogaol, both with scientifically proven pharmacological and nutritive actions. In addition to its essential oil, pharmacological properties are also reported and employed in the cosmetic and food industries. The main objective of this chapter is to establish some physicochemical characteristics of the species commercialized in Ecuador, as well as to extract and characterize their essential oils and alcoholic extracts.

Chapter 9 – In this chapter, authors have addressed Parkinson's disease, one of the neurodegenerative diseases whose incidence and prevalence has increased in recent decades. Different hypotheses about its origin - from age to the intestinal microbiota - are presented, accompanied by various advances in their diagnosis.

In: Medicinal Plants …
Editors: A. Cardador Martínez et al.
ISBN: 978-1-53618-061-9

Chapter 1

OBESITY: A METABOLIC DISORDER

Ulisses Moreno-Celis*[1,*]*, Teresa García-Gasca*[1]*,
***Miriam Aracely Anaya-Loyola*[1]**
***and Víctor Manuel Rodríguez-García*[2]**

[1]Facultad de Ciencias Naturales, Universidad Autónoma de Querétaro, Queretaro, Mexico

[2]Regional Department of Bioengineering, Tecnologico de Monterrey, Queretaro, Mexico

ABSTRACT

Obesity is a disease of multifactorial origin but it is well known that a sedentary lifestyle and consumption of high energy density food increase the probability to present this disease. Besides, obesity represents a risk factor for diabetes mellitus, hypertension, dyslipidemias, insulin resistance, cancer, and others. Lipotoxicity or metabolic obesity refers to the alteration of adipose tissue alters disturbing the production of adipocytokines, which leads to chronic systemic inflammation that causes a disorder in its endocrine function; thus multiple tissues can present different types of lipotoxicity which are explained in detailed in this chapter. Its increased prevalence in both, developed and underdeveloped countries, is recently related not only to lifestyle and food, but also to genetic elements that can cause this metabolic disorder.

---

[*] Corresponding Author's Email: ulisses.moreno@uaq.mx.

Keywords: obesity, lipotoxicity, adipose tissue, adipocytokines, endocrinology

Introduction

Obesity is common in the world population, has been increasing in adults and children, and is accompanied by severe diseases such as Type 2 Diabetes Mellitus, cardiovascular diseases, and certain types of cancer (Kazak et al. 2017). Obesity is a disease of multifactorial origin. It is generated by different circumstances that predispose the prevalence of this pathology as such. One of the most important factors is the environment in which the individual develops (obesogenic environment). Others are a sedentary lifestyle and high energy density food consumption that generate a high probability of having this disease (Yang et al. 2008; Al-Hasani and Joost 2005). This disease is heterogeneous and can be expressed depending on the activated genes presenting at an early and old age. There are a large number of studies about this disease, most of which frame prevention at the genetic level, treatment, and a few address the social-economic control that can be had in a whole country.

Obesity occurs mainly in developed countries, although there has also been a significant increase in underdeveloped countries lately (AR et al. 2018; Kazak et al. 2017). The World Health Organization estimates 1.9 million overweight adults with a BMI higher than or equal to 25 kg/m2 of which 32% are obese with a BMI higher than or similar to 30 kg/m2 (Organización Mundial de la Salud 2017). Childhood obesity has also increased significantly after the passage of only one generation, that is, in 2010 only 43 million children were overweight and obese in developed countries, obtaining a prevalence in the year 1990. In 2010 the prevalence was 4.2% to 6.7% which tells us that the amount will increase to 60 million children with problems of overweight and obesity obtaining 9.1% by 2020 (Ulloa, Armeno, and Mazza 2017). The increase in prevalence is due to different factors, among the most important is the current lifestyle where physical activity is not encouraged from a young age and high energy density foods known colloquially as "junk food or fast food". Another less common factor but with great importance of study in recent years is the genetic load of each person contributing to the problem of overweight and obesity of 40-60% of the population and the different mutations of these (Ulloa, Armeno, and Mazza 2017).

Obesity is a chronic noncommunicable disease (NCD) that is characterized by abnormal or excessive accumulation of body fat (Dirección General de

Epidemiologia 2015), generating mainly deposition of ectopic lipids in organs such as liver, muscle and pancreas, causing atrophy and organic dysfunction, which can be considered as lipotoxicity (Avalos-Soriano et al. 2015). Its etiology is considered multifactorial and may coexist with other factors and be itself a risk factor for diabetes mellitus, hypertension, dyslipidemias, insulin resistance, cancer, and others (Gómez et al. 2013). The genetic component is part of the pathogenesis, not only by activating multiple obesity-related genes activated by environmental components, as well as genes encoding peptides aimed at transmitting hunger and satiety signals, genes involved in the growth and differentiation of adipocyte and genes involved in the control of energy expenditure (González 2011); but also, from the hereditary point of view, genetics have a great weight in the predisposition of obesity (Locke et al. 2015). For its part, the adipocyte can accumulate fatty acids (AG) when the energy intake is excessive and to mobilize them when the body requires energy to, in this way, meet physiological needs (Gutiérrez, Velázquez, and Prieto 2011). At lipotoxicity or metabolic obesity, adipose tissue alters the production of adipocytokines, which leads to chronic systemic inflammation that causes a disorder in its endocrine function (Flores Lázaro, Rodríguez Martínez, and Rivas Arancibia 2013), leading to macrophage infiltration into adipose tissue, mainly in visceral adipose tissue (García 2012). Lipotoxicity promotes the inhibition of insulin secretion by chronic increase in free FA.

Importance of Adipogenesis in the Development of Obesity

Undoubtedly, the ability to store energy has been crucial for the evolution of organisms. We can understand that the generation of specialized cells for this purpose, somehow promoted the subsistence of species and in the case of humans, the decrease in periods of famine, resulting from harvesting and hunting, and the establishment of a standard diet covering the necessary energy and nutritional needs, and promoted brain growth and development. In this development, adipocytes are the protagonists of being able to store triglycerides, providing energy at the necessary time. This process can occur due to hypertrophy (adipocyte growth due to lipid accumulation) and hyperplasia (generation of new adipocytes from mesenchymal cells).

The differentiation process by which multipotential precursor mesenchymal cells give rise to mature fat cells is known as adipogenesis. This occurs by the activation of a coordinated gene expression program mediated by transcription factors (C/EBPα and the γ receptor activated by the peroxisome proliferator (PPARγ) (Reusch, Colton, and Klemm 2000; Rosen et al. 2000), which leads to changes in the activity, in the amount, or both, of key proteins in the physiology of the adipocyte, such as those involved in the homeostasis of lipids and glucose. Interestingly, in experiments performed on mouse fibroblasts which do not express C/EBPα and are not sensitive to the effects of insulin, but with normal PPARγ activity they achieve adipogenesis, otherwise when PPARγ activity is blocked, and C is added /EBPα cells fail to differentiate, indicating that PPARγ uses multiple pathways to initiate adipose differentiation independent of C/EBPα, while this depends on the activity of PPARγ (Rosen et al. 2000).

Lipotoxicity

The adipocyte is a specialized cell and adapted to store energy in the form of lipids, mainly in the form of triglycerides, and dispose of them when physiological energy levels are low. The AGs of the TGs are released by a process called lipolysis in which the TG is hydrolyzed by the action of lipase in Diacylglycerols (DG) and Monoacylglycerols. It is well known that lipolysis in visceral adipose tissue is more active compared to other regions of the body, responding, among many others, to the effects of insulin, catecholamines, and adenosine, which results in an exacerbated release of fatty acids during obesity. And these travel through the portal circulation to the liver, pancreas, heart, kidneys and even brain promoting the typical complications of obesity (Arner 1995).

Lipotoxicity is the term coined to the process by which AG and fat accumulate ectopically, causing alterations in the cellular environment that can trigger organic dysfunction (Rodriguez Cuenca and Vidal Puig 2015; Murea et al. 2010). A high energy intake from food passes over the storage capacity of AG through adipose tissue promoting an increase in AGLs that being in the bloodstream are mainly captured by liver, pancreas, and muscle, and in these tissues their excessive accumulation will trigger the process of lipotoxicity by the ceramide route, lysosomal pathway, endoplasmic reticulum stress, oxidative stress and by Toll-like receptors; mentioned below briefly.

PROCESSES THAT LEAD TO THE DEVELOPMENT OF LIPOTOXICITY

Ceramides and Metabolic Alterations

It is well known the important activity of ceramides on metabolism; they have been related to metabolic diseases such as diabetes, cardiomyopathy, diabetes mellitus, arterial hypertension, and hepatic steatosis (Chaurasia and Summers 2015). Ceramides are precursors of sphingolipids; these are mainly produced by the degradation of saturated fats and proteins in the endoplasmic reticulum, and synthesized by a family of six ceramides synthases (CerS), that continue to posterior modifications through the Golgi apparatus until achieving its structural specialization in sphingomyelins, glucoceramides, cerebrides, and gangleosides. Several studies have shown that a decrease in ceramide levels favors the metabolic response to insulin, promotes the oxidation of fatty acids and decreases the inflammation of obesity (Aburasayn, Al Batran, and Ussher 2016; Chaurasia and Summers 2015). In studies conducted in knock-out mice for CerS5 (indispensable for C16: 0 sphingolipids) and fed on an obesogenic diet, it was observed that weight gain was reduced and insulin sensitivity increased (Gosejacob et al. 2016); in another experiment in which the mice were knock-out for CerS1 (produces 18: 0 ceramide) similar effects on insulin sensitivity in skeletal muscle were observed although no effects were observed altering CerS5 and CerS6 (Turpin-Nolan et al. 2019).

On the other hand, a study in humans showed that when performing 1 hour of exercise for 12 weeks 5 days a week, plasma levels of ceramides C14: 0, C16: 0, C18: 0, C18: 1, C20 were reduced: 0, C24: 0 and C24: 1, improving insulin response in diabetic people and decreasing body weight in people with obesity (Kasumov et al. 2015). In the same way, other studies have reported that ceramides inhibit Akt-mediated anabolic signaling, which prevents translocation to the cell membrane of Glut4 avoiding glucose uptake, as well as an increase in muscle tissue promoting resistance to insulin and involved in the oxidation of fatty acids (Summers and Goodpaster 2016).

Lysosome Instability Induces Lipotoxicity

The endosomal-lysosomal apparatus is responsible for the intracellular digestion of carbohydrates, proteins, nucleic acids, and internalized lipids from outside by different types of endocytosis, and intracellular material generated mainly by the autophagic process. The distinction between the different compartments of this device is based on their pH. The lysosome is the most acidic compartment where degradation of macromolecules occurs and its role in lipid metabolism has been clearly described. The lysosome captures extracellular lipids carried by LDL, VLDL, and chylomicrons through the cell's endocytic apparatus thus promoting its degradation; on the other hand, endogenous lipids reach the lysosome from processes such as autophagy (Jaishy and Abel 2016).

In hepatocytes treated with high concentrations of free fatty acids (FFA) it was observed that the Bax protein (known to generate pores that destabilize the mitochondrial membrane in the apoptosis process) is capable of being located in the lysosomal membrane and inducing its instability by promoting the output of the content of said cell compartment causing physiological damage to the cell; as well as an inflamed cell microenvironment (Feldstein et al. 2004). In another study, it was observed that lysosome structure damage induced by the accumulation of hepatic fatty acids occurs initially, even before mitochondrial damage, as well as its dependence on cathepsin B (Li et al. 2008). On the other hand, in rats with a high-fat diet, it was observed that there was an accumulation of phospholipids in the lysosomes of the proximal tubules of the kidney, which triggered enlargement of these structures, in the cells a stagnant and related autophagy process was observed. pH decrease induced by damage to lysosomal structures, which has also been observed with obese patients, improves as the degree of obesity decreases (Yamamoto et al. 2017).

Endoplasmic Reticulum Stress-Induced Lipotoxicity

The endoplasmic reticulum (ER) is among many other functions responsible for lipid biosynthesis, and the alteration of its homeostasis is highly related to metabolic alterations producing what is considered ER stress. This condition is considered an indisputable marker of metabolic syndrome, related to obesity and non-alcoholic fatty liver. In studies in laboratory animals, it has been shown that obesity-induced inflammation causes stress in the ER which in turn leads to abnormalities in insulin signaling through the hyper-phosphorylation of the JNK protein that subsequently phosphorylates aberrantly to the substrate of the insulin receptor 1 (IRS-1) and thus inhibiting its function and producing insulin resistance (Ozcan 2004; Akazawa and Nakao 2016). It has been observed in pancreatic cells that the ER stress is associated with a depletion of Ca^{2+} induced by the increased production of oleate and palmitate. Furthermore, studies have reported that especially in pancreatic cells β (main insulin producers), free fatty acids, saturated and unsaturated, induce a different signaling pathway when there is ER stress (Cnop et al. 2010). On the other hand, in liver cells it has been observed that a chronic stress of the ER leads to alterations in the lipid composition of this promoting inhibition in the sarco/endoplasmic reticulum calcium ATPase (SERCA) and it was shown that correction in the amount of lipid intake or overexpression of SERCA improves chronic ER stress and glucose homeostasis. The authors concluded that abnormalities in the metabolism of lipids and calcium are factors of great influence in liver disorders triggered by obesity (Fu et al. 2011). In a study conducted on 78 healthy people, tests were performed to determine the stress of the ER where positive correlations of these markers with BMI and the percentage of body fat were observed and concluded that in human adipose tissue with obesity there is activation of multiple markers of ER stress as a 6α transcription factor and JNK phosphorylation (Sharma et al. 2008). The above shows the importance of the integrity and activity of ER in metabolic processes related mainly to insulin resistance of different tissues in the lipotoxicity process which is highly associated with metabolic obesity.

Oxidative Stress and Obesity

The relationship of nutrition with oxidative stress is an issue that has been approached from different points of view to such a degree that a positive influence has been observed when there is a decrease in caloric intake on oxidative stress markers such as systemic inflation, aging, and inclusive adiposity. In this regard, the different approaches to the relationship between these processes will be mentioned during this section. In several studies a correlation between the amount of fat and the oxidative stress present has been observed, in experimental times it was observed that in the obese there was a greater number of reactive oxygen species (ROS); while in adipocyte cell cultures an increase in the activity of NADPH oxidase is observed and when these markers are inhibited, ROS concentrations decreased considerably (Furukawa et al. 2017).

Much of the ROS promoting oxidative stress in obesity comes from the formation, by adipocytes, of pro-inflammatory molecules called cytokines (TNF-α, IL-1, and IL6, among many others). These participate in the stimulation of macrophages and monocytes (high producers of reactive oxygen and nitrogen) and an increase in angiotensin II which promotes the activity of NADPH oxidase which is the main producer of ROS in fat cells; on the other hand, in hepatic mitochondria an excess in the oxidation of fatty acids causes an excess in the formation of ROS. Likewise, in the myocardium, the increase in oxygen consumption derived from an increase in body volume leads to an increase in the oxygen-dependent metabolic pathways that have the purpose of generating energy, whose route leads to the production of ROS, which can increase in turn an increase in peroxynitrite which leads to an increase in blood pressure; promoting higher consumption of cardiac and systemic energy stimulating metabolic activation and generating a vicious circle in the production of ROS (Fernández-Sánchez et al. 2011).

Lipotoxicity in Specific Organs

Hepatic Lipotoxicity

Without a doubt, the most alarming result of hepatic lipotoxicity is the development of non-alcoholic liver steatosis, which has as an etiology the exacerbated accumulation of lipids, mainly triglycerides and free fatty acids, which may come from the diet or as a result of adipocyte overload. Such lipids lead to an increase in inflammation of the liver as a consequence, in hypothesis "of an increase in oxidative stress caused by the increase in lipid peroxidation, although there is also the hypothesis of the development of the pathology regardless of the accumulation of triglycerides" (Neuschwander-Tetri 2010). It has been observed that among the main mechanisms involved in the development of the non-alcoholic fatty liver are ER stress, the signaling pathway mediated by c-Jun, JNK, and BH3, which broadly trigger mitochondrial and lysosome dysfunction. On the other hand, alterations induced by high concentrations of carbohydrates (glucotoxicity) lead to an increase in lipogenic pathways such as those mediated by acetyl-CoA carboxylase (ACC), the enzyme fatty acid synthase (FAS) or stearoyl-CoA desaturase-1 (SCD-1) which will lead to an increase in fatty acids and triglycerides in the hepatocyte and promoting insulin resistance and ER stress. The primary mediators for the development of liver lipotoxicity are free fatty acids, triglycerides, lysophosphatidylcholine, ceramides, free cholesterol and bile acids (Cazanave and Sanyal 2015).

The fatty acids that have shown more significant hepatotoxic effects are palmitate and oleate. On the one hand, it has been observed that mitochondrial activity and oxygen consumption are increased when hepatocytes (H4IIEC3) are treated with palmitate as well as the production of ROS is increased and cell death induced by mitochondrial apoptosis (Egnatchik et al. 2014). In another study with 3 hepatocyte cell lines (HepG2, HuH7, WRL68) it was observed that the addition of palmitate decreases the ability of cells to metabolize glucose, by affecting the signaling of insulin, increases apoptotic activity unlike oleic acid-treated cells in which the response was lower with the same concentrations (Ricchi et al. 2009). Similarly, it has been observed that the treatment of hepatocytes with oleate, another free fatty acid, promotes insulin resistance through the decrease of the signaling pathway involving p38/Akt/IRS1, which leads to alterations that result in the loss of signaling for the outsourcing of Glut4 (Liu et al. 2007). This allows us to have a broad view of the implications on the lipotoxicity of free fatty acids, whether they come from the diet or the release of adipose tissue due to the excess of these inside the cell or by the high amount of energy from carbohydrates. On the other hand, lysophosphatidylcholine is a product resulting from the metabolism of palmitate and it has been observed that said metabolite increases linearly as the concentration of palmitate, stearate or exogenous lysophosphatidylcholine increases and has been found in *in vitro* models that in the presence of lysophosphatidylcholine Apoptosis and the generation of stress in ER, is given by signaling pathways equal to those observed in the presence of palmitate, which suggests that the metabolic effects induced by free fatty acids are indirectly caused after conversion into their metabolites as is the case of lysophosphatidylcholine (Kakisaka et al. 2012).

Triglycerides are another type of lipid involved in the development of hepatic lipotoxicity, some studies have shown that accumulation of these occurs during the early stages of non-alcoholic liver steatosis, as well as being the main suppliers of fatty acids that carry to liver cell damage (Neuschwander-Tetri 2010; Akazawa and Nakao 2016) and it has been observed that in mice the inhibition of diacylglycerol acyltransferase 2 (final enzyme in the synthesis of triglycerides), prevents the development of hepatic steatosis but promotes an increase of free fatty acids in the liver; as well as other markers of inflammation and liver damage (Yamaguchi et al. 2007; Liu et al. 2007).

Muscle Lipotoxicity

As mentioned previously, the high caloric load of current diets leads to alterations in the mobilization and storage of energy by adipocytes, which releases lipids that accumulate in other organs such as muscle tissue. It has been observed that intramuscular lipids combined with a decrease in mitochondrial function, promote insulin resistance in muscle cells, leading to an alteration in glucose metabolism generating a decrease in the production of energy necessary for the activity and this has been related to high fat and hypercaloric diets (Schrauwen 2007). In the genetically obese mouse model (ob/ob) and another obese one through diet it was observed that intramuscular lipid levels were increased, but there was no apoptosis induced by them (Turpin et al. 2009). In another study where the participation of the carbohydrate-rich diet (sucrose) was compared against a high-fat diet in Wistar rats for 24 weeks, it was observed that the rats with the high-fat diet had more significant infiltration of lipids in the tissue muscle compared to the high carbohydrate diet (Masgrau et al. 2012). It has also been observed that exogenous ceramides promote the under-expression of the myogenin transcription factor through the inhibition of phospholipase D, as well as an increase in the apoptosis of muscle cells and the overexpression of lysophosphatidylcholine promotes a defective differentiation thereof both *in vivo* and *in vitro*; although the mechanisms *in vivo* are not consistent (Akhmedov and Berdeaux 2013).

Mitochondria, the main providers of cellular energy, are also the result of their large ROS-producing processes. The fatty acids accumulated near the mitochondria are especially prone to oxidation by ROS, which commonly leads to their peroxidation, which in turn generates that if they come into contact with the mitochondrial membrane they cause oxidative damage and causing their dysfunction. On the other hand, it has been observed that interventions focused on decreasing the amount of corporal fat such as physical training, loss of body weight and decreased caloric intake by fat; promote the reduction of levels of the UCP3 protein which is related to the oxidation of fatty acids (Schrauwen et al. 2010). As in hepatocytes, lipotoxic muscle cells also suffer from insulin resistance, which is mainly attributed to the alterations caused by free fatty acids. In this sense, in *in vitro* experiments on myotubes different fatty acids were tested for the purpose of seeing the effects of these and it was observed that palmitic and stearic acids decrease the anabolism of insulin-mediated glycogen, via Akt as well as aerobic and anaerobic glycolysis. As in the liver cells mitochondrial damage was observed. While on the other hand the tested unsaturated fatty acids showed no significant metabolic alterations (Schrauwen et al. 2010; Hirabara, Curi, and Maechler 2010).

Lipotoxicity in Pancreatic Cells

It has been mentioned above how there may be fat infiltration in tissues not suitable for this purpose, in this sense the pancreas is not exempt from such a process and it has been observed that at a higher percentage of fat of the individual and increase in serum lipid levels there is a higher pancreatic lipid content as well as an increase in insulin production, but a decrease in organic sensitivity to its signaling. On the other hand, in experiments on islets isolated from the pancreas, it was observed that there is a lipotoxic effect when they are treated with free fatty acids for periods of 24 to 48 hours. Similarly, in obese male ZDF rats, it was observed that there was infiltration of adipocytes in the pancreatic tissue, and these were associated with structural damage in these cells, which improved by decreasing the dietary intake of lipids and improving serum triglyceride levels (van Herpen and Schrauwen-Hinderling 2008). In other experiments on isolated islets, it was observed again that palmitate is the fatty acid that has the most significant effects on pancreatic alterations related to insulin production, but not with the medium-chain fatty acids such as octanate (Briaud et al. 2001). This once again shows how the accumulation of saturated long-chain fatty acids has great implications for lipid infiltration in different organs. In insulin resistance resulting from pancreatic lipotoxicity it has been observed that proliferative receptor activated by peroxisome alpha (PPARα) has great implications in the development of such a condition; in knock out times for PPARα and in the obese, genotype dysfunction was observed in pancreatic β cells associated with decreased insulin secretion after glucose stimulation. These observations were replicated in *in vitro* models with PPARα inhibitors (Lalloyer et al. 2006). On the other hand, from the molecular point of view, it has also been observed that palmitate activates signaling pathways mediated by PERK (Cunha et al. 2008) has been associated with pancreatic degeneration, and with the loss of β cells and development of diabetes mellitus followed by loss of glucagon-secreting α cells as well as reduction of digestive enzymes in the exocrine pancreas (Zhang et al. 2002).

Cardiac Lipotoxicity

The energy expenditure necessary for the functioning of the heart is mainly solved by the metabolism of fatty acids in said organ, but an increase in their availability is associated with cardiac dysfunction. In the heart muscle, lipids reach through chylomicrons and very-low-density lipoproteins (VLDL), which travel through the bloodstream and in the heart their fatty acids are released by the action of lipoprotein lipase, which is bound to the endothelium; while endogenous lipids are released by the hormone-sensitive lipase and adipocyte triglyceride lipase. Both processes are the main ways to generate energy substrates that solve 70% of the energy necessary for the functioning of the heart. On the other hand, it has been observed that the uptake of free fatty acids is mainly given by the CD36 cell membrane receptor, and it has been shown that in its absence the amount of free fatty acids in the cardiac tissue decreases. Although triglycerides are a marker of cardiac lipid overload, they have not been directly associated with the damage caused by their accumulation and again palmitate is considered the most effective in inducing lipotoxicity in that organ. Like ceramides, they are considered a marker of lipotoxicity in the heart which, by inhibiting its activity with drugs, corrects cardiac toxicity induced by lipids. In animal models of obesity it has been observed that the increase in the bioavailability of lipids in the heart muscle is due to an increase in the enzymes that oxidize triglycerides and in those that produce ceramides; these processes trigger apoptotic cell death induced by lipids or lipopoptosis (Zhou et al. 2000). The above has been associated with non-ischemic heart failure and severe metabolic dysregulation characterized by increased triglycerides in the cardiac muscle associated with contractile dysfunction (Sharma et al. 2004).

Renal Lipotoxicity

In humans approximately 3% of the total weight of the kidney corresponds to lipids, the majority being phospholipids of cell membranes and those with metabolic activity that mainly come from triglycerides and to a lesser extent free fatty acids. These are not entirely free since they are usually bound to albumin, by means of which they are transported through the blood plasma and are released from them by specific enzymes, and oxidation of these are the main source of energy in structures such as the proximal tubule, in which the glycolytic pathway is low and in the oxidation of free fatty acids most of the renal oxygen is used. The excessively administered fatty acids in the kidney are most often esterified to form triglycerides and form intracellular reservoirs of these (Bobulescu 2010). It has been observed that chronic kidney disease is characteristic that there is a deficiency of high-density lipoproteins (HDL), and decreased antioxidant and anti-inflammatory abilities (Vaziri 2010). In studies conducted in laboratory rats it was observed that after the ingestion of a high-fat diet there was a decrease in the glomerular filtration rate, perhaps due to the glomerular retraction response observed in the histological results; as well as an increase in the deposition of renal lipids and inflammatory cytokines (Muller et al. 2019).

Brain Lipotoxicity

The role of lipids in brain aging has recently been evaluated and it has been observed that very-long-chain fatty acids promote the loss of calcium balance, increase oxidative stress and deregulate mitochondrial homeostasis, which promotes among other things cell death. Mainly it has been seen that phytanic acid induces an increase in ROS and inhibition of protonic activity which leads to mitochondrial deregulation, translated into decreased energy production (ATP). Chronic exposure to said compound can trigger neuronal damage by altering the transcription and epigenetics of exposed brain cells (Muller et al. 2019). In studies in rats with a high-fat diet, it was observed that mainly cholesterol and phospholipids accumulate in the brain, but not triglycerides. It is well known that there is a relationship between cholesterol and neurodegenerative diseases and that the concentrations of intracerebral cholesterol are independent of those of plasma cholesterol, and it has been observed that statins can modulate their cerebral accumulation (Charradi et al. 2012).

Conclusion

Traditional definitions of obesity mainly focus on describing excess weight and in some cases excess body fat, but it has been observed that there are differences in the metabolic activity of fat according to the site of accumulation, with abdominal and inter-organic fat being more active than subcutaneous fat and causing alterations such as insulin resistance, changes in blood pressure and in biochemical markers of lipid metabolism (Reyes-márquez et al. 2017; Osama, Porramatikul, and Al-Ozairi 2006). This is why the specific study of lipotoxicity markers in key organs is of great importance when determining to predict the impact that fat accumulation has on the organism.

REFERENCES

Aburasayn, Hanin, Rami Al Batran & John R. Ussher. (2016). "Targeting Ceramide Metabolism in Obesity." *American Journal of Physiology-Endocrinology and Metabolism*, *311* (2), E423–35. https://doi.org/10.1152/ajpendo.00133.2016.

Akazawa, Yuko & Kazuhiko Nakao. (2016). "Lipotoxicity Pathways Intersect in Hepatocytes: Endoplasmic Reticulum Stress, c-Jun N-Terminal Kinase-1, and Death Receptors." *Hepatology Research*, *46* (10), 977–84. https://doi.org/10.1111/hepr.12658.

Akhmedov, Dmitry & Rebecca Berdeaux. (2013). "The Effects of Obesity on Skeletal Muscle Regeneration." *Frontiers in Physiology*, 4, (December), 1–12. https://doi.org/10.3389/ fphys.2013.00371.

Al-Hasani, Hadi & Hans-Georg Joost. (2005). "Nutrition-/Diet-Induced Changes in Gene Expression in White Adipose Tissue." *Best Practice & Research Clinical Endocrinology & Metabolism*, *19* (4), 589–603. https://doi.org/10.1016/j.beem.2005.07.005.

Arner, Peter. (1995). "Differences in Lipolysis between Human Subcutaneous and Omental Adipose Tissues." *Annals of Medicine*, *27* (4), 435–38. https://doi.org/10.3109/ 07853899709002451.

Avalos-Soriano, Anaguiven, Ricardo De La Cruz-Cordero, Francisco Josue López-Martínez, Jorge L. Rosado, Miguel Ängel Duarte-Vázquez & Teresa Garcia-Gasca. (2015). "Effect of a B-Hydroxyphosphonate Analogue of L-Carnitine on Insulin-Sensitive and Insulin-Resistant 3T3-L1 Adipocytes." *Pharmacology*, *96* (3–4), 99–106. https://doi.org/ 10.1159/000430919.

Bobulescu, Ion Alexandru. (2010). "Renal Lipid Metabolism and Lipotoxicity." *Current Opinion in Nephrology and Hypertension*, *19* (4), 393–402. https://doi.org/10.1097/ MNH.0b013e32833aa4ac.

Briaud, Isabelle, Jamie S. Harmon, Cynthia L. Kelpe, Venkatesh Babu G. Segu & Vincent Poitout. (2001). "Lipotoxicity of the Pancreatic $^{N}{}_{L}$ -Cell Is Associated Acids Into Neutral Lipids." *Diabetes*, *50* (339), 315–21. http://diabetes.diabetesjournals.org/content/50/2/ 315.short.

Cazanave, Sophie C. & Arun J. Sanyal. (2015). "Molecular Mechanisms of Lipotoxicity in Nonalcoholic Fatty Liver Disease." *Hepatic De Novo Lipogenesis and Regulation of Metabolism*, *65* (8), 101–29. https://doi.org/ 10.1007/978-3-319-25065-6_5.

Charradi, Kamel, Salem Elkahoui, Ines Karkouch, Ferid Limam, Fethy Ben Hassine & Ezzedine Aouani. (2012). "Grape Seed and Skin Extract

Prevents High-Fat Diet-Induced Brain Lipotoxicity in Rat." *Neurochemical Research*, *37* (9), 2004–13. https://doi.org/10.1007/s11064-012-0821-2.

Chaurasia, Bhagirath & Scott A. Summers. (2015). "Ceramides – Lipotoxic Inducers of Metabolic Disorders." *Trends in Endocrinology & Metabolism*, *26* (10), 538–50. https://doi.org/10.1016/j.tem.2015.07.006.

Cnop, M., Ladrière, L., Igoillo-Esteve, M., Moura, R. F. & Cunha, D. A. (2010). "Causes and Cures for Endoplasmic Reticulum Stress in Lipotoxic β-Cell Dysfunction." *Diabetes, Obesity and Metabolism*, *12*, (SUPPL. 2), 76–82. https://doi.org/10.1111/j.1463-1326.2010.01279.x.

Cunha, D. A., Hekerman, P., Ladriere, L., Bazarra-Castro, A., Ortis, F., Wakeham, M. C., Moore, F., et al. (2008). "Initiation and Execution of Lipotoxic ER Stress in Pancreatic -Cells." *Journal of Cell Science*, *121* (14), 2308–18. https://doi.org/10.1242/jcs.026062.

Dirección General de Epidemiologia. (2015). "*Sistema Nacional De Vigilancia Epidemiológica.*," [*National Epidemiological Surveillance System*] *43*. México. 2015. http://www.epidemiologia.salud.gob.mx/dgae/sinave/sinave_04.html#.

Egnatchik, Robert A., Alexandra K. Leamy, Yasushi Noguchi, Masakazu Shiota & Jamey D. Young. (2014). "Palmitate-Induced Activation of Mitochondrial Metabolism Promotes Oxidative Stress and Apoptosis in H4IIEC3 Rat Hepatocytes." *Metabolism: Clinical and Experimental*, *63* (2), 283–95. https://doi.org/10.1016/j.metabol.2013.10.009.

Feldstein, Ariel E., Nathan W. Werneburg, Ali Canbay, Maria Eugenia Guicciardi, Steven F. Bronk, Robert Rydzewski, Laurence J. Burgart & Gregory J. Gores. (2004). "Free Fatty Acids Promote Hepatic Lipotoxicity by Stimulating TNF-α Expression via a Lysosomal Pathway." *Hepatology*, *40* (1), 185–94. https://doi.org/10.1002/hep.20283.

Fernández-Sánchez, Alba, Eduardo Madrigal-Santillán, Mirandeli Bautista, Jaime Esquivel-Soto, Ángel Morales-González, Cesar Esquivel-Chirino, Irene Durante-Montiel, Graciela Sánchez-Rivera, Carmen Valadez-Vega & José A. Morales-González. (2011). "Inflammation, Oxidative Stress, and Obesity." *International Journal of Molecular Sciences*, *12* (5), 3117–32. https://doi.org/10.3390/ijms12053117.

Flores Lázaro, José Rolando, Erika Rodríguez Martínez & Selva Rivas Arancibia. (2013). "Consecuencias Metabólicas de La Alteración Funcional Del Tejido Adiposo En El Paciente Con Obesidad." [Metabolic Consequences of the Functional Alteration of the Adipose Tissue in the Obese Patient]. *Revista Médica Del Hospital General de México*, *74* (3), 157–65.

Fu, Suneng, Ling Yang, Ping Li, Oliver Hofmann, Lee Dicker, Winston Hide, Xihong Lin, Steven M. Watkins, Alexander R. Ivanov & Gökhan S. Hotamisligil. (2011). "Aberrant Lipid Metabolism Disrupts Calcium Homeostasis Causing Liver Endoplasmic Reticulum Stress in Obesity." *Nature*, *473* (7348), 528–31. https://doi.org/10.1038/nature09968.

Furukawa, Shigetada, Morihiro Matsuda, Shigetada Furukawa, Takuya Fujita, Michio Shimabukuro & Masanori Iwaki. (2017). "Increased Oxidative Stress in Obesity and Its Impact on Metabolic Syndrome Find the Latest Version : Increased Oxidative Stress in Obesity and Its Impact on Metabolic Syndrome." *The Journal of Clinical Investigation*, *114* (12), 1752–61. https://doi.org/10.1172/JCI200421625.1752.

García, Edgar. (2012). "Obesidad, Tejido Adiposo y Resistencia a La Insulina." [Obesity, Adipose Tissue and Insulin Resistance]. *Bioqímica Clínica*, *46*(2).

Gómez, Almudena, Liliana Perdomo, Óscar Escribano & Manuel Benito. (2013). "Papel Del Tejido Adiposo Blanco En Las Complicaciones Vasculares Asociadas a La Obesidad. [Role of White Adipose Tissue in Vascular Complications Associated with Obesity] "*Clínica e Investigación En Arteriosclerosis*, *25* (1), 26–34.

González, Emilio. (2011). "Genes y Obesidad: Una Relación Causa-Consecuencia." [Genes and Obesity: A Cause-Consequence Relationship]. *Endocrinología y Nutrición : Órgano de La Sociedad Española de Endocrinología y Nutrición*, *58* (9), 492–96. https://doi.org/10.1016/j.endonu.2011.06.004.

Gosejacob, Dominic, Philipp S. Jäger, Katharina Vom Dorp, Martin Frejno, Anne C. Carstensen, Monika Köhnke, Joachim Degen, Peter Dörmann & Michael Hoch. (2016). "Ceramide Synthase 5 Is Essential to Maintain C16:0-Ceramide Pools and Contributes to the Development of Diet-Induced Obesity." *Journal of Biological Chemistry*, *291* (13), 6989–7003. https://doi.org/10.1074/jbc.M115.691212.

Gutiérrez, Josafat, Mireya Velázquez & Bertha Prieto. (2011). "El Tejido Adiposo Como Órgano Maestro En El Metabolismo. [Adipose Tissue As a Master Organ in Metabolism]. *Revista de Endocrinologia y Nutrición*, 2011.

Herpen, N. A. van & Schrauwen-Hinderling, V. B. (2008). "Lipid Accumulation in Non-Adipose Tissue and Lipotoxicity." *Physiology and Behavior*, *94* (2), 231–41. https://doi.org/10.1016/j.physbeh.2007.11.049.

Hirabara, Sandro M., Rui Curi & Pierre Maechler. (2010). "Saturated Fatty Acid-Induced Insulin Resistance Is Associated with Mitochondrial

Dysfunction in Skeletal Muscle Cells." *Journal of Cellular Physiology*, *222* (1), 187–94. https://doi.org/10.1002/ jcp.21936.

Jaishy, Bharat & Dale Abel, E. (2016). "Lipids, Lysosomes, and Autophagy." *Journal of Lipid Research*, *57* (9), 1619–35. https://doi.org/10.1194/ jlr.r067520.

Jones, A. R., Tovee, M. J., Cutler, L. R., Parkinson, K. N., Ells, L. J., Araujo-Soares, V., Pearce, M. S., et al. (2018). "Health Effects of Overweight and Obesity in 195 Countries over 25 Years." *Yearbook of Paediatric Endocrinology*, September, 13–27. https:// doi.org/10.1530/ey.15.15.2.

Kakisaka, Keisuke, Sophie C. Cazanave, Christian D. Fingas, Maria E. Guicciardi, Steven F. Bronk, Nathan W. Werneburg, Justin L. Mott & Gregory J. Gores. (2012). "Mechanisms of Lysophosphatidylcholine-Induced Hepatocyte Lipoapoptosis." *American Journal of Physiology-Gastrointestinal and Liver Physiology*, *302* (1), G77–84. https://doi.org/ 10.1152/ajpgi.00301.2011.

Kasumov, Takhar, Thomas P. J. Solomon, Calvin Hwang, Hazel Huang, Jacob M. Haus, Renliang Zhang & John P. Kirwan. (2015). "Improved Insulin Sensitivity after Exercise Training Is Linked to Reduced Plasma C14:0 Ceramide in Obesity and Type 2 Diabetes." *Obesity*, *23* (7), 1414–21. https://doi.org/10.1002/oby.21117.

Kazak, Lawrence, Edward T. Chouchani, Gina Z. Lu, Mark P. Jedrychowski, Curtis J. Bare, Amir I. Mina, Manju Kumari, et al. (2017). "Genetic Depletion of Adipocyte Creatine Metabolism Inhibits Diet-Induced Thermogenesis and Drives Obesity." *Cell Metabolism*, *26* (4), 660-671.e3. https://doi.org/10.1016/j.cmet.2017.08.009.

Lalloyer, Fanny, Brigitte Vandewalle, Frédéric Percevault, Gérard Torpier, Julie Kerr-Conte, Maaike Oosterveer, Réjane Paumelle, et al. (2006). "Peroxisome Proliferator-Activated Receptor α Improves Pancreatic Adaptation to Insulin Resistance in Obese Mice and Reduces Lipotoxicity in Human Islets." *Diabetes*, *55* (6), 1605–13. https://doi.org/ 10.2337/db06-0016.

Li, Zheng Zheng, Michael Berk, Thomas M. McIntyre, Gregory J. Gores & Ariel E. Feldstein. (2008). "The Lysosomal-Mitochondrial Axis in Free Fatty Acid-Induced Hepatic Lipotoxicity." *Hepatology*, *47* (5), 1495–1503. https://doi.org/10.1002/ hep.22183.

Liu, Hui Yu, Qu Fan Collins, Yan Xiong, Fatiha Moukdar, Edgar G. Lupo, Zhenqi Liu & Wenhong Cao. (2007). "Prolonged Treatment of Primary Hepatocytes with Oleate Induces Insulin Resistance through P38 Mitogen-

Activated Protein Kinase." *Journal of Biological Chemistry*, *282* (19), 14205–12. https://doi.org/10.1074/jbc.M609701200.

Locke, Adam E., Bratati Kahali, Sonja I. Berndt, Anne E. Justice, Tune H. Pers, Felix R. Day, Corey Powell, et al. (2015). "Genetic Studies of Body Mass Index Yield New Insights for Obesity Biology." *Nature*, *518* (7538), 197–206. https://doi.org/10.1038/nature14177.

Masgrau, Aurélie, Anne Mishellany-Dutour, Hitoshi Murakami, Anne-Marie Beaufrère, Stéphane Walrand, Christophe Giraudet, Carole Migné, et al. (2012). "Time-Course Changes of Muscle Protein Synthesis Associated with Obesity-Induced Lipotoxicity." *The Journal of Physiology*, *590* (20), 5199–5210. https://doi.org/10.1113/ jphysiol.2012.238576.

Muller, Cynthia R., Ana Paula O. Leite, Rodrigo Yokota, Renata O. Pereira, Anna Laura V. Americo, Nilberto R. F. Nascimento, Fabiana S. Evangelista, Vera Farah, Manasses C. Fonteles & Patricia Fiorino. (2019). "Post-Weaning Exposure to High-Fat Diet Induces Kidney Lipid Accumulation and Function Impairment in Adult Rats." *Frontiers in Nutrition*, *6* (May), 1–8. https://doi.org/10.3389/fnut.2019.00060.

Murea, Mariana, Barry I. Freedman, John S. Parks, Peter A. Antinozzi, Steven C. Elbein & Lijun Ma. (2010). "Lipotoxicity in Diabetic Nephropathy: The Potential Role of Fatty Acid Oxidation." *Clinical Journal of the American Society of Nephrology: CJASN*, *5* (12), 2373–79. https://doi.org/10.2215/ CJN.08160910.

Neuschwander-Tetri, Brent A. (2010). "Hepatic Lipotoxicity and the Pathogenesis of Nonalcoholic Steatohepatitis: The Central Role of Nontriglyceride Fatty Acid Metabolites." *Hepatology*, *52* (2), 774–88. https://doi.org/10.1002/hep.23719.

Organización Mundial de la Salud. (2017). "OMS | Las 10 Principales Causas de Defunción." Who. 2017. http://www.who.int/mediacentre/factsheets/ fs310/es/index1.html.

Osama, Hamdy, Sriurai Porramatikul & Ebaa Al-Ozairi. (2006). "Metabolic Obesity: The Paradox Between Visceral and Subcutaneous Fat." *Current Diabetes Reviews*, *2* (4), 367–73. https://doi.org/10.2174/1573399810 602040367.

Ozcan, U. (2004). "Endoplasmic Reticulum Stress Links Obesity, Insulin Action, and Type 2 Diabetes." *Science*, *306* (5695), 457–61. https://doi.org/ 10.1126/science.1103160.

Reusch, J. E., Colton, L. A. & Klemm, D. J. (2000). "CREB Activation Induces Adipogenesis in 3T3-L1 Cells." *Molecular and Cellular Biology*, *20* (3), 1008–20. https://doi.org/ 10.1128/MCB.20.3.1008-1020.2000.

Reyes-márquez, Roberto, Beatriz Adriana Aguilar-Galarza, Miriam Aracely Anaya-Loyola, Ulisses Moreno-, Juana Elizabeth Elton-Puente, Miguel Lloret, Carlos F Sosa-Ferreyra & Teresa García-Gasca. (2017). "Metabolic Alterations in Mexican Young Adults: Sensitivity and Specificity Approaches between Anthropometric Parameters and Biochemical Markers." *Obesity & Weight Management*, no. June: 1–9.

Rodriguez Cuenca, Sergio & Antonio Vidal Puig. (2015). "Lipotoxicidad, Obesidad y Enfermedades Metabólicas. [Lipotoxicity, Obesity and Metabolic Diseases]" *Bioquímica de La Obesidad*, *56*, 1–10. http://www.sebbm.es/revista/ articulo.php?id=322&url=lipotoxicidad-obesidad-y-enfermedades-metabolicas Página.

Rosen, Evan D., Christopher J Walkey, Pere Puigserver & Bruce M Spiegelman. (2000). "Transcriptional Regulation of Adipogenesis Transcriptional Regulation of Adipogenesis." *Genes & Development*, *14*, 1293–1307. https://doi.org/10.1101/ gad.14.11.1293.

Schrauwen, Patrick. (2007). "High-Fat Diet, Muscular Lipotoxicity and Insulin Resistance." *Proceedings of the Nutrition Society*, *66* (1), 33–41. https://doi.org/10.1017/ S0029665107005277.

Schrauwen, Patrick, Vera Schrauwen-Hinderling, Joris Hoeks & Matthijs K.C. Hesselink. (2010). "Mitochondrial Dysfunction and Lipotoxicity." *Biochimica et Biophysica Acta - Molecular and Cell Biology of Lipids*, *1801* (3), 266–71. https://doi.org/10.1016/ j.bbalip.2009.09.011.

Sharma, Neeraj K., Swapan K. Das, Ashis K. Mondal, Oksana G. Hackney, Winston S. Chu, Philip A. Kern, Neda Rasouli, Horace J. Spencer, Aiwei Yao-Borengasser & Steven C. Elbein. (2008). "Endoplasmic Reticulum Stress Markers Are Associated with Obesity in Nondiabetic Subjects." *Journal of Clinical Endocrinology and Metabolism*, *93* (11), 4532–41. https://doi.org/10.1210/jc.2008-1001.

Sharma, Saumya, Adrogue, J. V., Leonard Golfman, Ivan Uray, John Lemm, Keith Youker, George P. Noon, Frazier, O. H. & Heinrich Taegtmeyer. (2004). "Intramyocardial Lipid Accumulation in the Failing Human Heart Resembles the Lipotoxic Rat Heart." *The FASEB Journal*, *18* (14), 1692–1700. https://doi.org/10.1096/fj.04-2263com.

Summers, Scott A. & Bret H. Goodpaster. (2016). "CrossTalk Proposal: Intramyocellular Ceramide Accumulation Does Modulate Insulin Resistance." *The Journal of Physiology*, *594* (12), 3167–70. https://doi.org/10.1113/JP271676.

Turpin-Nolan, Sarah M., Philipp Hammerschmidt, Weiyi Chen, Alexander Jais, Katharina Timper, Motoharu Awazawa, Susanne Brodesser & Jens C.

Brüning. (2019). "CerS1-Derived C18:0 Ceramide in Skeletal Muscle Promotes Obesity-Induced Insulin Resistance." *Cell Reports*, *26* (1), 1-10.e7. https://doi.org/10.1016/j.celrep.2018.12.031.

Turpin, S. M., Ryall, J. G., Southgate, R., Darby, I., Hevener, A. L., Febbraio, M. A., Kemp, B. E., Lynch, G. S. & Matthew, J. Watt. (2009). "Examination of 'lipotoxicity' in Skeletal Muscle of High-Fat Fed and Ob/Ob Mice." *Journal of Physiology*, *587* (7), 1593–1605. https://doi.org/10.1113/jphysiol.2008.166033.

Ulloa, María Eugenia, Marisa L Armeno & Carmen S Mazza. (2017). "Obesidad Monogenica." [Monogenic obesity]. *Medicina Infantil*, XXIV, 294–302. http://www.medicinainfantil.org.ar/images/stories/volumen/2017/xxiv_3_294.pdf.

Vaziri, Nosratola D. (2010). "Lipotoxicity and Impaired High Density Lipoprotein-Mediated Reverse Cholesterol Transport in Chronic Kidney Disease." *Journal of Renal Nutrition*, *20* (5), S35–43. https://doi.org/10.1053/j.jrn.2010.05.010.

Yamaguchi, Kanji, Liu Yang, Shannon McCall, Jiawen Huang, Xian Yu Xing, Sanjay K. Pandey, Sanjay Bhanot, Brett P. Monia, Yin Xiong Li & Anna Mae Diehl. (2007). "Inhibiting Triglyceride Synthesis Improves Hepatic Steatosis but Exacerbates Liver Damage and Fibrosis in Obese Mice with Nonalcoholic Steatohepatitis." *Hepatology*, *45* (6), 1366–74. https://doi.org/10.1002/hep.21655.

Yamamoto, Takeshi, Yoshitsugu Takabatake, Atsushi Takahashi, Tomonori Kimura, Tomoko Namba, Jun Matsuda, Satoshi Minami, et al. (2017). "High-Fat Diet–Induced Lysosomal Dysfunction and Impaired Autophagic Flux Contribute to Lipotoxicity in the Kidney." *Journal of the American Society of Nephrology*, *28* (5), 1534–51. https://doi.org/10.1681/ ASN.2016070731.

Yang, Gonghuan, Lingzhi Kong, Wenhua Zhao, Xia Wan, Yi Zhai, Lincoln C. Chen & Jeffrey P. Koplan. (2008). "Emergence of Chronic Non-Communicable Diseases in China." *Lancet (London, England)*, *372* (9650), 1697–1705. https://doi.org/10.1016/ S0140-6736(08)61366-5.

Zhang, P., McGrath, B., Li, S.'a., Frank, A., Zambito, F., Reinert, J., Gannon, M., Ma, K., McNaughton, K. & Cavener, D. R. (2002). "The PERK Eukaryotic Initiation Factor 2 Kinase Is Required for the Development of the Skeletal System, Postnatal Growth, and the Function and Viability of the Pancreas." *Molecular and Cellular Biology*, *22* (11), 3864–74. https://doi.org/10.1128/mcb.22.11.3864-3874.2002.

Zhou, Y. T., Grayburn, P., Karim, A., Shimabukuro, M., Higa, M., Baetens, D., Orci, L. & Unger, R. H. (2000). "Lipotoxic Heart Disease in Obese Rats: Implications for Human Obesity." *Proceedings of the National Academy of Sciences*, *97* (4), 1784–89. https://doi.org/10.1073/pnas.97.4.1784.

In: Medicinal Plants …
Editors: A. Cardador Martínez et al.
ISBN: 978-1-53618-061-9

Chapter 2

Medicinal Plants with the Potential to Treat Hypertension: Studies That Were Done in the Last Decade

Anaberta Cardador-Martínez[*]
Regional Department of Bioengineering, Tecnologico de Monterrey, Queretaro, Mexico

Abstract

Hypertension or high blood pressure is a prevalent condition in the world. According to the World Health Organization, one out of five people is hypertensive. There are several drugs to treat hypertension, among them, vasorelaxants, diuretics, calcium modulators, and inhibitors of the angiotensin-converting enzyme are commonly used. The angiotensin-converting-enzyme is a key part of the system renin-angiotensin. The main role of this enzyme is to hydrolyze Angiotensin 1 into Angiotensin 2; the last is bond to blood vessel receptors causing vasoconstriction, then hypertension. Inhibitors of the angiotensin-converting enzyme are very effective, however, they present adverse effects such as cough. To substitute inhibitors, several plant extracts containing diverse phytochemicals have been proved. This book chapters focused on the description of medicinal plants with inhibitory activity of the angiotensin-converting enzyme. Besides, plant extracts have been proved as vasorelaxants. The potential of plant extracts for the treatment of

[*] Corresponding Author's Email: mcardador@tec.mx.

hypertension is continuously studied, and the possibility to find new hypertensive drugs is continuously increasing.

Keywords: hypertension, vasorelaxation, angiotensin enzyme, ACE inhibitors, plant extracts, phytochemicals

INTRODUCTION

Hypertension, also known as high or raised blood pressure, is a condition in which the blood vessels have persistently raised pressure. Each time the heartbeats, it pumps blood into the vessels. Blood pressure is created by the force of blood pushing against the walls of blood vessels (arteries) as the heart pumps it. The higher the pressure, the harder the heart must pump. Then, hypertension is defined as systolic blood pressure values ≥140 mmHg and/or diastolic blood pressure values ≥90 mmHg. The same values are used in younger, middle-aged, and older people. For children and teenagers, blood pressure centiles are used in children and teenagers, in whom data from interventional trials are not available.

According to WHO (2019) one out of five people suffers from hypertension, which means that 1.3 billion people in the world are hypertensive. The overall prevalence of hypertension among U.S. adults is 29.0%, and it increases to 64.9% in adults aged 60 years or older (Qaseem et al. 2017).

In the early 21st century, hypertension is a global public health issue; hypertension contributes to the burden of heart disease, stroke and kidney failure, and premature death and disability. Hypertension is known as a silent killer. Nearly one-third of people who have hypertension do not know it. On the other hand, hypertension is both preventable and treatable.

Causes of Hypertension

The exact causes of high blood pressure are not known, but several things may play a role, including smoking, overweight or obesity, lack of exercise, too much salt in the diet, stress, older age, among others. For many cases of hypertension, the underlying causes are unknown; then, this kind is called essential hypertension (Bilanda et al. 2017). Some risk factors have been linked to essential hypertension, such as familiarity, race, and age. For instance, blacks are more at risk to develop hypertension than whites.

Syndromes Associated with Hypertension

Atherosclerosis

One of the most severe health problems related to untreated high blood pressure is atherosclerosis or plaque build-up in the arteries. When those blockages occur in the arteries that supply blood to the heart muscle, the result is called coronary artery disease. People with high blood pressure are more likely to develop coronary artery disease because high blood pressure puts added force against the artery walls. Over time, this extra pressure can damage the arteries, making them more vulnerable to the narrowing and plaque buildup associated with atherosclerosis (Dzau 1990, Li and Chen 2005).

Stroke

Hypertension puts the arteries under constant stress. When there is too much force inside the blood vessels, damages the artery walls can occur and makes them weaker. After a wall vessel is more fragile, it can tear or burst causing bleeding, and then a hemorrhagic stroke. Stroke causes and hemodynamic consequences are heterogeneous which makes the management of blood pressure in stroke patients complex requiring accurate diagnosis and precise definition of therapeutic goals (Wajngarten and Silva 2019).

Heart Failure

This syndrome means that the heart's pumping power is weaker than normal, or the heart has become less elastic. With heart failure, blood moves through the heart's pumping chambers less effectively, and pressure in the heart increases, making it harder for the heart to deliver oxygen and nutrients to the body. As a response, the heart's chambers respond by stretching to hold more blood, keeping blood moving. But at last, the heart muscle walls may weaken and become unable to pump as strongly. Hypertension contributes to systolic and diastolic dysfunction. Activation of the sympathetic nervous system and the renin-angiotensin system is a key contributing factor of hypertension, and thus interventions that antagonize these systems promote regression of hypertrophy and heart failure (Kannan and Janardhanan 2014).

Kidney

Hypertension can cause damage to the blood vessels and filters in the kidney, making removal of waste from the body difficult. Once a person is diagnosed with end-stage renal disease, dialysis - a blood-cleansing process - or kidney transplantation is necessary. Hypertension is the second most common cause of chronic kidney disease and is a potentiator of kidney failure when accompanying disease. Chronic kidney disease is a common cause of resistant hypertension (Sternlicht and Bakris 2017).

Eye

Untreated high blood pressure can also affect the eyesight and lead to eye disease. Hypertension can cause damage to the blood vessels in the retina, the area at the back of the eye where images focus. This eye disease is known as hypertensive retinopathy. The damage can be serious if hypertension is not treated. Hypertensive retinopathy refers to retinal microvascular signs that develop in response to raised blood pressure. Signs of hypertensive retinopathy are frequently seen in adults 40 years and older, and are predictive of incident stroke, congestive heart failure, and cardiovascular mortality, independently of traditional risk factors. Hypertension is also a major risk factor for the development of other retinal vascular diseases, such as retinal vein and artery occlusion and ischemic optic neuropathy (Wong and Mitchell 2007).

Diabetes damages arteries and makes them targets for hardening, leading to atherosclerosis. That can cause high blood pressure, which, if not treated, can lead to troubles such as blood vessel damage, heart attack, and kidney failure. Hypertension and diabetes are two of the leading risk factors for atherosclerosis and its complications, including heart attacks and strokes. There is a substantial overlap between diabetes and hypertension, reflecting considerable overlap in their etiology and disease mechanisms (Cheung and Li 2012, Sun et al. 2019).

Pharmacological Treatment of Hypertension

Appropriate management of hypertension reduces the risk of cardiovascular disease, renal disease, cerebrovascular disease, and death (Qaseem et al. 2017).

Treatments for hypertension include lifestyle modifications, such as weight loss, dietary modification, and increased physical activity. Many therapeutic agents can be used for the pharmacologic management of hypertension. Some examples are thiazide-type diuretics, angiotensin-converting enzyme inhibitors (ACEIs), angiotensin-receptor blockers (ARBs), and calcium.

Loop diuretics favor water secretion at Henle loop, decreasing blood volume and therefore, reduces blood pressure. Several drugs act as loop diuretics, for instance, carbonic anhydrase inhibitors, which specific mechanism of action is the inhibition of proximal convoluted tubule sodium bicarbonate reabsorption, while thiazide-type diuretics inhibit Na/Cl cotransport in distal convoluted tubule (Jentzer, DeWald, and Hernandez 2010).

Angiotensin-converting enzyme inhibitors are high blood pressure drugs that widen or dilate the blood vessels to improve the amount of blood the heart pumps and to lower blood pressure. ACE inhibitors also increase blood flow, which helps to decrease the amount of work the heart must do and can help protect the kidneys from the effects of hypertension. However, ACE inhibitors show side effects such as cough, dizziness, itchy skin, among others.

HERBAL TREATMENT OF HYPERTENSION

The search for antihypertensive agents from plant origin has evolved in the last decades. Table 1 enlists several plants that have been used as a source for secondary metabolites to treat hypertension during the past decade.

Abdel-Zaher et al. (2018) and evaluated a standardize leaf extract of ginkgo biloba in hypertensive rats induced by L-NAME. The evaluated extract produced progressive reductions in the systolic, diastolic and mean arterial blood pressure. Moreover, the ginkgo biloba extract increased the progressive reductions in blood pressure induced by losartan, a competitive inhibitor of angiotensin II receptors. The final effect of ginkgo biloba extract was to protect against hypertension-induced renal injury. The same model of L-NAME hypertensive rats was used by Aekthammarat, Pannangpetch, and Tangsucharit (2019) to evaluate moringa leaf extracts. attenuated high BP, improved endothelium-dependent vasorelaxation and blunted adrenergic-mediated vasoconstriction in L-NAME hypertensive rats. Moringa extract treatment also reduced oxidative stress in both systemic and vascular compartments in hypertensive rats. Additionally, this extract exerted endothelium-dependent vasorelaxation in hypertensive resistance arteries.

Azadirachta indica is a plant with potential antioxidant and antihypertensive activity. In this sense, Omóbòwálé et al. (2019) evaluated a polyphenol-rich fraction of *A. indica* in L-NAME hypertensive rats. Their findings indicated that markers of oxidative stress (malondialdehyde, protein carbonyl) increased significantly while there was a reduction in glutathione level, activities of superoxide dismutase, glutathione peroxidase and glutathione-S-transferase as well nitric oxide bioavailability. All these activities were attributed to polyphenols.

Bidens pilosa is a plant that is used in traditional medicine to treat several diseases, for instance, hypertension. An ethyl acetate extract of *B. pilosa* was used in L-NAME hypertensive rats to decrease high arterial blood pressure from 166.18 to 110.03 mmHg. The antihypertensive activity of *B. pilosa* was related to its flavonoid content (Bilanda et al. 2017).

Table 1. Plants used in the treatment of hypertension

Plant	Kind of extract	Model	References
Ginko biloba	Leaf extract	hypertension-induced renal injury in rats	(Abdel-Zaher et al. 2018)
Moringa oleifera	Leaf extract	Hypertensive rats	(Aekthammarat, Pannangpetch, and Tangsucharit 2019)
Clove	Extract	streptozotocin-induced diabetic rats	(Akila et al. 2018)
Thymus linearis	Aqueous-methanolic extract of aerial parts	Vasorelaxation of coronary arteries	(Alamgeer et al. 2018)
Bidens pilosa	Ethylene acetate extract	L-NAME-induced hypertensive rats	(Bilanda et al. 2017)
Leersia hexandra	Aqueous Extract	Ethanol-Induced Hypertensive rats	(Bilanda et al. 2019)
Carthamus tinctorius	Extract	Improvement of hemodynamic and vascular alteration in rats	(Bunbupha et al. 2018)
Xenophyllum poposum	Hydroalcoholic extract	Hypertensive rats	(Cifuentes et al. 2018)
Euterpe oleraceas	Seeds Extract	Renovascular Hypertensive Rats	(Da Costa et al. 2017)
Polygonum hydropiper	Young leaves extract	High-salt induced hypertensive mice	(Devarajan et al. 2018)
Tartary buckwheat	Flavonoid extract	spontaneously hypertensive rats	(Hou et al. 2017)
Azadirachta indica	Polyphenol-Rich Fraction	Nω-Nitro-L-Arginine Methyl Ester-Induced Hypertension	(Omóbòwálé et al. 2019)
Citrus extracts	Flavonoids	Spontaneously hypertensive rats	(Paredes et al. 2018)

One of the most important complications of diabetes is diabetic nephropathy, which contributes to high blood pressure. Diabetic nephropathy is also related to oxidative stress. To treat diabetes, one of the must use drugs is metformin, not only because it improves the way the body uses insulin but also because it has antioxidant properties. Akila et al. (2018) evaluated clave extracts; their objective was to find a natural extract with similar properties to metformin. The model used was streptozotocin-diabetic rats, which after administration of clove extract or metformin, showed a reduction in renal injuries suggesting a neuroprotective effect attributed to modulation of oxidative status.

The decoction of *Thymus linearisas* herbal tea is traditionally used for the treatment of indigestion and hypertension. The aqueous-methanolic extract f *Thymus* elicited relaxation in coronary artery rings with and without endothelium in a dose-dependent way. The relaxation effect is attributed to thymol and carvacrol, the main constituents of *Thymus* extracts (Alamgeer et al. 2018).

Hypertension can be induced in rats by oral administration of ethanol. This model was used by Bilanda et al. (2019) to test *Leersia hexandra* aqueous extract of the leaves and stems. The administration of 100-200 mg aqueous extract /kg resulted in a reduction of systolic and diastolic blood pressure, comparable to that of nifedipine.

Renovascular hypertension due to one kidney ischemia is a widely used model of chronic hypertension that resembles secondary hypertension in humans. According to Bunbupha et al. (2018), the administration of 500mg/kg/day of *Carthamus tinctorius* L. extract to hypertensive rats decrease significantly blood pressure, in a similar way than captopril. It was suggested that *C. tinctorius* extract meliorated hemodynamic alteration and vascular remodeling in 2K-1C hypertensive rats. Using the same model of renovascular hypertension, da Costa et al. (2012) evaluated the hypotensive effect of polyphenols present in the seed of *Euterpe oleracea* Mart. a fruit commonly known as acai. Besides, acai extracts prevent the endothelial dysfunction and vascular structural changes in 2K-1C hypertension, probably through mechanisms involving antioxidant effects, and NOS activation.

Xenophyllum poposum is an endemic plant from The Andean mountains, it is used as a traditional treatment for altitude sickness. Based on this, (Cifuentes et al. 2018), evaluated an hydroalcoholic extract on hypertensive rats. Their results showed the ability of *X. poposum* to induce vasorelaxation, decrease blood pressure, heart rate and vascular response. The possible action mechanism may include action through the endothelial nitric oxide synthase, as well as calcium channel blocker (Da Costa et al. 2017).

MODELS USED TO EVALUATE THE ANTIHYPERTENSIVE EFFECT

Several models, both *in vitro* and *in vivo* have been used to test the hypertensive activity of plant extracts. *In vitro* models include the use of tissues such as the thoracic aortic ring. The aorta rings are usually isolated from Sprague Dawley rats (Ameer et al. 2009, Ch'ng et al. 2018, Senejoux et al. 2010).

The search for the antihypertensive activity of plants used *in vivo* models with both, animals and humans. Mice, rats, and guinea pigs have been used to assessed reduction in blood pressure, vasorelaxation, and prevention of infarction related to high blood pressure (Ameer et al. 2009, Fang et al. 2017, Haydari et al. 2017, Ibrar et al. 2019, Joukar et al. 2017, Salami et al. 2018).

Table 2 describes several models used to evaluate the antihypertensive activity of plant extracts.

Table 2. Different models used to evaluate plant extracts for antihypertensive activity

Model	Extract Source	Reference
Two-kidney one-clip (2K1C) Goldblatt model	*Gastrodia elata*	(Fang et al. 2017)
	Crataegus azarolus	(Haydari et al. 2017)
Thoracic aortic ring from Sprague Dawley rat	*Swietenia macrophylla*	(Ch'ng et al. 2018)
	Inula viscosa	(Hakkou et al. 2017)
	Angelica decursiva	(Kim et al. 2017)
	Ziziphora clinopodioides	(Senejoux et al. 2010)
	Canarium odontophyllum	(Basri et al. 2018)
	Macrosolen cochinchinensis	(Ameer et al. 2009)
Spontaneously hypertensive rats	*Tartary buckwheat*	(Hou et al. 2017)
	Swietenia macrophylla	(Ch'ng et al. 2018)
	Artemisia afra	(Tata et al. 2018)
	Leonotis leonurus	(Tata et al. 2018)
	Urtica dioica	(Vajic et al. 2018)

Model	Extract Source	Reference
Guinea pig	*Holarrhena floribunda*	(Kpegba et al. 2018)
Ethanol-Induced Hypertension in Wistar rat	*Leersia hexandra*	(Bilanda et al. 2019)
L-NAME-hypertensive rats	*Bidens pilosa*	(Bilanda et al. 2017)
	Artemisia campestris	(Dib et al. 2017)
	Inula viscosa	(Hakkou et al. 2017)
	Parkia speciosa	(Kamisah et al. 2017)
	Tridax procumbens	(Salami et al. 2018)
	Senecio serratuloides	(Tata et al. 2019)
High-salt induced hypertensive mice	*Polygonum hydropiper*	(Devarajan et al. 2018)
	Moringa stenopetala	(Fekadu et al. 2017)
Fructose-induced hypertensive rats	*Monascus purpureus*	(Hsieh and Tai 2003)
Isoproterenol hydrochloride myocardial infarction in rats	*Paeonia emodi*	(Ibrar et al. 2019)
Dexamethasone-induced hypertension in Male Wistar rats	*Juglans regia*	(Joukar et al. 2017)
Administration of angiotensin II in mice	*Malva parviflora*	(Lagunas-Herrera et al. 2019)
Human model	*Lycopersicon esculentum*	(Krasińska et al. 2018, Krasinska et al. 2018)
	Gastrodia elata-notoginseng	(Dengqin et al. 2018)

Thoracic Aortic Ring

The seeds of *Swietenia macrophylla* King are used in traditional medicine against hypertension. Ch'ng et al. (2018) demonstrated that a 50% ethanolic extract was able to reduce hypertension in a thoracic aortic ring isolated from Sprague-Dawley rat model. The reduction of blood pressure was related to vasorelaxation of the aorta.

Ziziphora clinopodioides Lam. (ZC) is widely used in Uyghur folk medicine for the treatment of hypertension diseases in Xinjiang, an autonomous region of China. An extract of *Ziziphora clinopodioides* as evaluated in the thoracic aortic ring model, exhibited endothelium-independent vasodilating properties that are mediated by inhibition of extracellular Ca^{2+} influx through the voltage and receptor-operated Ca^{2+} channels; therefore *Ziziphora clinopodioides* Lam. is a source of vasoactive compounds (Senejoux et al. 2010).

Another plant that has been tested in the thoracic aorta ring model is *Canarium odontophyllum*. The aqueous extract of this plant had a vasorelaxant effect in an endothelium-independent way, possibly mediated through the blockade of voltage-dependent calcium channel and receptor-operated calcium channel, suggesting that *C. odontophyllum* could be an alternative treatment for hypertension and other cardiovascular diseases (Basri et al. 2018).

Methanol and water extracts from the fresh aerial parts *Macrosolen cochinchinensis* had the ability to relax the vascular smooth muscle at a concentration of 0.5, 1 and 2 mg/mL. extracts obtained from *M. cochinchinensis*. Moreover, polar and non-polar extracts of *M. conchinchinesis* contains enough levels of active constituents that can inhibit isolated rat aortic rings contraction (Ameer et al. 2009).

Spontaneously Hypertensive Rat

Spontaneously hypertensive rat strains have been used to study heart failure for many years. The spontaneously hypertensive-heart failure strain is one of the more commonly used strains, with progressive left ventricular hypertrophy evident over the first 9 months of life, progressing to systolic dysfunction by 12 or more months. In such a model, *Tartary buckwheat* flavonoids fraction was tested, and blood pressure, mesenteric arteriolar vasorelaxation, superoxide anion (O2-) generation, NAD(P)H oxidase activity, and insulin-stimulated Akt/endothelial nitric oxide synthase activation and nitric oxide (NO) production were determined. A group of normotensive rats was used as a control. The treatment with buckwheat extract, at a dosage of 100 mg/kg/day significantly reduced systolic blood pressure and increased vasodilator response to insulin in the spontaneously hypertensive rats. Moreover, buckwheat flavonoids reduced the overproduction of basal O^{2-} in association with a reduction of NAD(P)H oxidase activity in mesenteric arterioles of the spontaneously hypertensive rats (Hou et al. 2017).

Artemisia afra and *Leonotis leonurus* are common plants used in African traditional medicine. Tata et al. (2018) evaluated hydro-ethanolic extracts of these plants in Sprague-Dawley rats. The administered doses varied between 10-1000 mg/kg. Both plants extracts reduced blood pressure significantly.

Furthermore, *A. afra* and *L. leonorus*, reduced the heart rate, suggesting an interaction of phytochemicals with β-adrenergic receptors.

Among other plant extracts evaluated in the spontaneously hypertensive rat model is *Urtica dioica.* This plant is commonly used to obtain fibers, but also phytochemicals such as phenolics can be obtained. Aerial parts and rhizome of *U. dioica* were evaluated by Vajic et al. (2018), their results showed that extracts reduced systolic and diastolic blood pressure, as well as the cardiac index. Additionally, extracts showed high antioxidant activity, increasing the activity of superoxide dismutase and catalase, without changing the concentration of the enzymes.

L-NAME Hypertensive Rats

N omega-Nitro-L-arginine methyl ester hydrochloride (L-NAME) is a widely used inhibitor of nitric oxide synthase (NOS) activity both *in vitro* and *in vivo.* Acute and chronic L-NAME treatment leads to changes in blood pressure and vascular reactivity due to decreased nitric oxide (NO) bioavailability (Kopincova, Puzserova, and Bernatova 2012). A usual dose of L-NAME to induce hypertension in rats is 50 mg/kg/day, orally (Abdel-Rahman et al. 2017).

A Roselle-Olive combination consisting of 226 mg hydro alcoholic powdered extract from calyxes of *Hibiscus sabdariffa* and 113 mg hydro alcoholic powdered extract from leaves of *Olea europaea* as active ingredients were administered to L-NAME hypertensive rats. The blood pressure of rats decreased significantly in treated rats in a similar way than lisinopril (Abdel-Rahman et al. 2017).

Reduction in blood pressure in L-NAME rats was achieved by the administration of *Artemisia campestris* due to its hypotensive and vasorelaxant effect, which is mediated via calmodulin-NO-cGC-PKG pathway, and via inhibition of calcium influx through voltage-operated calcium channels and activation of intracellular calcium mobilization into the sarcoplasmic reticulum (Dib et al. 2017).

Hakkou et al. (2017) proved that an extract of *Inula viscosa* is able to reduce blood pressure, its antihypertensive effect is predominantly mediated by an endothelium-dependent vasodilatory effect.

Parkia speciosa Hassk is a plant found abundantly in the Southeast Asia region, in which pods are used in traditional medicine to treat hypertension. On the other hand, nicardipine is a drug with antihypertensive activity. *Parkia speciosa* methanolic extract and nicardipine treatments had significantly prevented the elevations of blood pressure, angiotensin-converting enzyme, NADPH oxidase activities and lipid peroxidation in the heart induced by the L-NAME. *Parkia speciosa* extract but not nicardipine prevented the reduction in plasma nitric oxide level caused by L-NAME (Kamisah et al. 2017).

Other plants that had been tested for antihypertensive activity in L-NAME hypertensive rats are *Tridax procumbens* (Salami et al. 2018) and *Senecio serratuloides* (Tata et al. 2019). Aqueous leaf extract of *Tridax procumbens* reduced the mean arterial blood pressure of L-NAME treated rats significantly and also enhanced cavernosal tissue relaxation. This relaxation activity may be mediated partly through the NO pathway (Salami et al. 2018). On the other hand, *Senecio serratuloides*, a plant used in folk medicine for treating hypertension, skin disorders, internal and external sores, rashes, burns, and wounds, not only reduces systolic and diastolic blood pressure but also low-density lipoprotein cholesterol and triglycerides levels. Furthermore, the hydroethanolic extract of *S. serratuloides* was able to prevent a decrease in high-density lipoprotein cholesterol and serum nitric oxide concentrations in L-NAME treated rats (Tata et al. 2019).

Other Animal Models

The aforementioned models are more frequently used to evaluate the antihypertensive activity of extract plants. However, there are other less used such as the high-salt induced hypertensive mice model, which was used to evaluate the biological activity of *Polygonum hydropiper* (Devarajan et al. 2018) and *Moringa stenopetala* (Fekadu et al. 2017). *Monascus purpureus* extract was evaluated on fructose-induced hypertensive rats reversed the elevated blood pressure to normal level (Hsieh and Tai 2003).

Lagunas-Herrera et al. (2019) assessed the anti-hypertensive activity of extracts and fractions from *Malva parviflora* by using a chronic model of hypertension induced by angiotensin II and in this same assay was measured the capacity of the plant to modify the concentration of cytokines in kidneys, as well as the lipid peroxidation. Their results showed a dose-dependent effect in the reduction of blood pressure. Also, the aqueous extract of *M. parviflora* reduce oxidative stress and tissue damage caused by inflammation, which is the cause of hypertension (Lagunas-Herrera et al. 2019).

Human Models

Human models have also been used to evaluate the antihypertensive effects of plants. For instance, 80 hypertensive patients were administered with *Gastrodia elatanotoginseng* decoction along with a 2.5 mg Lamlodipine tablet. Patients who received the combined treatment showed a significant reduction in diastolic and systolic blood pressure compared to the Lamlodipine control group (Dengqin et al. 2018). Moreover, the decoction of *G. elatanotoginseng* has multiple anti-inflammatory effects on hypertensive patients such as harmful factors suppression and protective factors enhancement.

The consumption of tomatoes can potentially reduce or delay the development of the cardiovascular disease by anti-aggregation, anti-hypertensive, antidiabetic, antioxidative, antiangiogenic, and protective endothelial effects. Mediterranean diet includes high consumption of tomatoes, which results in cardiovascular risk reduction. The consumption of a tomato extract can influence the anti-platelet effect, which is heterogeneous and may be weight-dependent. The mechanism involved in the reduction of blood pressure and anti-aggregating platelet could be related to a decrease in the expression of renin and angiotensin-converting enzyme. Also, tomato extract can increase nitric oxide production, which subsequently leads to vasodilation (Krasińska et al. 2018, Krasinska et al. 2018).

Mechanisms of Action Identified for Plant Extracts

Table 3. Mechanism of action identified in antihypertensive extract plants

Mechanism of action	Plant understudy	Reference
Vasorelaxation	*Thymus linearis*	(Alamgeer et al. 2018)
	Leersia hexandra	(Bilanda et al. 2019)
	Xenophyllum poposum	(Cifuentes et al. 2018)
	Swietenia macrophylla	(Ch'ng et al. 2018)
	Artemisia campestris	(Dib et al. 2017)
ACE inhibition	*Carthamus tinctorius L.*	(Bunbupha et al. 2018)
	Pine needle	(He 2017)
	Saururus chinensis	(Lee et al. 2018)
	Senna garrettiana	(Madaka and Charoonratana 2018)
	Asparagus officinalis	(Sanae and Yasuo 2013)
	Coccinia indica	(Vinothkumar et al. 2019)

Anti-hypertensive agents have different mechanisms of action. Five major pharmacological classes of antihypertensive drugs are beta-blockers, diuretics, angiotensin-converting enzyme inhibitors, angiotensin II receptor antagonists, and calcium channel blockers. Other mechanisms include renin inhibitors, alpha-adrenergic receptor blockers, centrally acting agents, and direct-acting vasodilators (Laurent 2017). However, plant extracts had shown two main mechanisms to inhibit the angiotensin-converting enzyme (Table 3).

Vasorelaxation

Vasodilators are highly effective antihypertensive agents that dominated the management of hypertension in the 1950s and 1960s. However, treatment with these agents is associated with an unacceptable level of adverse reactions. With the advent of newer and better-tolerated antihypertensive agents, their use has declined dramatically. Many vasodilators can now be considered only of historical interest.

Vasodilators such as nitrates and hydralazine reduce the load on the heart, improve tissue perfusion in heart failure, and increase survival rates in patients. Because of their adverse effects, the alternative to using plants is being studied.

Thymus linearis possesses endothelium-independent vasorelaxant effects in a coronary artery by direct-acting on the smooth muscles. These effects involve the elevation of the cyclic AMP and cyclic GMP, possibly through the inhibition of various vascular isoforms of phosphodiesterase (Alamgeer et al. 2018).

The vasodilation properties of hexane extract of *Xenophyllum poposum* extract and its isolated compounds may act through the endothelial nitric oxide synthase, as well as calcium channel blocker mechanisms (Cifuentes et al. 2018). A similar mechanism of blocking channel-linked receptors pathways through the obstruction of voltage-operated calcium channels is reported for *Swietenia macrophylla* (Mahogany) seed extract. Moreover, *S. macrophylla* also acts as both potassium channels opener and inositol triphosphate receptor (IP_3R) inhibitor, followed by β_2-adrenergic pathway, and ultimately mediated through the nitric oxide/soluble guanylyl cyclase/cyclic 3',5'-guanosine monophosphate signaling pathways (Ch'ng et al. 2018). The vasorelaxant effect of *Artemisia campestris* is mediated via calmodulin-NO-cGC-PKG pathway and via inhibition of calcium influx through voltage-operated calcium channels and activation of intracellular calcium mobilization into the sarcoplasmic reticulum (Dib et al. 2017).

Angiotensin-Converting Enzyme inhibition

Angiotensin-converting enzyme inhibitors play a critical role in treating hypertension. Drugs used to inhibit angiotensin-converting enzyme are a competitive inhibitor of the natural substrate, for instance, captopril. The benefits of captopril in hypertension and heart failure result primarily from suppression of the renin-angiotensin-aldosterone system. As an angiotensin-converting enzyme inhibitor, it prevents the conversion of angiotensin I to angiotensin II. Side effects of captopril include dose-dependent rash, taste alterations, hypotension, gastric irritation, cough, and angioedema. Because of this, the look for plants that can inhibit angiotensin-converting enzyme has arisen in the last decades.

The extract *Carthamus tinctorius* had antihypertensive activity by suppressing renin-angiotensin system activation, including elevated serum ACE activity, and plasma Angiotensin II level and up-regulated aortic AT1R protein expression in 2K-1C rats (Bunbupha et al. 2018).

Other plants that had shown inhibition of the angiotensin-converting enzyme are *Saururus chinensis S. garrettiana, Berberis integerrima, Crataegus microphylla*, *Nymphaea alba*, *Onopordon acanthium*, *Quercus infectoria* and *Rubus* sp. (Lee et al. 2018, Madaka and Charoonratana 2018, Sharifi et al. 2013, Jalahalli Mariswamy, D'Souza, and Vishwanath 2010). ACE inhibition of these plants varied from 51 to 94%, being *Q. infectoria* the most potent inhibitor (Sharifi et al. 2013). Similar percent ACE inhibition was obtained with the whole leaf extract as well as the ethyl acetate and hexane fractions of *Eleusine indica* (Tutor and Chichioco-Hernandez 2018).

On the other hand, extracts of *Tacca integrifolia* prevented the formation of angiotensin II but stimulated the synthesis and releasing of aldosterone from the adrenal cortex that leads to increasing sodium, water retention, and blood pressure. However, the reduction in angiotensin II production could lead to a decrease in blood pressure (Jamaludin and Mohamad 2016).

Phytochemicals are Responsible for the Hypotensive Activity

Several mechanisms could mediate the hypotensive activity of plant extracts, including reduction of diastolic and systolic blood pressure, vasorelaxation and calcium channel blocking effects, and ACE inhibition.

The major class of compounds showing ACE inhibition is found to be flavonoids followed by peptides, alkaloids, phenylpropanoid glycosides, terpenes, iridoids, lipids, polyphenols, tannins and xanthones (Jalahalli Mariswamy, D'Souza, and Vishwanath 2010). Some studies on ACE inhibition mediated by phytochemicals are described in Table 4.

Polyphenols are secondary plant metabolites that had shown several effects on hypertension, including inhibition of the angiotensin-converting enzyme. For instance, the methanolic, ethanolic and aqueous leaf extracts of *Catharanthus roseus*, *Pongamia pinnata* and *Azadirachta indica*, as well as that of *Tamarindus indicus* seed coat, showed good ACE inhibition compared to acetone extracts, suggesting the benefit of polar compounds as potent ACE inhibitors. (Jalahalli Mariswamy, D'Souza, and Vishwanath 2010).

Table 4. Phytochemicals with antihypertensive activity

Phytochemical	Source	Reference
Polyphenols	*Azadirachta indica*	(Omóbòwálé et al. 2019)
	Urtica dioica	(Vajic et al. 2018)
Flavonoids	*Tartary buckwheat*	(Hou et al. 2017)
	Citrus extracts	(Paredes et al. 2018)
	Macrosolen cochinchinensis	(Ameer et al. 2009)
	Pine needle	(He 2017)
	Green tea	(Kanlaya and Thongboonkerd 2019)
Fatty acids	*Seabuckthorn seed oil*	(Vashishtha et al. 2017)
Sterols	*Macrosolen cochinchinensis*	(Ameer et al. 2009)

Polyphenols from *Azadirachta indica* could restore high blood pressure, reduced markers of oxidative stress, normalized serum NO bioavailability in L-NAME hypertensive rats (Omóbòwálé et al. 2019).

Urtica dioica polyphenols, showed strong antioxidant capacity and were able to reduce systolic and diastolic blood pressure, as well as the cardiac index, and to improve the antioxidative defense by increasing the activity of superoxide dismutase and catalase, without changing the concentration of the enzymes. Moreover, UE supplementation increased plasma antioxidant capacity and reduced systemic oxidative stress in rats (Vajic et al. 2018).

Tartary buckwheat flavonoid extracts significantly reduced systolic blood pressure and increased vasodilator response to insulin in the spontaneously hypertensive rats. Additionally, the extract treatment significantly reduced phosphorylation of insulin receptor substrate 1 (IRS-1) at serine 307 and increased insulin-stimulated Akt/eNOS activation in the SHRs. Furthermore, TBF treatment reduced the overproduction of basal O2 - in association with a reduction of NAD(P)H oxidase activity in mesenteric arterioles of the spontaneously hypertensive rats (Hou et al. 2017).

Different citrus extracts, as well as citric isolated compounds, improved aortic vascular relaxation, and increased plasma and urinary excretion of nitrites in spontaneously hypertensive rats (Paredes et al. 2018).

The rhizome water extract *of Tacca integrifolia* showed strong ACE inhibition which could be due to the presence of gypenoside (Jamaludin and Mohamad 2016).

Conclusion

Hypertension is a widely distributed health problem, which could lead to heart disease, stroke, and death. A person can have high blood pressure for years without any symptoms. Even without symptoms, damage to blood vessels, and heart continues and can be detected. Uncontrolled high blood pressure increases the risk of severe health problems, including heart attack and stroke. Drugs usually employed to treat hypertension have adverse effects. That is why the look for alternative treatments had evolved lately. Plants are a good source of diverse phytochemicals that can decrease blood pressure through several mechanisms such as reducing systolic and diastolic blood pressure, vasorelaxation and inhibition of the angiotensin-converting enzyme. Although there are many studies on this topic, more research is needed to generate more information about the in vivo effect and the possible mechanisms of action of phytochemicals.

References

Abdel-Rahman, R. F., A. F. Hessin, M. Abdelbaset, H. A. Ogaly, R. M. Abd-Elsalam, and S. M. Hassan. 2017. "Antihypertensive Effects of Roselle-Olive Combination in L-NAME-Induced Hypertensive Rats." *Oxidative Medicine and Cellular Longevity* 2017:9460653. doi: 10.1155/2017/9460653.

Abdel-Zaher, A. O., H. S. M. Farghaly, A. E. M. El-Refaiy, and A. M. Abd-Eldayem. 2018. "Protective effect of the standardized leaf extract of *Ginkgo biloba* (EGb761) against hypertension-induced renal injury in rats." *Clinical and Experimental Hypertension* 40 (8):703-714. doi: 10.1080/10641963.2018.1425421.

Aekthammarat, D., P. Pannangpetch, and P. Tangsucharit. 2019. "*Moringa oleifera* leaf extract lowers high blood pressure by alleviating vascular dysfunction and decreasing oxidative stress in L-NAME hypertensive rats." *Phytomedicine* 54:9-16. doi: 10.1016/j.phymed.2018.10.023.

Akila, G., K. Djamil, D. Nawal, and B. Saadia. 2018. "Comparative study of antihypertensive and antioxidant effects of clove and metformin on renal dysfunction in streptozotocin-induced diabetic rats." *PharmaNutrition* 6 (1):37-44. doi: 10.1016/j.phanu.2018.01.001.

Alamgeer, C. Auger, P. Chabert, C. Lugnier, M. N. Mushtaq, and V. B. Schini-Kerth. 2018. "Mechanisms underlying vasorelaxation induced in the porcine coronary arteries by *Thymus linearis*, Benth." *Journal of Ethnopharmacology* 225:211-219. doi: 10.1016/j.jep.2018.07.010.

Ameer, OZ, IM Salman, Md JA Siddiqui, MF Yam, RN Sriramaneni, AF Mutee, A Sadikun, Z Ismail, and MZ Asmawi. 2009. "Vascular responsiveness to *Macrosolen cochinchinensis* extracts in isolated rat thoracic aorta." *IJP-International Journal of Pharmacology* 5 (3):191-199.

Basri, Dayang Fredalina, Nur Sa'adah Abdul Rahman, Shafreena Shaukat Ali, and Satirah Zainalabidin. 2018. "The vasorelaxant effect of *Canarium odontophyllum* Miq. (Dabai) extract in rat thoracic aorta." *Egyptian Journal of Basic and Applied Sciences* 5 (1):75-79. doi: 10.1016/j.ejbas.2017.11.004.

Bilanda, D. C., P. D. D. Dzeufiet, L. Kouakep, B. F. O. Aboubakar, L. Tedong, P. Kamtchouing, and T. Dimo. 2017. "*Bidens pilosa* ethylene acetate extract can protect against L-NAME-induced hypertension on rats." *BMC Complementary and Alternative Medicine* 17 (1). doi: 10.1186/s12906-017-1972-0.

Bilanda, D. C., Y. C. Tcheutchoua, P. D. Djomeni Dzeufiet, D. L. D. Fokou, Y. B. Fouda, T. Dimo, and P. Kamtchouing. 2019. "Antihypertensive Activity of *Leersia hexandra* Sw. (Poaceae) Aqueous Extract on Ethanol-Induced Hypertension in Wistar Rat." *Evidence-based Complementary and Alternative Medicine* 2019. doi: 10.1155/2019/2897867.

Bunbupha, S., C. Wunpathe, P. Maneesai, T. Berkban, U. Kukongviriyapan, V. Kukongviriyapan, P. Prachaney, and P. Pakdeechote. 2018. "*Carthamus tinctorius* L. extract improves hemodynamic and vascular alterations in a rat model of renovascular hypertension through Ang II-AT_1R-NADPH oxidase pathway." *Annals of Anatomy* 216:82-89. doi: 10.1016/j.aanat. 2017.11.005.

Ch'ng, Y. S., Y. C. Loh, C. S. Tan, M. Ahmad, M. Z. Asmawi, W. M. Wan Omar, and M. F. Yam. 2018. "Vasodilation and Antihypertensive Activities of *Swietenia macrophylla* (Mahogany) Seed Extract." *Journal of Medicinal Food* 21 (3):289-301. doi: 10.1089/jmf.2017.4008.

Cheung, Bernard M. Y., and Chao Li. 2012. "Diabetes and hypertension: is there a common metabolic pathway?" *Current atherosclerosis reports* 14 (2):160-166. doi: 10.1007/s11883-012-0227-2.

Cifuentes, F., J. Palacios, J. Kuzmicic, L. Carvajal, F. Muñoz, C. Quispe, C. R. Nwokocha, G. Morales, I. Norambuena-Soto, M. Chiong, and A. Paredes. 2018. "Vasodilator and hypotensive effects of pure compounds and hydroalcoholic extract of *Xenophyllum poposum* (Phil) V. A Funk (Compositae) on rats." *Phytomedicine* 50:99-108. doi: 10.1016/j.phymed. 2018.09.226.

da Costa, C. A., P. R. de Oliveira, G. F. de Bem, L. C. de Cavalho, D. T. Ognibene, A. F. da Silva, S. Dos Santos Valenca, K. M. Pires, P. J. da Cunha Sousa, R. S. de Moura, and A. C. Resende. 2012. "*Euterpe oleracea* Mart.-derived polyphenols prevent endothelial dysfunction and vascular structural changes in renovascular hypertensive rats: role of oxidative stress." *Naunyn Schmiedebergs Arch Pharmacol* 385 (12):1199-209. doi: 10.1007/s00210-012-0798-z.

Da Costa, C. A., D. T. Ognibene, V. S. C. Cordeiro, G. F. De Bem, I. B. Santos, R. A. Soares, L. L. De Melo Cunha, L. C. R. M. Carvalho, R. S. De Moura, and A. C. Resende. 2017. "Effect of *Euterpe oleracea* Mart. Seeds Extract on Chronic Ischemic Renal Injury in Renovascular Hypertensive Rats." *Journal of Medicinal Food* 20 (10):1002-1010. doi: 10.1089/jmf. 2017.0011.

Dengqin, W., Z. Xiaoxue, S. Guohong, L. Lei, and S. Bing. 2018. "Effect of Gastrodia elata-notoginseng decoction on blood pressure variability and inflammatory factors in old hypertensive patients with yin-deficiency and yang-hyperactivity syndrome." *Biomedical Research (India)* 2018:S156-S160.

Devarajan, S., E. Yahiro, Y. Uehara, R. Kuroda, Y. Hirano, K. Nagata, S. Miura, K. Saku, and H. Urata. 2018. "Depressor effect of the young leaves of *Polygonum hydropiper* Linn. In high-salt induced hypertensive mice." *Biomedicine and Pharmacotherapy* 102:1182-1187. doi: 10.1016/j.biopha. 2018.03.055.

Dib, I., M. Tits, L. Angenot, J. N. Wauters, A. Assaidi, H. Mekhfi, M. Aziz, M. Bnouham, A. Legssyer, M. Frederich, and A. Ziyyat. 2017. "Antihypertensive and vasorelaxant effects of aqueous extract of *Artemisia campestris* L. from Eastern Morocco." *Journal of Ethnopharmacology* 206:224-235. doi: 10.1016/j.jep.2017.05.036.

Dzau, V. J. 1990. "Atherosclerosis and hypertension: mechanisms and interrelationships." *Journal of Cardiovascular Pharmacology* 15 Suppl 5:S59-64.

Fang, Hua, Wei-jing Zhang, Jing-chao Zhang, Miao Yang, Fang-xiang Zhang, and Jian-ping Zhang. 2017. "Anti-hypertensive effect of *Gastrodia elata* Bl leaf extract in rats." *Tropical Journal of Pharmaceutical Research* 16 (8):1887-1891.

Fekadu, N., H. Basha, A. Meresa, S. Degu, B. Girma, and B. Geleta. 2017. "Diuretic activity of the aqueous crude extract and hot tea infusion of *Moringa stenopetala* (Baker f.) Cufod. leaves in rats." *Journal of Experimental Pharmacology* 9:73-80. doi: 10.2147/JEP.S133778.

Hakkou, Z., A. Maciuk, V. Leblais, N. E. Bouanani, H. Mekhfi, M. Bnouham, M. Aziz, A. Ziyyat, A. Rauf, T. B. Hadda, U. Shaheen, S. Patel, R. Fischmeister, and A. Legssyer. 2017. "Antihypertensive and vasodilator effects of methanolic extract of *Inula viscosa:* Biological evaluation and POM analysis of cynarin, chlorogenic acid as potential hypertensive." *Biomedicine and Pharmacotherapy* 93:62-69. doi: 10.1016/j.biopha.2017.06.015.

Haydari, M. R., M. R. Panjeshahin, E. Mashghoolozekr, and A. A. Nekooeian. 2017. "Antihypertensive effects of hydroalcoholic extract of *Crataegus azarolus* subspecies aronia fruit in rats with renovascular hypertension: An experimental mechanistic study." *Iranian Journal of Medical Sciences* 42 (3):266-274.

He, J. 2017. "Bioactivity-Guided Fractionation of Pine Needle Reveals Catechin as an Anti-hypertension Agent via Inhibiting Angiotensin-Converting Enzyme." *Scientific Reports* 7 (1). doi: 10.1038/s41598-017-07748-x.

Hou, Z., Y. Hu, X. Yang, and W. Chen. 2017. "Antihypertensive effects of *Tartary buckwheat* flavonoids by improvement of vascular insulin sensitivity in spontaneously hypertensive rats." *Food and Function* 8 (11):4217-4228. doi: 10.1039/c7fo00975e.

Hsieh, Po-Shiuan, and Yueh-Hua Tai. 2003. "Aqueous Extract of *Monascus purpureus* M9011 Prevents and Reverses Fructose-Induced Hypertension in Rats." *Journal of Agricultural and Food Chemistry* 51 (14):3945-3950. doi: 10.1021/jf026157n.

Ibrar, M., M. A. Khan, Abdullah, M. Nisar, and M. Khan. 2019. "Evaluation of *Paeonia emodi* for its cardioprotective potentials: An investigative study towards possible mechanism." *Journal of Ethnopharmacology* 231:57-65. doi: 10.1016/j.jep.2018.10.041.

Jalahalli Mariswamy, Siddesha, Cletus D'Souza, and B. S. Vishwanath. 2010. "*Inhibition of Angiotensin Converting Enzyme (ACE) by medicinal plants exhibiting antihypertensive activity.*" In, 269-308.

Jamaludin, Farah Liyana, and Jamaludin Mohamad. 2016. "Antihypertension Activity of Water Extract of *Tacca integrifolia*." *Sains Malaysiana* 45 (3):425-433.

Jentzer, J. C., T. A. DeWald, and A. F. Hernandez. 2010. "Combination of loop diuretics with thiazide-type diuretics in heart failure." *Journal of the American College of Cardiology* 56 (19):1527-34. doi: 10.1016/j.jacc.2010.06.034.

Joukar, S., S. Ebrahimi, M. Khazaei, A. Bashiri, M. R. Shakibi, V. Naderi, B. Shahouzehi, and M. Alasvand. 2017. "Co-administration of walnut (*Juglans Regia*) prevents systemic hypertension induced by long-term use of dexamethasone: A promising strategy for steroid consumers." *Pharmaceutical Biology* 55 (1):184-189. doi: 10.1080/13880209.2016.1233570.

Kamisah, Y., J. S. F. Zuhair, A. H. Juliana, and K. Jaarin. 2017. "*Parkia speciosa* empty pod prevents hypertension and cardiac damage in rats given N(G)-nitro-L-arginine methyl ester." *Biomedicine and Pharmacotherapy* 96:291-298. doi: 10.1016/j.biopha.2017.09.095.

Kanlaya, R., and V. Thongboonkerd. 2019. "Protective Effects of Epigallocatechin-3-Gallate from Green Tea in Various Kidney Diseases." *Advances in Nutrition* 10 (1):112-121. doi: 10.1093/advances/nmy077.

Kannan, A., and R. Janardhanan. 2014. "Hypertension as a risk factor for heart failure." *Curr Hypertens Rep* 16 (7):447. doi: 10.1007/s11906-014-0447-7.

Kim, B., Y. Kwon, S. Lee, K. Lee, I. Ham, and H. Y. Choi. 2017. "Vasorelaxant effects of *Angelica decursiva* root on isolated rat aortic rings." *BMC Complementary and Alternative Medicine* 17 (1). doi: 10.1186/s12906-017-1965-z.

Kopincova, J., A. Puzserova, and I. Bernatova. 2012. "L-NAME in the cardiovascular system - nitric oxide synthase activator?" *Pharmacology Reports* 64 (3):511-20. doi: 10.1016/s1734-1140(12)70846-0.

Kpegba, K., E. T. Kondo, O. Simalou, K. Togbenou, P. Boyode, O. Toundou, N. Y. Gbandjaba, A. Agbonon, and M. Gbeassor. 2018. "A significant antihypertensive effect of *Holarrhena floribunda* supported by an exploratory phytochemical study." *Journal of HerbMed Pharmacology* 7 (3):160-167. doi: 10.15171/jhp.2018.27.

Krasińska, B., A. Osińska, A. Krasińska, M. Osiński, P. Rzymski, A. Tykarski, and Z. Krasiński. 2018. "Favourable hypotensive effect after standardised tomato extract treatment in hypertensive subjects at high cardiovascular risk: A randomised controlled trial." *Kardiologia Polska* 76 (2):388-395. doi: 10.5603/KP.a2017.0215.

Krasinska, B., A. Osińska, M. Osinski, A. Krasinska, P. Rzymski, A. Tykarski, and Z. Krasiński. 2018. "Standardised tomato extract as an alternative to acetylsalicylic acid in patients with primary hypertension and high cardiovascular risk – a randomised, controlled trial." *Archives of Medical Science* 14 (4):773-780. doi: 10.5114/aoms.2017.69864.

Lagunas-Herrera, H., J. Tortoriello, M. Herrera-Ruiz, G. B. Martínez-Henández, A. Zamilpa, L. A. Santamaría, M. G. Lorenzana, G. Lombardo-Earl, and E. Jiménez-Ferrer. 2019. "Acute and chronic antihypertensive effect of fractions, tiliroside and scopoletin from malva parviflora." *Biological and Pharmaceutical Bulletin* 42 (1):18-25. doi: 10.1248/bpb.b18-00355.

Laurent, Stéphane. 2017. "Antihypertensive drugs." *Pharmacological Research* 124:116-125. doi: 10.1016/j.phrs.2017.07.026.

Lee, E. H., H. J. Park, J. B. Jo, Y. J. Kim, M. U. Kim, D. H. Ahn, H. Y. Jung, and Y. J. Cho. 2018. "Elevation of anti-oxidative and inhibitory activities against xanthine oxidase and angiotensin-converting enzyme and anti-microbial activities of extracts from saururus chinensis by elicitor treatment." *Journal of the Korean Society of Food Science and Nutrition* 47 (10):988-994. doi: 10.3746/jkfn.2018.47.10.988.

Li, J. J., and J. L. Chen. 2005. "Inflammation may be a bridge connecting hypertension and atherosclerosis." *Medical Hypotheses* 64 (5):925-9. doi: 10.1016/j.mehy.2004.10.016.

Madaka, F., and T. Charoonratana. 2018. "Angiotensin-converting enzyme inhibitory activity of Senna garrettiana active compounds: Potential markers for standardized herbal medicines." *Pharmacognosy Magazine* 14 (57):S335-S339. doi: 10.4103/pm.pm_325_17.

Omóbòwálé, T. O., A. A. Oyagbemi, B. S. Ogunpolu, O. E. Ola-Davies, J. O. Olukunle, E. R. Asenuga, T. O. Ajibade, O. A. Adejumobi, J. M. Afolabi, O. O. Falayi, A. Ashafa, A. A. Adedapo, and M. A. Yakubu. 2019. "Antihypertensive Effect of Polyphenol-Rich Fraction of *Azadirachta indica* on Nω-Nitro-L-Arginine Methyl Ester-Induced Hypertension and

Cardiorenal Dysfunction." *Drug Research* 69 (1):12-22. doi: 10.1055/a-0635-0638.

Paredes, M. D., P. Romecín, N. M. Atucha, F. O'Valle, J. Castillo, M. C. Ortiz, and J. García-Estañ. 2018. "Moderate effect of flavonoids on vascular and renal function in spontaneously hypertensive rats." *Nutrients* 10 (8). doi: 10.3390/nu10081107.

Qaseem, Amir, Timothy J. Wilt, Robert Rich, Linda L. Humphrey, Jennifer Frost, Mary Ann Forciea, for the Clinical Guidelines Committee of the American College of Physicians, the Commission on Health of the Public, and Science of the American Academy of Family Physicians. 2017. "Pharmacologic Treatment of Hypertension in Adults Aged 60 Years or Older to Higher Versus Lower Blood Pressure Targets: A Clinical Practice Guideline From the American College of Physicians and the American Academy of Family Physicians." *Annals of Internal Medicine* 166 (6):430-437. doi: 10.7326/m16-1785.

Salami, S. A., H. M. Salahdeen, E. C. Ugbebor, B. A. Murtala, and Y. Raji. 2018. "Effects of aqueous leaf extract of *Tridax procumbens* on contractile activity of corpus cavernosum in N-nitro-l-arginine methyl ester-induced hypertensive male rats." *Journal of Integrative Medicine* 16 (1):51-56. doi: 10.1016/j.joim.2017.11.001.

Sanae, Matsuda, and Aoyagi Yasuo. 2013. "Green Asparagus (Asparagus officinalis) Prevented Hypertension by an Inhibitory Effect on Angiotensin-Converting Enzyme Activity in the Kidney of Spontaneously Hypertensive Rats." *Journal of Agricultural and Food Chemistry* 61 (23):5520-5525. doi: 10.1021/jf3041066.

Senejoux, François, Corine Girard, Parhat Kerram, Haji Aisa, Berthelot Alain, Françoise Bévalot, and Céline Demougeot. 2010. "Mechanisms of vasorelaxation induced by *Ziziphora clinopodioides* Lam. (Lamiaceae) extract in rat thoracic aorta." *Journal of ethnopharmacology* 132:268-73. doi: 10.1016/j.jep.2010.08.028.

Sharifi, Niusha, Effat Souri, Seyed Ali Ziai, Gholamreza Amin, and Massoud Amanlou. 2013. "Discovery of new angiotensin converting enzyme (ACE) inhibitors from medicinal plants to treat hypertension using an in vitro assay." *Daru: journal of Faculty of Pharmacy, Tehran University of Medical Sciences* 21 (1):74-74. doi: 10.1186/2008-2231-21-74.

Sternlicht, H., and G. L. Bakris. 2017. "The Kidney in Hypertension." *Medical Clinics of North America* 101 (1):207-217. doi: 10.1016/j.mcna.2016.08.001.

Sun, Dianjianyi, Tao Zhou, Yoriko Heianza, Xiang Li, Mengyu Fan, Vivian A. Fonseca, and Lu Qi. 2019. "Type 2 Diabetes and Hypertension." *Circulation Research* 124 (6):930-937. doi: doi:10.1161/CIRCRESAHA. 118.314487.

Tata, C. M., C. R. Sewani-Rusike, O. O. Oyedeji, E. T. Gwebu, F. Mahlakata, and B. N. Nkeh-Chungag. 2019. "Antihypertensive effects of the hydro-ethanol extract of *Senecio serratuloides* DC in rats." *BMC Complementary and Alternative Medicine* 19 (1). doi: 10.1186/s12906-019-2463-2.

Tata, Charlotte, Gwebu Tobela, Olukayode Aremu, Sewani-Rusike Rufaro, Oyedeji Omowumi, Oyedeji Oyehan, and Benedicta Nkeh-Chungag. 2018. "Acute Toxicity and Antihypertensive Effects of *Artemisia afra* and *Leonotis leonurus* in Spontaneously Hypertensive Rats." *Research Journal of Biotechnology* 13:20-25.

Tutor, Jasmin T, and Christine L Chichioco-Hernandez. 2018. "Angiotensin-Converting Enzyme Inhibition of Fractions from *Eleusine indica* Leaf Extracts." *Pharmacognosy Journal* 10 (1).

Vajic, U. J., J. Grujic-Milanovic, Z. Miloradovic, D. Jovovic, M. Ivanov, D. Karanovic, K. Savikin, B. Bugarski, and N. Mihailovic-Stanojevic. 2018. "*Urtica dioica* L. leaf extract modulates blood pressure and oxidative stress in spontaneously hypertensive rats." *Phytomedicine* 46:39-45. doi: 10.1016/j.phymed.2018.04.037.

Vashishtha, V., K. Barhwal, A. Kumar, S. K. Hota, O. P. Chaurasia, and B. Kumar. 2017. "Effect of seabuckthorn seed oil in reducing cardiovascular risk factors: A longitudinal controlled trial on hypertensive subjects." *Clinical Nutrition* 36 (5):1231-1238. doi: 10.1016/j.clnu.2016.07.013.

Vinothkumar, G., P. Venkataraman, V. M. Vinodhini, R. Lavanya, and D. Sathishkumar. 2019. "Effect of *Coccinia indica* leaf extract on angiotensin converting enzyme (ACE) inhibitor induced hepatotoxicity in wistar albino rats." *Clinical Nutrition Experimental* 24:24-33. doi: 10.1016/j.yclnex. 2019.01.004.

Wajngarten, Mauricio, and Gisele Sampaio Silva. 2019. "Hypertension and Stroke: Update on Treatment." *European cardiology* 14 (2):111-115. doi: 10.15420/ecr.2019.11.1.

WHO. 2019. "*Hypertension.*" https://www.who.int/health-topics/hypertension/.

Wong, T. Y., and P. Mitchell. 2007. "The eye in hypertension." *Lancet* 369 (9559):425-35. doi: 10.1016/s0140-6736(07)60198-6.

In: Medicinal Plants …
Editors: A. Cardador Martínez et al.
ISBN: 978-1-53618-061-9

Chapter 3

METABOLIC PROCESSES IN CANCER

Ulisses Moreno-Celis * ***and Teresa García-Gasca***
Facultad de Ciencias Naturales, Universidad Autónoma de Querétaro, Queretaro, Mexico

ABSTRACT

From the point of view of public health, cancer is considered as a group of diseases whose primary feature is disorderly growth and dysfunction of the affected tissue, but these physiological and anatomical characteristics are regulated by the metabolism which is adapted to allow cell survival. This can be seen in the increase in levels of lactic acid in tumor cells which have a normal supply of energy from carbohydrates, as well as in experiments where mitochondria are transferred from tumor cells to non-tumor cells. Throughout this review, the main metabolic alterations in the main types of cancer will be analyzed from the epidemiological point of view, focusing on specific metabolic or molecular markers of each, as well as the differences and/or similarities that characterize them. On the other hand, the main compounds of plant extracts are also addressed, as well as promising natural therapies that are currently in clinical or pre-clinical evaluations that could add to current cancer therapies.

Keywords: cancer, phenolic compounds, lectins, carcinoma, medicinal plants

* Corresponding Author's Email: ulisses.moreno@uaq.mx.

INTRODUCTION

Cancer is a global public health problem. In 2012, 8.2 million deaths and 14.1 million new cases were reported worldwide. Affecting countries of any economic level, with those located in North America, Europe and Oceania most affected (Torre et al., 2016). Although cancer is not a disease itself, but a group of them, it shares similar pathophysiological mechanisms among most types of cancer, in which the loss of sensitivity to signs of cell death can be observed, as well as signs of growth arrest, evasion of apoptosis, increase of replicative capacity, promotion of angiogenesis and gain of migratory capacity and metastasis (Hanahan and Weinberg 2000), as well as the promotion of a microenvironment that stimulates metabolic changes, immunological modulation and an altered response to stress (Likis 2010).

CANCER AS A METABOLIC DISORDER

Cancer is classically seen as a genetic pathology characterized by the loss of proliferative control, as well as cell function and structure, but without a doubt the cancer cell must adapt its metabolism to the new energy requirements necessary to carry out the new rhythms of growth demanded. In this sense it was observed that unlike normal cells cancer cells increase their glucose and glutamine consumption, and increased glycolysis as well as the release of lactic acid despite having normal oxygen conditions (Coller 2014; Seyfried et al. 2014).

While it is true that nuclear injury is considered the most important effect for the initiation of carcinogenesis, some studies have demonstrated the importance of mitochondrial health in this process and important issues have been discussed, such as: the nuclear genome that triggers carcinogenesis or only directs the process of tumor development; or if cancer could be considered as a mitochondrial disease. Given the evidence of important alterations in tumor cells, it has been found that nuclear injury encourages the loss of mitochondrial function, as well as a significant decrease in the number of mitochondria present in these cells. In studies with diploid frog anucleate oocytes, which were transferred to a nucleus of a triploid tumor cell, the oocytes conserved the diploid phenotype suggesting that the tumor development depends not only on the genetic content but also on alternative mechanisms that complement the process (Figure 1A) (McKinnell, Deggins, and Labat 1969). On the other hand, to determine the role of mitochondria in the carcinogenesis process, mammary benign cancer cells were performed to a highly aggressive osteosarcoma cell line (Figure 1B), producing a decrease of the malignant phenotype, turning off important oncogenic pathways (evaluated by micro-arrangements), as well as improving the effect of chemotherapeutic drugs (Kaipparettu et al., 2013). The preceding makes us note the importance of mitochondrial activity and above all of the metabolic activity resulting from its structural integrity, giving relevance to the structure and mitochondrial activity as a fundamental entity in the appearance and tumor development.

On the other hand, it has been observed that when important mitochondrial lesions exist, the signaling pathways that promote the transcription of MYC, TP53, KRAS, and BRAF1 are deregulated, which are highly involved in different types of cancer (Seyfried et al., 2014). According to the mortality, the main types of cancer are those of the lung, liver, stomach, colon, and breast.

Lung Cancer

The lungs are two spongy organs located in the thorax responsible for the ventilation of the body. They are responsible for entering the oxygen into the blood and excreting carbon dioxide from the energy metabolism. Lung cancer ranks first in the causes of death from cancer worldwide. Although the reasons are multiple, the habit of smoking implies a higher risk to develop it (Dela Cruz, Tanoue, and Matthay 2011). Lung cancer can be classified into two main types depending on the appearance of the lung cancer cells seen under the microscope. Small cell lung cancer occurs almost exclusively in people who smoke a lot and is less common than non-small cell lung cancer (Mountain and Dresler 1997). Non-small cell lung cancer refers to several types of lung cancer that behave similarly, such as squamous cell carcinoma, adenocarcinoma, and large cell carcinoma, whose specific mechanisms differ, as well as its development (Lynch et al., 2004). From the genetic point of view lung cancer develops from alterations in tumor suppressor genes and proto-oncogenes, which are altered in the different stages of tumor development. In this sense we have Ras proto-oncogenes, Myc and ERBB2, tumor suppressors, p53, Rb, p16, and anti-apoptotic genes such as Bcl-2, and enzymatic factors such as polymerase activity mainly (Volm et al., 2002).

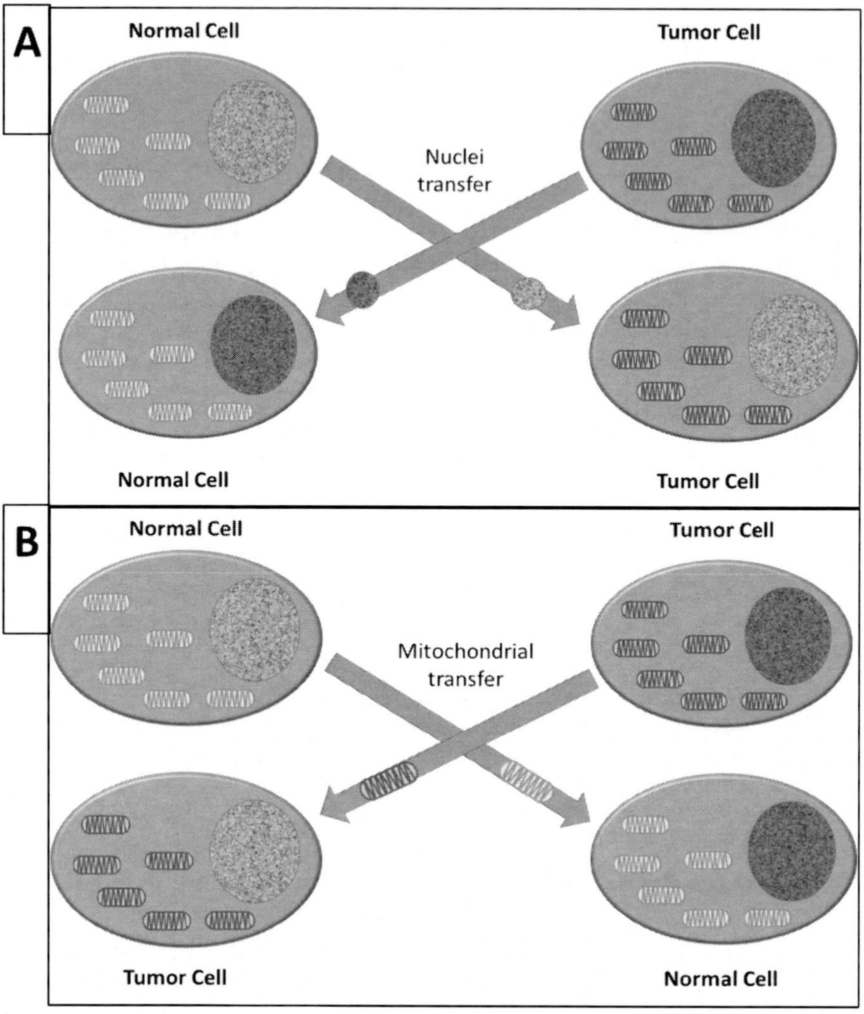

Figure 1. Summary of the experiments of (A) transfer of frog oocyte nuclei. (B) transfer of mitochondria from benign epithelial cancer cells of the breast to osteosarcoma cells.

Liver Cancer

Liver cancer is the fifth most common cancer worldwide, and within this group of diseases, hepatocellular carcinoma is the leading cause, mainly due to metastasis from cancer of other organs, due to hepatic lesions that cause cirrhosis, such as infection by hepatitis B or C, non-alcoholic fatty liver or habitual alcohol consumption (El-Serag and Mason 2000).

In liver tumor cells it has been seen that lipid metabolism is different between non-tumor cells and cells adjacent to the tumor; what has been seen is that the tumor cells increase their capacity to capture free fatty acids and triglycerides (C. R. Santos and Schulze 2012), while decreasing the capacity of cholesterol synthesis. The mechanism is thought to be through microsomal alterations of said cells. When *in vitro* models, it has been observed that a high level of inflammatory cytokines such as tumor necrosis factor-alpha (TNF-α) and interleukin 6 (IL-6) can alter the concentration of serum lipids, mainly causing a decrease in serum concentrations of triglycerides. On the other hand, high levels of interleukin 2 (IL-2) can reduce cholesterol and increase levels of IL-6 and IL-1, and promote the decrease of the microsomal triglyceride transfer protein (Grivennikov and Karin 2011). It should be mentioned that inflammation is present and to varying degrees during the process of liver carcinogenesis. Although these findings have been measured in the tumor environment, they have also been observed in blood markers (Ahaneku et al., 1992), which indicates the significant influence they can have on the metabolism.

Stomach Cancer

The most common stomach cancer in the population is gastric adenocarcinoma (90 to 95% of cases), followed by lymphoma, benign gastrointestinal tumors, carcinoid tumors and others such as squamous cell carcinoma, small cell carcinoma, and leiomyosarcoma (D. Schrijvers 2010). The primary source of energy is anaerobic fermentation given the failure to metabolize available glucose (Yuan, Yamashita, and Seto 2016). It has been observed that there are at least 95 different metabolites related to energy metabolism in gastric cancer (Hirayama et al. 2009). On the other hand, deficiencies in folate metabolism have been associated with the development of stomach cancer (Zhang et al., 2007). Likewise, changes in protein metabolism have been observed that lead to changes in the tumor matrix, promoting the disruption of the tissue to favor the establishment of the tumor (Guszczyn and Sobolewski 2004).

COLON CANCER

Colorectal cancer (CRC) has an annual incidence of approximately one million cases and an annual mortality of more than 500,000 people (Ferlay et al., 2015; Rafiemanesh et al., 2016). It is expected that the absolute number of cases will increase in the next two decades as a result of aging and population expansion, both in developed and developing countries (GMO 2007). In Mexico, in a period of 10 years between 1998 and 2007, there was an increase of 80% of registered cases of colon cancer according to a study conducted at the General Hospital of Mexico in 2009 (Charúa-Guindic et al., 2009; Rafiemanesh et al., 2016; Tirado-Gómez and Betancourt 2008). The previous shows the significant increase in this condition and the importance of discovering new preventive therapies as well as efficient treatments. Current therapies to fight cancer, i.e., resection, radiation and chemotherapy, are not as effective as they often cannot rid the patient of all cancer cells (Silva 2008, Monteverde 2008). Experimental therapy strategies and study protocols include immunotherapy, gene therapy, inhibition of the activity of proteins promoters of cancer, and the inhibition of the formation of new blood vessels (angiogenesis) (Torrecillas-Torres 2008).

The process of carcinogenesis is long-term and is caused by a series of damages that affect DNA repairing genes (Gatenby and Vincent 2003). The accumulation of these genetic alterations in the colonic epithelium requires some years, usually decades, which coincides with the average age of patients diagnosed with CRC (around 65-70 years) (Jackson and Loeb 2001). In addition to mutations, other genetic changes are involved in tumorigenesis: DNA methylation, amplification, overexpression and deletions (Campo Alegria and Garcia Garrido 1997).

For the above and considering that cancer can have several determinants and although the cited evidence points to the origin of cancer from a point of view of alterations in mitochondria, we consider that a pathology of such magnitude of processes cannot be considered an only cause, but the sum of various factors such as cytoplasmic and mitochondrial alterations, as well as nuclear and genetic alterations. Especially in colon cancer it has been observed that there are mitochondrial alterations that trigger metabolic changes related to the way of obtaining energy by tumor cells, it has been observed that caloric restriction decreases the increase of the tumor mass, while in people with high caloric intake progression is promoted. In the same way, the presence of high amounts of free radicals has been considered a risk factor and promoter of cancer progression (Sanchez-Pino 2007). Likewise, damage has been observed in mitochondrial complexes I and IV in cells adjacent to the tumor and could indicate that this phenomenon is related to the transformation to tumor cells of non-tumor tissue (Guerra et al., 2017).

BREAST CANCER

Breast cancer is the most prevalent in women worldwide, and at least 4 types are considered: hormonal which are sub-classified in luminaries, A and B, positive to the HER2 oncogene, and triple-negative, of which the hormone-dependent are the most frequent. Breast cancer is considered a socio-epidemiological problem since it has been observed that it is more frequent in developed countries, related to a delayed or null start of conception, and affecting mainly women between 35 and 60 years of age. Currently, early detection campaigns have had great effects and make it a treatable disease, although it is still considered to have a mortality rate of around 20% in developed countries. Specific metabolic disorders such as obesity and insulin resistance have been widely associated with the development of breast cancer, as well as with a low response to treatment. The proposed mechanisms for this assertion are those related to the increase of adipocytokines, increased synthesis of lipogenic hormones and deregulation in the production of leptin (Pasanisi et al. 2006, Vona-Davis, Howard-McNatt, and Rose 2007).

PI3K/Akt, one of the commonly deregulated pathways in several types of cancer, has great inferences in the metabolic activity of breast cancer, as well as in the protection of the oxidative stress of said pathology, promoting the activity of glutathione (GSH) considered a major promoter of cell survival in breast cancer (Clish et al., 2017; Lien et al., 2016). On the other hand, it has been observed that there is a tumor regulation by the adipocytes adjacent to the breast cancer cells, by means of the liberation of free fatty acids (FFA) which are captured by the tumor cells and stored in triglycerides (TG), promoting β-oxidation which is not a process that takes place in normal breast epithelial cells. This leads to an imbalance in the production of energy through a sustained activation of the MAPK pathway (Wang et al., 2017), which is largely related to cell growth, proliferation and survival (Hanahan and Weinberg 2000).

DRUGS DERIVED FROM PLANTS CURRENTLY USED WITH ANTI-CANCER EFFECTS

Important and complex cancer therapies have been developed based on the classic physiopathological approach, which addresses the solution of the problem by attacking the cells of rapid reproductive capacity from the point of view of the cell cycle or replication. This causes tumor cells to be attacked, as well as cells of organs and systems that have a high rate of reproduction due to their nature and biological specificity, such as epithelia and cells of the hematopoietic system, and thus the cells of the immune system. For this reason, several studies point to the search for therapies against colon cancer, which are more specific and less aggressive for the organism (Monteverde 2008, Torrecillas-Torres 2008, Silva 2008).

The use of traditional medicine has been a watershed for major research focused on the discovery and development of new therapies not only for cancer but for various pathologies. In this sense it is worth mentioning that the use of traditional medicine is due to knowledge of empirical and plants used for medicinal purposes; those that gave effect at the time of use, doses, ways to use, the appropriate harvest time for the use of the active compound, the proper variety, genetics, pesticides and contaminants, among other factors that can affect the desired outcome (Alonso-Castro et al., 2011).

In Mexico alone, there are more than 4 thousand plants used for medicinal purposes, of which about 300 are known to be useful in cancer patients and 88 of which have been found to affect cell lines *in vitro*. In these plant extracts, 187 different metabolites were identified, of which 41% were found cytotoxic effects in cells (Loraine and Mendoza-Espinoza 2010, Alonso-Castro et al., 2011).

Currently, various products or extracts obtained from plants are used in the clinical field, such as the *Catharanthus roseus alcamis* (pink vinca), which were proposed as anticancer therapy for some decades (El-Sayed and Cordell 1981), for its effects on the cell cycle of tumor cells (Gajalakshmi, Vijayalakshmi, and Rajeswari 2013). On the other hand, the use of taxane derivative chemotherapeutics obtained from *Taxus brevifolia* (Paclitaxel and Docetaxel) has been shown to have effects on mitosis by inhibiting the depolymerization of microtubules. They have been widely used in the treatment of breast and ovarian cancers but mainly lung cancer, although serious side effects are reported such as cardiotoxicity, neutropenia, arthralgia, and myalgia (Kilic et al., 2015). The toxin from *Podophyllum peltatum*, Podphyllotoxin, is also clinically used, which is the basis for synthesizing the etoposide and teniposide drugs that effect the assembly of microtubules and are used to treat lung cancer, testicular cancer, neuroblastoma, and hepatoma (Giri and Lakshmi Narasu 2000; Clark and Slevin 1987). On the other hand, the camtopthecin and topotecan, compounds extracted from *Camptotheca acuminate*, show effects on the cell cycle in various types of cancer and on cancers of the central nervous system respectively (Gallo 1971, Lamond, Mehta, and Boothman 1996). Lectins extracted from *Viscum album coloratum*, have also been widely studied and used as an adjuvant of cancer therapy. Recent studies show good subcutaneous tolerability and improvement in the quality of life of patients with breast cancer (Semiglasov et al., 2004).

Active Compounds from Plants with Anti-Cancer Properties

Currently, the properties of various phytochemicals and/or nutraceuticals are known primarily from plants, which are mostly produced in the secondary metabolism of plants; however, a few are part of the primary metabolism. Resulting from primary metabolism are the flavonoids, carotenes, thromboxanes, alkamides, cyanidins, lycopenes, sulforaphanes among others that have been studied extensively but still do not have conclusive results due to the lack of reproducibility as well as the costs in obtaining them. On the other hand, the main players among the primary metabolites of plants are protease inhibitors and lectins, which have shown to induce cell death and impede angiogenesis and metastasis. Throughout this section we will focus on providing specific, detailed and updated information on those compounds with the highest pharmaceutical potential in cancer therapy.

Phenolic Compounds

Phenolic compounds are products of the secondary metabolism of plants. They are not considered to have any activity on the physiology of plants and can be synthesized mainly by two routes: the shikimic acid route and/or the malonic acid pathway. We can divide them in flavonoids and flavones. In the first are the flavonols, flavones, flavonones, isoflavones, isoflavins and chalcones, while in the flavones we will find tannins, phenolic acids and stilbenes (Aguilera, Martin-Cabrejas, González de Mejia 2016). These compounds have been widely studied for their antioxidant properties in different chronic noncommunicable diseases (Ambriz-Pérez et al., 2016). The main activity of these compounds has to do with their anti-inflammatory effect. It has been seen that both extracts are rich in specific flavonols (Ortega et al., 2017); as well as diets high in these, decrease the inflammatory activity (Cassidy et al., 2015). In the same way, isoflavones (Yu et al., 2016) and some related compounds also have analgesic effects (Verri et al., 2012). A great variety of plant extracts and phenolic compound isolates have been evaluated on different types of cancer. Both *in vitro* and *in vivo*, these compounds usually have anticancer, chemotherapeutic or adjuvant properties, due to a diversity of mechanisms, such as inhibiting cell growth and proliferation, promoting cell death, inhibiting angiogenesis; mutagenic inhibition and the aforementioned anti-inflammatory properties via various signaling pathways.

Lectins in Cancer

The term Lectins is applied to a group of non-immunological glycoproteins or proteins with the ability to bind specifically and reversibly to carbohydrates, either free or forming part of more complex structures (Goldstein and Hayes 1978; Estrada-Martínez et al., 2017; Freed 1999). These proteins usually have at least two binding sites per molecule (AFS Santos et al., 2014) and, as a particular feature, tend to bind to common cells (Kim, Isaacs, and Perdomo 1974, Rüdiger and Gabius 2001)). The ability of these proteins to interact with cells of the immune response allows them to exert immunosuppressive effects. Others are toxic and some of them inhibit the growth of tumor cells and may participate in cell adhesion (Lichtenstein and Rabinovich 2013; Kiss et al., 1997). All of the biological activities reported for the lectins have in common the recognition of an oligosaccharide receptor (Castillo-Villanueva and Abdullaev 2005).

In plants, most lectins are found in reserve organs, which is indirect evidence of their role as defense proteins (Mendoza et al., 2007). A large variety of lectins from different organisms have been isolated and evaluated. (Fu et al., 2011) and it has been found that there is similarity between lectins from related families and, in some cases, it has been shown that lectins are capable of recognizing carbohydrates in a certain configuration or carbohydrate sequence; that is, the characteristics of specificity by saccharide structures are also highly conserved among proteins of the same species (Castillo-Villanueva and Abdullaev 2005).

The lectins have been used for some years as differential markers in the detection of cancer of the esophagus and stomach. These have been conjugated with fluorescent markers for easy identification (Mechref et al., 2009; Fardini et al., 2013). Stomach cancer is the fifth cause of cancer death in the world, while the cancer of esophagus is the sixth. Invasive cancer of the esophagus and stomach is a progressive multi-stage process that involves the conversion of the normal epithelium to basal cell hyperplasia (BHC), dysplasia (DIS) or carcinoma *in situ* (CIS), and then to invasive squamous cell carcinoma. (Labenz et al., 2015).

Recently, some attention has been paid to the expression of TF antigen in carcinomas, and it has been proposed as a possible marker in cancer of the esophagus and stomach (Kannan et al., 2003). The lectins have been used as diagnostic tools for esophageal cancer and gastric cancer, since it has been shown that there are alterations in the expression of the TF antigen in the case of the esophagus and of N-glycans in the case of the stomach, which facilitates the recognition by lectins (Yau et al., 2015, Singh et al. 2006, Medina and Quesada 2014, Aricigil and Pryme 2015). These lectins are used mainly as markers for immunohistochemistry, either with fluorochromes or enzymatic reaction molecules for colorimetry, giving excellent results (Castaño-Rodríguez, Kaakoush, and Mitchell 2014, Baintner et al., 2000).

Malignant tumors of the small intestine are rare, accounting for only 2% of all tumors of the gastrointestinal tract and less than 0.4% of all malignant tumors. For this reason, our knowledge of lectins in this organ is based on the etiology of colon or gastric cancer, depending on the type and location affected (Bowcutt et al., 2014). Several studies indicate the effect of lectins from different plants on the inhibition of growth, proliferation and promotion of cell death in colon cancer cell lines (Sasaki et al. 2002, López-Sánchez et al. 2009, Ma et al. 2008 Singh et al., 2006). Currently, it is known that there are differences in the glycosylations of various structures of normal cell membranes (NCs) and colon cancers (CCs), both in lipids (Shida et al., 2009), and in glycoproteins (Kim, Isaacs, and Perdomo 1974) such certain receptors (Hung et al., 2014), and what makes CCs more susceptible to recognition by lectins. In 1999, Jordinson reported that *Vicia faba* agglutinin increase the cellular differentiation of different lines of CCs, decreasing the malignant phenotype (Jordinson et al., 1999). Such is the case of lectins of some fungi such as *Agrocybe aegerita* (AAL), *Algaricus bisporus* (ABL) as well as plants such as *Arisaema helleborifolium* (AHL), *Arisaema tortuosum* (ATL), *Arachis hypogaea* (PNA), *Viscum album* (VAL, VAA, VAA-1), *Sauromatum venosum* (SVA), *Phaseolus acutifolius* (García-Gasca et al., 2012; Valadez-Vega et al.,

2014), *Phaseolus vulgaris* (PVA) (Cruz-Bravo et al., 2011), and mainly *Vicia. faba* (VFA) (Fu et al., 2011; (Ferriz-Martinez et al., 2010).

Globally, liver cancer represents more than one million cases diagnosed each year worldwide, while it is estimated that each year about 233,000 new cases of pancreatic cancer are diagnosed, 60% of them in developed countries Including Europe, the Americas, and Australia (WHO 2011). The lectins have been used in the treatment and diagnosis of these pathologies; it was demonstrated that recombinant lectins of *Viscum album* induce apoptosis in cells of hepatic carcinoma (Yang et al., 2012), while it has been shown that peanut lectins (PNA) are capable of diagnosing pancreatic cancer with a sensitivity of 77% and a specificity of 82% compared to a radioimmunoassay. For their part, wheat germ lectins (WGA) were found to be toxic to pancreatic cancer compared to other lectins such as Concavalin A and common bean lectins (PHA), which were found to have a dose-response effect several times lower (Schwarz et al., 1999).

In the same sense, tepary bean lectins (FCL) have been studied in *in vitro* and *in vivo* studies. In cells in culture it has been shown to have a differential cytotoxic effect between untransformed cells (3T3-L1) and cells transformed with a malignant phenotype (3T3-L1 / Vmos) studies the same way that the lectins showed differential cytotoxic effects between different types of cancer such as breast and cervical cancers, and most effectively in colon cancer (Garcia-Gasca et al., 2012). On the other hand, in *in vivo* studies, low toxic was observed related to slight weight loss (approximately 10%), increase in the amount of blood granulocytes, and a decrease in lymphocytes, without altering liver and renal markers of nutritional status (Ferriz-Martinez et al., 2015). In the same way, the damage resulting from the administration of FCL in the intestinal villi and tissues related to the immune system was recently evaluated. Damage was seen, but recovery was achieved after the suspension thereof (A la Torre-Cruz et al., 2018)

Although the specific mechanism by which lectins act metabolically and molecularly is uncertain, they appear to have a great capacity to affect certain cancer cells. Our working group has determined that FCL differentially recognizes cancer cells from their non-cancerous counterparts as well as between cells of different types of cancer (García-Gasca et al., 2012).

References

Aguilera, Yolanda, Maria Angeles Martin-Cabrejas & Elvira González de Mejia. (2016). "Phenolic Compounds in Fruits and Beverages Consumed as Part of the Mediterranean Diet: Their Role in Prevention of Chronic Diseases." *Phytochemistry Reviews*, *15* (3), 405–23. https://doi.org/10.1007/s11101-015-9443-z.

Ahaneku, J. E., Taylor, G. O., Olubuyide, I. O. & Agbedana, E. O. (1992). "Abnormal Lipid and Lipoprotein Patterns in Liver Cirrhosis with and without Hepatocellular Carcinoma." JPMA. *The Journal of the Pakistan Medical Association*, *42* (11), 260–63. http://www.ncbi.nlm.nih.gov/pubmed/1336073.

Alonso-Castro, Angel Josabad, Maria Luisa Villarreal, Luis A. Salazar-Olivo, Maricela Gomez-Sanchez, Fabiola Dominguez & Alejandro Garcia-Carranca. (2011). "Mexican Medicinal Plants Used for Cancer Treatment: Pharmacological, Phytochemical and Ethnobotanical Studies." *Journal of Ethnopharmacology*, *133* (3), 945–72. https:// doi.org/10.1016/j.jep.2010.11.055.

Ambriz-Pérez, Dulce L., Nayely Leyva-López, Erick P. Gutierrez-Grijalva & Basilio Heredia, J. (2016). "Phenolic Compounds: Natural Alternative in Inflammation Treatment. A Review." Edited by Fatih Yildiz. *Cogent Food & Agriculture*, *2* (1). https://doi.org/10.1080/23311932.2015.1131412.

Aricigil, Selma & Ian F Pryme. (2015). "Potential Beneficial Effects of Dietary Plant Lectins on Health." *Natural Products: Research Reviews*, *2*, (November).

Baintner, K., Jakab, G., Gyôri, Z. & Kiss, P. (2000). "Binding of FITC-Labelled Lectins to the Gastrointestinal Epithelium of the Rat." *Pathology Oncology Research : POR*, *6* (3), 179–83. https://doi.org/10.1007/BF03032370.

Bowcutt, Rowann, Ruth Forman, Maria Glymenaki, Simon Richard Carding, Kathryn Jane Else, Rowann Bowcutt, Ruth Forman, et al. (2014). "Heterogeneity across the Murine Small and Large Intestine." *World Journal of Gastroenterology*, *20* (41), 15216–32. https://doi.org/10.3748/wjg.v20.i41.15216.

Campo Alegria, Lorena & Ana B. Garcia Garrido. (1997). "Fisiopatología y Patogenia Del Cáncer Colorrectal." [Physiopathology and patogeny of colorectal cancer] *Colorectal Cancer*, *1* (1), 1–19.

Cassidy, Aedin, Gail Rogers, Julia J. Peterson, Johanna T. Dwyer, Honghuang Lin & Paul F. Jacques. (2015). "Higher Dietary Anthocyanin and Flavonol Intakes Are Associated with Anti-Inflammatory Effects in a Population of

US Adults." *American Journal of Clinical Nutrition*, *102* (1), 172–81. https://doi.org/10.3945/ajcn.115.108555.

Castaño-Rodríguez, Natalia, Nadeem O. Kaakoush & Hazel M. Mitchell. (2014). "Pattern-Recognition Receptors and Gastric Cancer." *Frontiers in Immunology*, *5* (JUL), 1–23. https://doi.org/10.3389/fimmu.2014.00336.

Castillo-villanueva, Adriana & Fikrat Abdullaev. (2005). "Lectinas Vegetales y Sus Efectos En El Cáncer." [Plant lectins and their effects on cancer]. *Revista de Investigación Clínica*, *57* (1), 55–64.

Charúa-Guindic, L., Lagunes-Gasca, A. A., Villanueva-Herrero, J. A., Jiménez-Bobadilla, B., Avendaño-Espinosa, O. & Charúa-Levy, E. (2009). "Comportamiento Epidemiológico Del Cáncer de Colon y Recto En El Hospital General de México. Análisis de 20 Años: 1988-2007." [Epidemiologic development of colorectal cancer at the General Hospital of Mexico. 20 years analysis]. *Revista de Gastroenterologia de Mexico*, *74* (2), 99–104.

Clark, Peter I. & Maurice L. Slevin. (1987). "The Clinical Pharmacology of Etoposide and Teniposide." *Clinical Pharmacokinetics*, *12* (4), 223–52. https://doi.org/10.2165/ 00003088-198712040-00001.

Clish, Clary B., Sarah Jeanfavre, Haejin Yoon, Jessica B. Spinelli, Alison E. Ringel & Marcia C. Haigis. (2017). "Metabolic Recycling of Ammonia via Glutamate Dehydrogenase Supports Breast Cancer Biomass." *Science*, *358* (6365), 941–46. https://doi.org/ 10.1126/science.aam9305.

Coller, Hilary A. (2014). "Is Cancer a Metabolic Disease?" *The American Journal of Pathology*, *184* (1), 4–17. https://doi.org/10.1016/j.ajpath. 2013.07.035.

Cruz-Bravo, R. K., Guevara-Gonzalez, R., Ramos-Gomez, M., Garcia-Gasca, T., Campos-Vega, R., Oomah, B. D. & Loarca-Piña, G. (2011). "Fermented Nondigestible Fraction from Common Bean (*Phaseolus vulgaris* L.) Cultivar Negro 8025 Modulates HT-29 Cell Behavior." *Journal of Food Science*, *76* (2), T41-7. https://doi.org/10.1111/j.1750-3841.2010.02025.x.

Cruz, Charles S. Dela, Lynn T. Tanoue & Richard A. Matthay. (2011). "Lung Cancer: Epidemiology, Etiology, and Prevention." *Clinics in Chest Medicine*, *32* (4), 605–44. https://doi.org/10.1016/j.ccm.2011.09.001.

El-Sayed, Aly & Geoffrey A. Cordell. (1981). "Catharanthus Alkaloids. XXXIV. Catharanthamine, A New Antitumor Bisindole Alkaloid From *Catharanthus roseus*." *Journal of Natural Products*, *44* (3), 289–93. https://doi.org/10.1021/np50015a009.

El-Serag, Hashem B. & Andrew, C. Mason. (2000). "Risk Factors for the Rising Rates of Hepatocellular Carcinoma in the United States." *Gastroenterology, 118* (4), A693. https://doi.org/10.1016/S0016-5085(00)84904-5.

Estrada-Martínez, Laura Elena, Ulisses Moreno-Celis, Ricardo Cervantes-Jiménez, Roberto Augusto Ferriz-Martínez, Alejandro Blanco-Labra & Teresa García-Gasca. (2017). "Plant Lectins as Medical Tools against Digestive System Cancers." *International Journal of Molecular Sciences, 18* (7). https://doi.org/10.3390/ijms18071403.

Fardini, Yann, Vanessa Dehennaut, Tony Lefebvre & Tarik Issad. (2013). "O-GlcNAcylation: A New Cancer Hallmark?" *Frontiers in Endocrinology*, *4*, (AUG), 1–14. https://doi.org/10.3389/fendo.2013.00099.

Ferlay, Jacques, Isabelle Soerjomataram, Rajesh Dikshit, Sultan Eser, Colin Mathers, Marise Rebelo, Donald Maxwell Parkin, David Forman & Freddie Bray. (2015). "Cancer Incidence and Mortality Worldwide: Sources, Methods and Major Patterns in GLOBOCAN 2012." *International Journal of Cancer*, *136* (5), E359-86. https://doi.org/10.1002/ijc.29210.

Ferriz-Martinez, R. A., Torres-Arteaga, I. C., Blanco-Labra, A. & Garcia-Gasca, T. (2010). "The Role of Plant Lectins in Cancer Treatment." *Uaq. Mx*, 71–89.

Freed, D L. (1999). "Do Dietary Lectins Cause Disease?" *BMJ* (Clinical Research Ed.). https://doi.org/10.1136/bmj.318.7190.1023.

Fu, Lei-lei, Cheng-cheng Zhou, Shun Yao, Jia-Ying Yu, Bo Liu & Jin-Ku Bao. (2011). "Plant Lectins: Targeting Programmed Cell Death Pathways as Antitumor Agents." *The International Journal of Biochemistry & Cell Biology*, *43* (10), 1442–49. https://doi.org/ 10.1016/j.biocel.2011.07.004.

Gajalakshmi, S., Vijayalakshmi, S. & Devi, V. Rajeswari. (2013). "Pharmacological Activities of Catharanthus Roseus: A Perspective Review." *International Journal of Pharma and Bio Sciences*, *4* (2).

Gallo, Robert C. (1971). "Studies on the Antitumor Activity, Mechanism of Action, and Cell Cycle Effects of Camptothecin1." *Journal of the National Cancer Institute*, *46* (4), 789–95. https://doi.org/10.1093/jnci/46.4.789.

García-Gasca, Teresa, Marlen García-Cruz, Elisa Hernandez-Rivera, Josue López-Matínez, Ana L Castañeda-Cuevas, Lorena Yllescas-Gasca, Adriana J Rodríguez-Méndez, Elizabeth Mendiola-Olaya, José L Castro-Guillén & Alejandro Blanco-Labra. (2012). "Effects of Tepary Bean (Phaseolus Acutifolius) Protease Inhibitor and Semipure Lectin Fractions on Cancer Cells." *Nutrition and Cancer*, *64* (8), 1269–78. https://doi.org/ 10.1080/01635581.2012.722246.

Gatenby, Robert A. & Thomas L Vincent. (2003). "An Evolutionary Model of Carcinogenesis." *Cancer Research, 63* (19), 6212–20. https://doi.org/ 10.1038/421321a.

Giri, Archana & Lakshmi Narasu, M. (2000). "Production of Podophyllotoxin from Podophyllum Hexandrum: A Potential Natural Product for Clinically Useful Anticancer Drugs." *Cytotechnology* 34 (1–2): 17–26. https://doi. org/10.1023/A:1008138230896.

Goldstein, Irwin J. & Colleen E. Hayes. (1978). "The Lectins: Carbohydrate-Binding Proteins of Plants and Animals." *Advances in Carbohydrate Chemistry and Biochemistry, 35* (C), 127–340. https://doi.org/10.1016/ S0065-2318(08)60220-6.

Grivennikov, Sergei I. & Michael Karin. (2011). "Inflammatory Cytokines in Cancer: Tumour Necrosis Factor and Interleukin 6 Take the Stage." *Annals of the Rheumatic Diseases, 70*, (Suppl 1), i104–8. https://doi.org/10.1136/ ard.2010.140145.

Guerra, Flora, Nicoletta Guaragnella, Arnaldo A. Arbini, Cecilia Bucci, Sergio Giannattasio & Loredana Moro. (2017). "Mitochondrial Dysfunction: A Novel Potential Driver of Epithelial-to-Mesenchymal Transition in Cancer." *Frontiers in Oncology, 7*, (December). https://doi.org/10.3389/ fonc.2017.00295.

Guszczyn, Tomasz & Krzysztof Sobolewski. (2004). "Deregulation of Collagen Metabolism in Human Stomach Cancer." *Pathobiology, 71* (6), 308–13. https://doi.org/10.1159/ 000081726.

Hanahan, D. & Weinberg, R. A. (2000). "The Hallmarks of Cancer." *Cell, 100* (1), 57–70. https://doi.org/10.1007/s00262-010-0968-0.

Hirayama, Akiyoshi, Kenjiro Kami, Masahiro Sugimoto, Maki Sugawara, Naoko Toki, Hiroko Onozuka, Taira Kinoshita, et al. (2009). "Quantitative Metabolome Profiling of Colon and Stomach Cancer Microenvironment by Capillary Electrophoresis Time-of-Flight Mass Spectrometry." *Cancer Research, 69* (11), 4918–25. https://doi.org/ 10.1158/0008-5472.CAN-08-4806.

Hung, Js., Huang, J., Lin, Yc., Huang, Mj., Lee, Ph., Lai, Hs., Liang, Jt. & Huang, Mc. (2014). "C1GALT1 Overexpression Promotes the Invasive Behavior of Colon Cancer Cells through Modifying O-Glycosylation of FGFR2." *Oncotarget, 5* (8), 2096–2106.

Jackson, Aimee L. & Lawrence A. Loeb. (2001). "The Contribution of Endogenous Sources of DNA Damage to the Multiple Mutations in Cancer." *Mutation Research - Fundamental and Molecular Mechanisms of*

Mutagenesis, *477* (1–2), 7–21. https:// doi.org/10.1016/S0027-5107(01) 00091-4.

Jordinson, M., El-Hariry, I., Calnan, D., Calam, J. & Pignatelli, M. (1999). "Vicia Faba Agglutinin, the Lectin Present in Broad Beans, Stimulates Differentiation of Undifferentiated Colon Cancer Cells." *Gut*, *44* (5), 709–14. https://doi.org/10.1136/ gut.44.5.709.

Kaipparettu, Benny Abraham, Yewei Ma, Jun Hyoung Park, Tin-Lap Lee, Yiqun Zhang, Patricia Yotnda, Chad J. Creighton, Wai-Yee Chan & Lee-Jun C. Wong. (2013). "Crosstalk from Non-Cancerous Mitochondria Can Inhibit Tumor Properties of Metastatic Cells by Suppressing Oncogenic Pathways." Edited by Dhyan Chandra. *PLoS ONE*, *8* (5), e61747. https://doi.org/10.1371/journal.pone.0061747.

Kannan, Sankaranarayanan, Reddi a Lakku, Devaraj Niranjali, Kamala Jayakumar, Arulraj H Steven, V V Taralakshmi, S Chandramohan, Ramathilakam Balakrishnan, Christian Schmidt & Devaraj Halagowder. (2003). "Expression of Peanut Agglutinin-Binding Mucin-Type Glycoprotein in Human Esophageal Squamous Cell Carcinoma as a Marker." *Molecular Cancer*, *2*, 38. https://doi.org/10.1186/1476-4598-2-38.

Kilic, Murat Ozgur, Metin Yalaza, Celal Ismail Bilgic & Cenap Dener. (2015). "Docetaxel-Induced Scleroderma in A Breast Cancer Patient: A Case Report." *Journal of Breast Health*, *11* (2), 95–97. https://doi.org/10.5152/ tjbh.2015.1879.

Kim, Y. S., Isaacs, R. & Perdomo, J. M. (1974). "Alterations of Membrane Glycopeptides in Human Colonic Adenocarcinoma." *Proceedings of the National Academy of Sciences of the United States of America*, *71* (12), 4869–73. https://doi.org/10.1073/pnas.71.12.4869.

Kiss, R., Camby, I., Duckworth, C., De Decker, R., Salmon, I., Pasteels, J. L., Danguy, a. & Yeaton, P. (1997). "*In Vitro* Influence of *Phaseolus Vulgaris*, *Griffonia Simplicifolia*, Concanavalin A, Wheat Germ, and Peanut Agglutinins on HCT-15, LoVo, and SW837 Human Colorectal Cancer Cell Growth." *Gut*, *40* (2), 253–61.

Labenz, Joachim, Herbert Koop, Andrea Tannapfel, Ralf Kiesslich & Arnulf H Hölscher. (2015). "*The Epidemiology , Diagnosis , and Treatment of Barrett's Carcinoma*," 224–35. https://doi.org/10.3238/arztebl.2015.0224.

Lamond, John P., Minesh P. Mehta & David A. Boothman. (1996). "The Potential of Topoisomerase I Inhibitors in the Treatment of CNS Malignancies: Report of a Synergistic Effect between Topotecan and

Radiation." *Journal of Neuro-Oncology, 30* (1), 1–6. https://doi.org/10.1007/BF00177437.

Lichtenstein, R. G. & Rabinovich, G. A. (2013). "Glycobiology of Cell Death: When Glycans and Lectins Govern Cell Fate." *Cell Death and Differentiation*, *20* (8), 976–86. https://doi.org/10.1038/cdd.2013.50.

Lien, Evan C., Costas A. Lyssiotis, Ashish Juvekar, Hai Hu, John M. Asara, Lewis C. Cantley & Alex Toker. (2016). "Glutathione Biosynthesis Is a Metabolic Vulnerability in PI(3)K/Akt-Driven Breast Cancer." *Nature Cell Biology*, *18* (5), 572–78. https:// doi.org/10.1038/ncb3341.

Likis, Frances E. (2010). "Revisiting the Hallmarks of Midwifery." *Journal of Midwifery & Women's Health*, *55* (1), 1–1. https://doi.org/10.1016/j.jmwh.2009.11.004.

López-Sánchez, C., López-Martínez, F. J., Castañeda-Cuevas, A. L., Yllescas-Gasca, L., Ferriz-Martínez, R. A., Torres-Arteaga, I. C. & García-Gasca, T. (2009). *"Evaluación de La Toxicidad In Vitro e In Vivo de Lectinas de Frijol Tépari,"* [*Evaluation of in vitro and in vivo toxicity of lectins tepary bean*], 3–13.

Loraine, Schlaepfer & José Alberto Mendoza-Espinoza. (2010). "Medicinal Plants as Potential Agents against Cancer, Relevance for Mexico." *Revista Mexicana de Ciencias Farmacéuticas*, *41*, 18–27. http://www.redalyc.org/articulo.oa?id=57916060003.

Lynch, Thomas J., Daphne W. Bell, Raffaella Sordella, Sarada Gurubhagavatula, Ross A Okimoto, Brian W Brannigan, Patricia L Harris, et al. (2004). "Activating Mutations in the Epidermal Growth Factor Receptor Underlying Responsiveness of Non–Small-Cell Lung Cancer to Gefitinib." *New England Journal of Medicine*, *350* (21), 2129–39. https://doi.org/10.1056/NEJMoa040938.

Ma, Yan Hui, Wei Zhi Cheng, Fang Gong, An Lun Ma, Qi Wen Yu, Ji Ying Zhang, Chao Ying Hu, Xue Hua Chen & Dong Qing Zhang. (2008). "Active Chinese Mistletoe Lectin-55 Enhances Colon Cancer Surveillance through Regulating Innate and Adaptive Immune Responses." *World Journal of Gastroenterology*, *14* (34), 5274–81. https://doi.org/10.3748/wjg.14.5274.

McKinnell, R. G., Deggins, B. A. & Labat, D. D. (1969). "Transplantation of Pluripotential Nuclei from Triploid Frog Tumors." *Science*, *165* (3891), 394–96. https://doi.org/ 10.1126/science.165.3891.394.

Mechref, Yehia, Ahmed Hussein, Slavka Bekesova, Vitara Pungpapong, Min Zhang, Lacey E. Dobrolecki, Robert J. Hickey, Zane T. Hammoud & Milos V. Novotny. (2009). "Quantitative Serum Glycomics of Esophageal

Adenocarcinoma and Other Esophageal Disease Onsets." *Journal of Proteome Research*, *8* (6), 2656–66. https://doi.org/ 10.1021/pr8008385.

Medina, Miguel Ángel & Ana R. Quesada. (2014). "Dietary Proteins and Angiogenesis." *Nutrients*, *6*(1),371–81.https://doi.org/10.3390/nu6010371.

Mendoza, Werner, Laura Gandolfo, Luis Ponce, José Novello & Sergio Marangoni. (2007). "Estudios Estructura y Función de una Lectina Aislada de Semillas de *Caesalpinia spinosa* Kuntze (Tara)." [Structure and Function Studies of a Lectin From *Caesalpinia spinosa* Kuntze (Tara) Seeds]. *Idesia (Arica)*, *25* (2), 49–58. https://doi.org/10.4067/ S0718-34292007000200006.

Monteverde, Enrique Ávila. (2008). "Tratameinto Quirúrgico En Colon" [Colon Surgical Treatment]. *Gaceta Mexicana de Oncología*, *7* (01662), 31–33.

Mountain, Clifton F. & Carolyn M. Dresler. (1997). "Regional Lymph Node Classification for Lung Cancer Staging." *Chest*, *111* (6), 1718–23. https://doi.org/10.1378/ chest.111.6.1718.

OMG. (2007). "Tamizaje Del Cáncer Colorrectal." [Colorectal Cancer Screening]. Organización Mundial de Gastroenterologia. 2007.

OMS. (2011). "*OMS Cáncer*." Http://Www.Who.Int/Topics/Cancer/Es/. 2011.

Ortega, Yannarys Hernández, Kenn Foubert, Wim Vanden Berghe, Chandra Sekhar Chirumamilla, Luc Pieters, Dulce María González Mosquera & Sandra Apers. (2017). "Flavonol Glycosides from the Leaves of Boldoa Purpurascens and Their Anti-Inflammatory Properties." *Phytochemistry Letters*, *19* (March), 71–76. https://doi.org/ 10.1016/j.phytol.2016.12.002.

Pasanisi, Patrizia, Franco Berrino, Michela De Petris, Elisabetta Venturelli, Antonio Mastroianni & Salvatore Panico. (2006). "Metabolic Syndrome as a Prognostic Factor for Breast Cancer Recurrences." *International Journal of Cancer*, *119* (1), 236–38. https://doi.org/10.1002/ijc.21812.

Rafiemanesh, H., Mohammadian-Hafshejani, A., Ghoncheh, M., Sepehri, Z., Shamlou, R., Salehiniya, H., Towhidi, F. & Makhsosi, B. R. (2016). "Incidence and Mortality of Colorectal Cancer and Relationships with the Human Development Index across the World." *Asian Pacific Journal of Cancer Prevention*, *17* (5), 2465–73. http://www.ncbi.nlm.nih.gov/ pubmed/27268615.

Rüdiger, H. & Gabius, H. J. (2001). "Plant Lectins: Occurrence, Biochemistry, Functions and Applications." *Glycoconjugate Journal*, *18* (8), 589–613.

Sanchez-Pino, Maria-Jesus. (2007). "Mitocondrial Dysfunction in Human Colorectal Cancer Progression." *Frontiers in Bioscience*, *12* (1), 1190. https://doi.org/10.2741/2137.

Santos, A. F. S., da Silva, M. D. C., Thiago Henrique Napoleão, Patrícia Maria Guedes Paiva, Maria Tereza dos Santos Correia & Luana Cassandra Breitenbach Barroso Coelho. (2014). "Lectins: Function, Structure, Biological Properties and Potential Applications." *Current Topies in Peptide and Protein Research*, *15* (April).

Santos, Claudio R. & Almut Schulze. (2012). "Lipid Metabolism in Cancer." *FEBS Journal*, *279* (15), 2610–23. https://doi.org/10.1111/j.1742-4658.2012.08644.x.

Sasaki, M., Fitzgerald, a. J., Grant, G., Ghatei, M. a., Wright, N. a. & Goodlad, R. a. (2002). "Lectins Can Reverse the Distal Intestinal Atrophy Associated with Elemental Diets in Mice." *Alimentary Pharmacology and Therapeutics*, *16* (3), 633–42. https://doi.org/ 10.1046/j.1365-2036.2002.01160.x.

Schrijvers, D. (2010). ESMO Handbook of Cancer in the Senior Patient. Edited by Dirk Schrijvers, Matti Aapro, Branko Zakotnik, and Riccardo Audisio. *ESMO Handbook of Cancer in the Senior Patient.*, Vol. *472*. CRC Press. https://doi.org/10.3109/ 9781841847481.

Schwarz, R. E., Wojciechowicz, D. C., Picon, a. I., Schwarz, M. a. & Paty, P. B. (1999). "Wheatgerm Agglutinin-Mediated Toxicity in Pancreatic Cancer Cells." *British Journal of Cancer*, *80* (11), 1754–62. https://doi.org/ 10.1038/sj.bjc.6690593.

Semiglasov, V. F., Stepula, V. V., Dudov, A., Lehmacher, W. & Ulrich Mengs. (2004). "The Standardised Mistletoe Extract PS76A2 Improves QoL in Patients with Breast Cancer Receiving Adjuvant CMF Chemotherapy: A Randomised, Placebo-Controlled, Double-Blind, Multicentre Clinical Trial." *Anticancer Research*, *24* (2 C), 1293–1302.

Seyfried, T. N., Flores, R. E., Poff, A. M. & D'Agostino, D. P. (2014). "Cancer as a Metabolic Disease: Implications for Novel Therapeutics." *Carcinogenesis*, *35* (3), 515–27. https://doi.org/10.1093/carcin/bgt480.

Shida, Kyoko, Yoshiko Misonou, Hiroaki Korekane, Yosuke Seki, Shingo Noura, Masayuki Ohue, Koichi Honke & Yasuhide Miyamoto. (2009). "Unusual Accumulation of Sulfated Glycosphingolipids in Colon Cancer Cells." *Glycobiology*, *19* (9), 1018–33. https:// doi.org/10.1093/glycob/cwp083.

Silva, Juan Alejandro. (2008). "Quimioprotección En Cáncer de Colon." [Chemoprotection in colon cancer]. *Gaceta Mexicana de Oncología*, *7*, 20–21.

Singh, Ravinder, Sreedhar Subramanian, Jonathan M Rhodes & Barry J Campbell. (2006). "Peanut Lectin Stimulates Proliferation of Colon Cancer

Cells by Interaction with Glycosylated CD44v6 Isoforms and Consequential Activation of C-Met and MAPK: Functional Implications for Disease-Associated Glycosylation Changes" *Glycobiology*, *16* (7), 594–601. https://doi.org/10.1093/glycob/cwj108.

Tirado-gómez, Laura L. & Alejandro Mohar Betancourt. (2008). "Epidemiología Del Cáncer de Colon y Recto." [Epidemiology of colorectal cancer]. *Gaceta Mexicana de Oncología*, *7* (4), 9–17. http://www.smeo.org.mx/images/gamo2/2008/SUPLEMENTO_V7_No4-2008.pdf#page=9.

Torre, Lindsey A., Rebecca L. Siegel, Elizabeth M. Ward & Ahmedin Jemal. (2016). "Global Cancer Incidence and Mortality Rates and Trends--An Update." *Cancer Epidemiology Biomarkers & Prevention*, *25* (1), 16–27. https://doi.org/10.1158/1055-9965.EPI-15-0578.

Torrecillas-Torres, L. (2008). "Terapias Dirigidas En El Cáncer de Colon y Recto Therapies Directed in the Colon and Rectum Cancer." *Gaceta Mexicana de Oncología*, *7*, 42–47.

Valadez-vega, Carmen, José A Morales-gonzález, María Teresa Sumaya-martínez, Luis Delgado-olivares, Areli Cruz-castañeda, Mirandeli Bautista & Manuel Sánchez-gutiérrez Clara Zuñiga-pérez. (2014). "*Cytotoxic and Antiproliferative Effect of Tepary Bean Lectins on C33-A, MCF-7, SKNSH, and SW480 Cell Lines*," 9610–27. https://doi.org/10.3390/molecules 19079610.

Verri, Waldiceu A., Fabiana T. M. C. Vicentini, Marcela M. Baracat, Sandra R. Georgetti, Renato D. R. Cardoso, Thiago M. Cunha, Sergio H. Ferreira, Fernando Q. Cunha, Maria J. V. Fonseca & Rubia Casagrande. (2012). "Flavonoids as Anti-Inflammatory and Analgesic Drugs: Mechanisms of Action and Perspectives in the Development of Pharmaceutical Forms." In *Studies in Natural Products Chemistry*, 1st ed., 36:297–330. Elsevier B.V. https://doi.org/10.1016/B978-0-444-53836-9.00026-8.

Volm, Manfred, Reet Koomägi, Jürgen Mattern & Thomas Efferth. (2002). "Expression Profile of Genes in Non-Small Cell Lung Carcinomas from Long-Term Surviving Patients." *Clinical Cancer Research*, *8* (6), 1843–48.

Vona-Davis, L., Howard-McNatt, M. & Rose, D. P. (2007). "Adiposity, Type 2 Diabetes and the Metabolic Syndrome in Breast Cancer." *Obesity Reviews*, *8* (5), 395–408. https://doi.org/10.1111/j.1467-789X.2007.00396.x.

Wang, Yuan Yuan, Camille Attané, Delphine Milhas, Béatrice Dirat, Stéphanie Dauvillier, Adrien Guerard, Julia Gilhodes, et al. (2017). "Mammary Adipocytes Stimulate Breast Cancer Invasion through Metabolic

Remodeling of Tumor Cells." *JCI Insight*, *2* (4), (7), 1–20. https://doi.org/10.1172/jci.insight.87489.

Yang, Xueliang, Shuang Jiang, Yahui Liu, Ping Zhang, Shuli Xie & Guangyi Wang. (2012). "Recombinant VAA-I from Viscum Album Induces Apoptotic Cell Death of Hepatocellular Carcinoma SMMC7721 Cells." *Molecules*, *17* (10), 11435–46. https://doi.org/10.3390/molecules171011435.

Yau, Tammy, Xiuli Dan, Charlene Cheuk Wing Ng & Tzi Bun Ng. (2015). "Lectins with Potential for Anti-Cancer Therapy." *Molecules* (Basel, Switzerland), *20* (3), 3791–3810. https://doi.org/10.3390/molecules20033791.

Yu, Jie, Xiaojuan Bi, Bing Yu & Daiwen Chen. (2016). "Isoflavones: Anti-Inflammatory Benefit and Possible Caveats." *Nutrients*, *8* (6), 361. https://doi.org/10.3390/nu8060361.

Yuan, Lian Wen, Hiroharu Yamashita & Yasuyuki Seto. (2016). "Glucose Metabolism in Gastric Cancer: The Cutting-Edge." *World Journal of Gastroenterology*, *22* (6), 2046–59. https://doi.org/10.3748/wjg.v22.i6.2046.

Zhang, Fang Fang, Mary Beth Terry, Lifang Hou, Jinbo Chen, Jolanta Lissowska, Meredith Yeager, Witold Zatonski, Stephen Chanock, Alfredo Morabia & Wong Ho Chow. (2007). "Genetic Polymorphisms in Folate Metabolism and the Risk of Stomach Cancer." *Cancer Epidemiology Biomarkers and Prevention*, *16* (1), 115–21. https://doi.org/10.1158/1055-9965.EPI-06-0513.

In: Medicinal Plants …
Editors: A. Cardador Martínez et al.
ISBN: 978-1-53618-061-9

Chapter 4

Alzheimer's Disease: Causes and Possible Alternative Herbal Treatment

Gabriel Alfonso Gutiérrez Rebolledo, PhD
Natural Products Toxicology Laboratory, Pharmacy Department, National School of Biological Sciences, National Polytechnic Institute, Mexico City, Mexico

Abstract

Alzheimer is a chronic-generative neurological syndrome which affects mainly the central nervous system, however late experimental, epidemiological and clinical data had shown that the illness also affects nerve endings beyond the brain and cerebellum. The current panorama of the fight against Alzheimer's disease, although it has made great advances in terms of its early diagnosis, has been halted due to the complex of its physiopathology, so that although there is not yet a cure for this condition, if it has been possible to establish and develop therapies focused on decreasing its progression and its impact on the quality of life of patients. However, the current allopathic therapy available, in addition to being expensive and of little access, also brings a diversity of adverse side effects due to the interaction between medications and the prolonged term of these treatments. The study of medicinal plants still today, offers possible pharmacological agents for treatments of chronic degenerative diseases such as Alzheimer's, in the search for new therapies with greater therapeutic effect and lower toxic effects than conventional therapies. However, the greatest limitation that still exists is to transpose the results obtained in the pre-clinical phase into the clinical phase, which implies time and investment funds, which is why bio-directed studies and semi-synthesis changes in the chemical structure of metabolites are viable tools that allow us to facilitate research and production. It was also concluded that those natural compounds that have amphipathic characteristics and a small molecular weight are the most viable candidates as anti-Alzheimer agents, such as modified alkaloids and flavonoids, which exert a therapeutic multi-effect at various levels of the disease, mainly in the inhibition of key enzymes like acetyl and butyrylcholine esterase.

INTRODUCTION

Physiopathology

In the last decades, an increase in the incidence and prevalence of chronic degenerative or non-communicable diseases have been observed all around the world, this could be due to the interaction of diverse exogenous and endogenous factors, that allows the appearance of these illness in the worldwide population. These medical cases increasing from 562 million to 853 million from 1990 to 2017, also all these chronic illnesses are accounted for 39.5 million of the 54.7 million deaths (72%) reported for 2016 (Lancet, 2018). Among the exogenous factors, there are the increasing rates of pollution and bad diet, and for the endogenous factor there are age, epigenetics, genetic charge (clinical incidence in the family), and co-morbility (Marabotti et al., 2017). World Health Organization (WHO) estimate that between 16 to 57% of adults in developed countries suffer from a chronic illness, and also declare that the increase in the incidence and prevalence of these diseases are closely related to the economic, educational and geographical characteristics of each country, being the third world countries the most affected (Hajat and Stein, 2018).

On the other hand, the healthcare of these illnesses increased so much in the last years that in some countries (first, in development and of third world), they have allocated from their annual total budget a 19.5% for uninsured population and 12.5% for the population with healthcare (Arredondo and Aviles, 2015). WHO and US-based studies, developed a list of almost 20 known chronic-degenerative diseases, within which, the ones with major incidence and prevalence, are cancer, diabetes, cardiovascular and lung affectations, Parkinson, autoimmune illness and Alzheimer (Hajat and Stein, 2018).

Alzheimer is a neurological chronic-degenerative syndrome, which affects mainly the central nervous system, however late experimental, epidemiological and clinical data had shown that the illness extents even to affect nerve endings beyond the brain and cerebellum (Wang et al., 2017). This disease is characterized by three well-known stages: the earlier one, also known as pre-clinical, in which a discrete memory loss is perceived caused by a 25% hippocampus's shrinking; then occurs the intermediate phase, characterized by the difficult to recognize persons and to speak, related with a decreasing in the acetylcholine levels in neurons responsible for the storage of information; and finally, the last stage, in which the patient becomes dependent as the peripheral nervous system neurons are affected by decreasing mobility, and there is also an increase in dementia and disorientation until the day of death (dos Santos Picanço et al., 2018). In this context, the most important clinical features of this neurological syndrome are mild cognitive impairment, which includes a change in cognition compared to the patient's previous levels, and dementia when the neuropsychological symptoms interfere with the ability to function in usual activities (Escher et al., 2019).

Its etiology is related, in past years, mostly to heritage; however, recent data had demonstrated that the physiopathology of Alzheimer is more complex than the scientist thought. In the last years, more factors that help to the appearance and maintenance of this illness besides genetics were discover, such as physiological and metabolic mechanisms that involve apo-lipoprotein E, oxidative stress (dos Santos Picanço et al., 2018), abnormal amyloid-β metabolism, as well hyper-phosporilation of tau protein, and thus accumulation and formation of plaques from both altered proteins in the brain (Wang et al., 2017); authors also suggested that this neurological syndrome is provoked by a decrease in the acetylcholine brain levels, mostly in the cortex and hippocampus regions (dos Santos Picanço et al., 2018), associated to memory loss, because of the death of cholinergic neurons in these brain's areas in the affected patients.

From all these discover causes, two of them are the most studied: genetics and the amyloid-β plaques formation, where for the first one Deture and Dickson (2019) describe that this disease is dominantly inherited familiar, occurring mutations in the amyloid precursor protein, presenilin 1 and 2 coding genes, important in the metabolism of amyloid-β produced in the brain (mostly isoform 42), and also in other parts of the body, which contributes to its final accumulation (plaque formation), altering normal neural function and causing inflammation, loss of synapsis and oxidative stress (Wang et al., 2017). Authors also described that another genetic abnormality found in late onset of Alzheimer, is related to apo-lipoprotein E polymorphism (APOE 4), which has been associated to vascular dementia, Lewy body dementia, Down's syndrome and traumatic brain injury (Deture and Dickson, 2019).

Alzheimer's disease causes in the patient macroscopic and microscopic pathological alterations, the most notorious are moderate cortical atrophy mostly in the cortex and limbic lobe structures, as well enlarged spaces with atrophy in the gyri and posterior cortical areas, as a result of this atrophy, there is often enlargement of the frontal and temporal horns of the lateral ventricles; this loss of volume is also observed in lower total weight of the affected brain. Other neuronal structures that present atrophy are the amygdala and hippocampus, where the emotions and memory are processed. Unless these structural changes are strongly associated to Alzheimer, they are also observed in other neuropathies and aging; however, they could be co-morbidity illnesses. For the microscopic alterations, the most important parameter is the formation of β-amyloid plaques and aggregated tau protein (Deture and Dickson, 2019).

Diagnosis of this neurological illness it is not always successful, since it is only detected when it is already in the intermediate or final stages (Femminella et al., 2018); so in recent years, the search of early stage biomarkers for Alzheimer's disease is an important research focus. For many years in the past, the only possible diagnosis of this illness was through confirmatory histopathological evidence in post-mortem brains of patients, where β-amyloid plaques and neurofibrillary tangles (aggregated tau protein) were confirmed (Escher et al., 2019). The search for Alzheimer related biomarkers in peripheral blood or plasma that reflects brain damage result almost impossible, due to blood complexity and the low sensibility of past laboratory instruments, because in these two biological matrix amyloid-β_{42} and tau proteins concentrations are very low (Wang et al., 2017); nonetheless in recent years, an early detection of this disease could be achieve by measure these biomarkers in the cerebrospinal liquid, however, this is still waiting the completion of many studies in patients for clinical validation (Femminella et al., 2018). Normal neuronal, psychometric and cognitive test are carried out in addition to structural neuroimaging, molecular and functional neuroimaging, electroencephalogram and genetic studies, all of them are important complementary tests that can integrate a more complete diagnosis of Alzheimer (dos Santos Picanço et al., 2018).

Today, most advanced techniques with higher sensibility ratio are now performed, for example, molecular test such as cerebrospinal liquid amyloid-β_{42} concentration, and cortical binding of amyloid measured by positron emission tomography ligands as biomarkers for cerebral amyloid plaques, as well elevated phosphorylated tau and cortical binding of tau positron emission tomography ligands for fibrillary tau. All these tests allow the diagnosis of

Alzheimer in living patients with pre-clinical stage of the disease, in which pathological processes are already developing in the brain, but no clinical symptoms are present (Escher et al., 2019).

Epidemiology: Worldwide and in Mexico

Alzheimer's disease consequences such as dementia, affect in 2015 an estimate of 47 million people worldwide, and WHO has estimated that this number will increase to 75 million affected people in 2030, and up to 135 million in 2050 (Chen et al., 2019); WHO has reported for 2019, that dementia associated to Alzheimer's disease has showed 7.7 million new cases worldwide (one case every four seconds) annually, where most cases has been reported in Asia (3.6 million, 46%), Europe (2.3 million, 31%), America (1.2 million, 16%), and finally Africa (0.5 million, 7%). Previous analyses (1980-2009), have demonstrated that dementia associated to Alzheimer's disease, showed prevalence between 5-8% for > 60 years, with a two-fold exponential increase related to aging every 5 years (Brito-Aguilar, 2019). Also, as for the prevalence of this disease, women, African-American, and Hispanics ethnics are more likely to develop it; one of six women are diagnosed with Alzheimer's dementia compared to one of eleven men, as well compared to Caucasians, African-American and Hispanic ethnics have 4 and 2.7 times greater risk of developing it (Sherzai and Sherzai, 2019). Projections estimate that for 2060, only in the United States of America, Alzheimer will affect 3.6 million of Hispanic, follow by 2.7 million of African-American and finally 6.3 million cases for the Caucasian population (Wu et al., 2018).

For 2015, the worldwide cost destined to treat Alzheimer's disease and its consequences such as dementia, was estimated at US$ 818 billion (Takeda, 2019), and WHO expects that this number increase in the coming years, along with the world life expectancy, however, this also implies an increase in the worldwide healthcare costs for each country to almost 35% for 2010 (Chen et al., 2019). A previous study described that only in the United States of America, in 2018 the Alzheimer has surpassed all other diseases in healthcare costs around US$ 277 billion in combined spending, compared to other illness such as heart diseases and all cancers, and for 2050 year healthcare costs will arise to almost US$ 20 trillion worldwide, and US$ 1.1 trillion in the United States of America only (Sherzai and Sherzai, 2019). Finally, in 2010 the total estimated global costs fordementia were US$ 604 000 million, which corresponds to 1.0% of the gross domestic product (GDP) aggregated worldwide, while in 2016 total payments for healthcare, long-term care and hospice were US$ 236 000 million, for people with Alzheimer and other dementias (Aranda and Calabria, 2019).

In Mexico, dementia cases associated to Alzheimer's disease in 2015 were 7% of total Mexican population (Valencia-González et al., 2017), exhibited minor cognitive deterioration and 3.3% major cognitive problems with functional dependence; also, previous studies has showed similar prevalence in urban and rural regions as well (≈7.35%), while incidence was found to be for urban areas of 16.9 per 1000 person/years, and 34.2 per 1000 person/years for rural areas, with a mean of 25.55 per 1000 person/years. Studies have described also its strong association to other factors such as illiteracy, economic status, diabetes, brain-vascular and heart diseases, as well depression (Gutiérrez-Robledo and Arrieta-Cruz, 2015). Other risk factors found to be relate to Alzheimer's prevalence, incidence and development in Mexico City were air pollution and the presence of iron-rich magnetic nanoparticles accumulated in affected Alzheimer's patients brains (Brito-Aguilar, 2019).

Despite the serious public health problem that this disease represents for Mexico, in the last years, one of the biggest challenges to treat this kind of illness is the under-reporting of dementia cases or associated deaths. In 2014, was reported 86 000 new cases in all the country, and health authorities and institutions expect for 2050 an increase of almost 3.5 million affected persons (Gutiérrez-Robledo and Arrieta-Cruz, 2015). This lack of control is due to the poor preparation of health professionals, which is reflected in 150 cases reported for Alzheimer in 2015 and 227 cases of this disease in 2017 only in Mexico City, which has an approximate total population of almost 9 million people (Secretary Mexican Health, 2018).

In 2013 the economic impact of Alzheimer's disease in Mexico was estimated nearly to US$ 6 157, being this amount an approximated that a family has to spend in the treatment and care of a person with dementia, from which almost 60% of it comes directly from the family economic in-come when they assume the care of a person affected by Alzheimer, the rest 40% comes from government healthcare, however, not all the elder Mexican people are insured by the system (Gutiérrez-Robledo and Arrieta-Cruz, 2015).

Elderly population in Mexico affronts a very uncertain future, due to the fact that Alzheimer, and its latter dementia incidence and prevalence, will grow in the next 30 years in all Latin America among the population; however, experts state that the amount of population that is insured within the public health system will not increase as well (Brito-Aguilar, 2019); in 2017, 10% of Mexican population with healthcare received theirs Alzheimer's treatment in hospitals (81 900 beneficiaries of >65 years old), nonetheless, the total of diagnosed patients did not match those of the reported statistics, which means that only a 14.3% of the supposed total are detected and treated successfully (Valencia-González et al., 2017).

Allopathic Treatment

Despite the great growth in pharmaceutical research in recent years, and decades of studies to know in depth the etiological mechanisms of Alzheimer's disease, due to its role of an incipient and growing public health problem worldwide, the pharmaceutical industry has not yet been able to develop effective therapies or discovered its cure, but has achieved to discover treatments aimed at reducing its impact on normal brain functions (Graham et al., 2017).

In the last decade since 1998, more than 100 novel compounds to treat Alzheimer have failed to prevent its development in its early stages, when the first clinically symptoms appear, this due to the complexity of its etiology, as well as the multifactorial external and internal changes that occur for this illness to appear in patients, and also the potency and ability of each drug to trespass the blood brain barrier (Folch et al., 2018). In addition today, although there is no cure for Alzheimer, most of its allopathic therapies are focus to delay its progression disease during late stage, with the final goal to attenuate the global burden expenses (Frozza et al., 2018). Even though a lot of tests were carried out in the past years by the US Food and Drug Administration, from all these experiments only a few novel molecules achieve to arrive at clinic testing in healthy humans and Alzheimer's patients in risk populations, shifting the focus of this illness research to prevention and treatment in the early stages of this neurophatology (Graham et al., 2017).

To date, there are a few possibilities of allopathic treatment for Alzheimer, from all the disease-modifying therapies a few has been approved by the US Food and Drug Administration until 2018 year: 1) cholinesterase inhibitors, and 2) N-methyl-D-aspartate receptor antagonists (Lou Diana et al., 2019), however since 2019 another compounds with other pharmacological action mechanism were considered such as: secretase inhibitors, reducing of amyloid-β_{42} isoform plaque formation, tau protein phosphorylation, microglial activation inhibitors, and glycogen synthase kinase inhibitors, as well antioxidants and anti-inflammatory agents (Cummings et al., 2018; do Santos Picanço et al., 2018; Weller and Budson, 2018).

Next, we will mention examples of each of the types of Alzheimer's treatments that are already approved, or are still in clinical research stage in patients: *Cholinesterase inhibitors* (donepezil, galantamine, tacrine, and rivastigmine), *N-methyl-D-aspartate receptor antagonists or glutamatergic agents* (memantine, B3C, and riluzole), *secretase inhibitors* (EVP-062, and LY45013A), *β-site amyloid precursor protein cleaving enzyme* (LY2811376, OMM99-2, HEA, E2609, AZD3293, CNP520, JNJ-54861911, and Verubecestat), *amyloid-β_{42} isoform clearance* (AAB-003, Solanezumab, Crenezumab, Gantenerumab, BAN2401, and Aducanumab), *tau aggregation inhibitor* (TRx0237), *tau clearance* (AADvc-1 and ACI-35), *microglial activation inhibitor* (Azeliragon), *glycogen synthase kinase inhibitors* (Bis-indole, Aniline, Indirubin, and Hymenialdisin), *anti-inflammatory agents* (Indomethacin, Ibuprofen, Infliximab, and adalimumab) (Cummings et al., 2019; do Santos Picanço et al., 2018; Folch et al., 2018; Graham et al., 2017; Lou Diana et al., 2019).

From all these approved drugs to treat Alzheimer, there are 5 standard treatments approved also by European Union to treat symptoms of mild-moderate cases, but not to slow down the illness progression (Lou Diana et al., 2019), such as: three cholinesterase inhibitors (donepezil, galantamine and rivastigmine), and N-methyl-D-aspartate receptor antagonists (memantine); finally in 2014, a fifth treatment consists in the combination of each group donepezil and memantine was approved to treat patient with moderate to severe Alzheimer's disease stages (Cummings et al., 2019).

However, despite the few treatment options available for Alzheimer's disease, these therapies could exert in the patients severe secondary adverse effects due polypharmacy and long-term administrations, such as: hepatotoxicity, drug interaction by hepatic metabolism through cytochrome P_{450}, nephrotoxicity, appearance of gastric ulcers and hemorrhages by prolonged cyclooxygenase inhibition, protein synthesis alteration, and other clinical symptoms such as nausea, dizziness, muscle pain, headache and arrhythmias (do Santos Picanço et al., 2018; Folch et al., 2018).

Aim of This Chapter

The current panorama of the fight against Alzheimer's disease, although it has made great advances in terms of its early diagnosis by identifying other biomarkers *in vivo* using non-invasive techniques, has been halted as to the investigation of its possible future treatments, due to the complex of its physiopathology, which has not yet been fully understood; so that although there is not yet a cure for this condition, if it has been possible to establish and develop therapies focused on decreasing its progression and impact on the life quality of patients. However, the current allopathic therapy available, in addition to being expensive and of little access for the most affected sectors of the population, also brings a series of adverse side effects, due to the interaction between medications (polypharmacy), and the prolonged term of these treatments. In this context, scientists have focused their research on the discover of new molecules with beneficial activity over Alzheimer's disease, and with fewer toxic effects. Because of this, the study of medicinal plants, and secondary metabolites isolated from them, has resulted in a viable alternative in the search of new treatments with a greater pharmacological effect than the approved allopathic conventional therapies.

Methodology

Various scientific text search engines were used such as: *PubMed, SCOPUS* and *Google Scholar* using as key words: *Alzheimer's alternative therapy, Mexican medicinal plants used for Alzheimer, Natural products for Alzheimer, Secondary metabolites with anti-Alzheimer potential, Alzheimer's novel treatment*, and 67 published articles were found among the years of 2017-2019, and used as references to make up this chapter related to new therapy possibilities based on medicinal plants and its isolated molecules, as well herbal remedies used in the treatment of Alzheimer's disease.

Results

Anti-Alzheimer's Mexican Medicinal Plants

Mexico has over 3,000 medicinal plants used by ethno-medicinal folk knowledge to treat several chronic diseases, nonetheless, very few of these species have been studied through scientific experiments to support their pharmacological effect, hence, the true health benefits of these plants remain still unknown (Gutiérrez-Rebolledo et al., 2016). In relation, their activity over Alzheimer's disease is even less known, and scarce works of these medicinal plants were published.

Malva parviflora, commonly known as "malva de quesitos (cheese weed)", dichloromethane fraction, obtained from the standardized hydroalcoholic extract of its aerial parts, showed beneficial effects in CD-1 mice neuro-inflammation induced by lipopolysaccharides (LPS), where the treatment at doses of 5, 10 and 20 mg/kg administered by intragastric route by 7 days, exerted a beneficial effect over the spatial learning and memory impairment, and also a decrease in IL-1β and TNF-α levels in brain tissue at the lowest tested dose, which agrees with what has been reported that only low concentration of molecules reach the brain tissue to perform its effect. Authors adjudicated this biological activity to the presence of the secondary metabolite daucosterol, contained in this dichloromethane fraction, and which showed the same effect by itself, and also both inhibited the expression of NF-κB factor in macrophages *in vitro* (Ramírez-Serrano et al., 2019).

Other Mexican medicinal plant used by the ethno-medicinal folk tradition to treat inflammatory processes is *Iresine celosia*, commonly known as "hierba de la rodilla (knee grass)"; authors decided to study its possible beneficial activity, of the ethanolic extract made of its aerial parts has, over neuro-inflammation induced by LPS in male ICR mice, when the extract was administered by intragastric route daily by 2 days at dose of 30 and 100 mg/kg before the LPS-induction, and they observed that it generated an amelioration of the translocation of NF-κB factor, and also attenuated behavioral disturbances through the inactivation of microglia and astrocytes in the brain tissue. Authors suggested that this extract's activity was exerted by the presence of secondary metabolites such as iresin (Kim et al., 2019).

Another medicinal plant used in herbal medicine in Mexico is *Plectranthus scutellarioides*, commonly known as "coleo (coleus)", used to treat inflammatory illnesses. Kubínová et al. (2018), evaluated the isolated compounds from ethyl acetate fraction obtained from hydroalcoholic extract of its aerial parts over the *in vitro* inhibition of butyrylcholinesterase, and observed that two compounds, apigenin derivatives, exerted at 100 μM an inhibition better than the reference dug galanthamine at the same concentration. Due to these facts, authors proposed this medicinal plant, and its secondary metabolites, as an alternative treatment of Alzheimer's disease.

Aloe vera, commonly known as "sabila (burn aloe)", is a shrubby plant used in the Mexican traditional medicine to cure burns and open wounds, as well as gastric ulcer and inflammation. Shakir (2018), studied the effect of the ethanolic extract obtained from the parenchymatous internal tissue of its leaves to evaluate its possible inhibition over acetylcholine esterase *in vitro*, and they observed that at a concentration 0.1 M the extract exerted 89.82% of inhibition; due to these results, author suggested that the chemical compounds contained in the mucilage, could be a possible future option in the treatment of chronic neuropathology's.

Bauhinia blakeana, commonly known as "orquídea de árbol (orchid tree)", is used in Mexico to treat loss of appetite, lack of motivation, and paleness, occurring in persons with sadness, disappointment, and bad mood, so scientists decided to study its effects over Alzheimer's disease, due to all these behavior's alterations are related to this neurological illness. Ethanolic extract obtained from its leaves, and its later methanolic fraction, was tested in behavioral pre-clinical tests using male ICR mice with neuro-inflammation induced by LPS. Animals were administered at doses of 100, 250 and 500 mg/kg with the complete extract, and doses of 5, 25 and 200 mg/kg of the methanolic fraction, by the same intragastric route both by 8 days after LPS-induction. Authors observed that both, the complete ethanolic extract and its methanolic fraction, exerted and anti-depressant effect at 500 mg/kg and 5 mg/kg, respectively. And finally, both complete extract and its fraction, showed a decrease in brain tissue of all the cytokines at the doses of 500 and 25 mg/kg. Authors suggested this beneficial effect over neuro-inflammation was due to the presence in both of secondary metabolites such as rutin, which is a well-known inhibitor of NF-κB factor, a genetic inductor for the expression of all these cytokines (Herrera-Ruiz et al., 2019).

Other Mexican medicinal plant used for the ethno-medicinal treatment of inflammation is *Larrea tridentata*, commonly known as "La gobernadora (creosote bush)"; authors chose this medicinal plant, due to its proven biological activities such as anti-inflammatory and antioxidant, since it is expected that through them a beneficial effect on Alzheimer's disease will be exerted, as is known to have a high oxidative component that causes neuro-degeneration. Morán-Santibañez et al. (2019), used the ethanolic, aqueous and hydroalcoholic leaf extracts of this plant to test they effect over the cytotoxicity provoked by hydrogen peroxide (H_2O_2) *in vitro* over human neuroblastoma cells culture; they found that the hydroalcoholic extract generated a decrease in the levels of H_2O_2-provoked reactive oxidative species (ROS) accumulation in a concentration-dependent manner (0.96 to 15 μg/ml), mitochondrial depolarization (7.5 and 15 μg/ml), phosphatidylserine externalization, caspase-3/7 activation (7.5 and 15 μg/ml), and poly (ADP-ribose) polymerase (PARP) cleavage significantly, which are hallmarks of apoptosis, cellular process related to neurodegenerative illnesses. Through HPLC analysis of this extract, authors observed the presence of polyphenolic compounds, glycosylated flavonoids, sapogenins, halogenic alkaloids, and lignans.

Inside Mexican herbal medicine, we also found *Liquidambar styraciflua*, commonly known as "liquidambar (sweet gum)", is used in Mexico as a traditional herbal remedy to treat wounds, diarrhea, dysentery, coughs and skin inflammation; previous works have demonstrated its inhibitor effect over acetylcholine esterase enzyme which suggest its potential in the treatment of Alzheimer. Mancarz et al. (2019), study the effect that hydroalcoholic extract from its leaves and stems, as well its consecutive fractions, could exert over hyaluronidase activity *in vitro*, key enzyme related to inflammatory processes observed in neurodegenerative illness. Authors observed that only the complete stem hydroalcoholic extract, and its butanol fraction, showed the greatest median inhibitory concentration (IC_{50}) over hyaluronidase activity *in vitro* (38.11±0.04 mg/ml), same as the complete hydroalcoholic extract; authors suggested that this anti-inflammatory effect is due to the presence in both of hydrolyzable tannins and gallotannins.

In 2017, Vázquez-García et al. have demonstrated the inhibitor activity over acetylcholine esterase enzyme *in vitro* of three Mexican medicinal plants used in the ethnomedicinal knowledge to treat neuro-degenerative diseases such as Parkinson and Alzheimer: *Huperzia cuernavacensis, Huperzia dichotoma* and *Huperzia linifolia*, and they are commonly known in central Mexico as "licopodios". Aerial parts of the three species were used to elaborate methanolic extracts after a de-fatty process with n-hexane, and then alkaloid fraction was obtained using chloroform to isolated the alkaloid huperzine A. Results showed that of the complete methanolic extracts the one obtained from *H. cuernavacensis* exerted the most notorious IC_{50} value over acetylcholine esterase activity (5.32±0.8 μg/ml), followed by *H. dichotoma* (14.11±2.1 μg/ml), and finally by *H. linifolia* (158.37±8.7 μg/ml). Alkaloid fractions of each plant showed even a greater inhibitory effect over this enzyme, with the same behavior that the complete extracts (0.74±0.05, 0.64±0.09, and 4.2±1.24 μg/ml). Alkaloid huperzine A was only found and detected in *H. dichotoma*, so authors suggested that *H. cuernavacensis* possible has other kind of alkaloids with possible anti-Alzheimer's effect.

Other medicinal plant used to treat neuro-inflammation in Mexican traditional medicine is *Agastache Mexicana,* which contains the secondary metabolite known as acacetin which confers neuro-protection by inhibiting the activation of the NLRP3 inflammasome, through microglia mediated inflammation in a stroke mouse model. Another medicinal specie used in Mexico is *Galphimia glauca*, used in traditional medicine to treat anxiety and inflammatory processes, and scientists have found that its methanolic and ethyl acetate leaf extracts contain quercetin, a flavonoid that reduces caspase-1 protein levels resulting in low systemic IL-1ß and IL-18 levels, pro-inflammatory cytokines related to neuro-degenerative processes; as well both extracts showed the presence of galphimines, which are triterpenes with anxiolytic and sedative properties. Finally, the aqueous extract from the Mexican tree *Ternstroemia pringlei*, which has sedative and antioxidant properties awarded to the presence of the benzoquinone jacaranone (Pedraza-Alva et al., 2019).

In 2019, Castillo-Bautista et al. have studied the effect of diverse ethanolic extracts from medicinal plants used in traditional Mayan ethno-medicine to treat headache, epilepsy, neuralgia, convulsions, alteration of nerves, depression, dementia, loss of orientation, and loss of speech as possible neuro-protective agents over glutamate-induced toxicity in human neuroblastoma cell line and isolated Wistar rat cortical neurons *in vitro*. Results showed that from 34 plant species identified, only six ethanolic extracts showed neuro-protective effect over glutamate toxicity in human neuroblastoma cells with the following half maximal effective concentration (EC_{50}): *Schwenckia americana* roots (11.3 ± 2.9 µg/ml), *Isotoma longiflora* roots (13.1 ± 1.6 µg/ml), *Mimosa bahamensis* stems (15.4 ± 3.0 µg/ml), *Schwenckia americana* aerial parts (16.7 ± 2.2 µg/ml), *Elytraria imbricata* aerial parts (18.4 ± 2.3 µg/ml), and finally *Zanthoxylum caribaeum* stems (23.9 ± 2.1 µg/ml). In the other hand, neuro-protective effect of these ethanolic extracts over glutamate-induced toxicity in rat cortical neurons the EC_{50} values were for each: *Elytraria imbricate* aerial parts (6.8 ± 3.1 µg/ml), *Zanthoxylum caribaeum* stems (8.6 ± 2.4 µg/ml), *Isotoma longiflora* roots (12.4 ± 1.8 µg/ml), and finally *Mimosa bahamensis* stems, *Schwenckia americana* aerial parts and roots (> 25 µg/ml). Authors suggested that these neuro-protective effects were exerted due to the presence of secondary metabolites, such as piperidine and tetrahydropyiridine alkaloids, saponins, glycosides, tannins, phenols, flavonoids, saponins, terpenoids, steroids, and phytosteroids through their antioxidant and anti-inflammatory activities.

Isolated Secondary Metabolites with Anti-Alzheimer Activity

In the scientific study of medicinal plants, bio-directed studies must be carried out, in which the first step is to conduct an ethno-pharmacological inquiry to choose pre-clinical models and clinical studies where a human illness is mimic and related with the traditional use of these medicinal species. Latter, select the part of the plant used by the population and emulate the type of extract that will be studied with scientific bases, as well the way of preparation by the indigenous groups. Subsequently, the complete extract should be characterized, and also perform a chemical fractionation, to put together the secondary metabolites according to their polarity, and be able to perform their possible isolation. After all of these steps, authors must carry out first *in vitro* tests, and then in laboratory animals to elucidate which metabolite is responsible of the observed pharmacological activity by the complete extract.

Eugenol (1) belongs to the secondary metabolite family of carboxylic acids, and found to be a potent inhibitor of acetylcholine esterase enzyme activity, which is related to the development of Alzheimer's disease. Zhao et al. (2019), have demonstrated its potency as an inhibitor agent of this enzyme *in vitro,* and neuro-protective effect in an aluminum chloride induced dementia model in Wistar rats, which were treated with eugenol orally at doses of 50 mg/kg in a single administration, also rats with dementia received eugenol at the same dose mixed up with an approved anti-Alzheimer's drug rivastigmine by oral route at dose of 1.25 mg/kg. Authors observed that eugenol showed an IC_{50} value of 5.52 mg/l, even a greater potency than that showed by reference drug rivastigmine (7.52 mg/l), in relation to the inhibition of acetylcholine esterase activity *in vitro*.. Next test was the escape latency in the Morris water maze to evaluate memory and results showed that eugenol alone and the mix treatment with rivastigmine decrease the time latency (≈ 6 seconds), compared to dementia control group without treatment (22 seconds), a beneficial effect over memory. Also, acetylcholine esterase activity was quantified in the brain tissue of rats with dementia and same behavior than in the *in vitro* test was observed. Finally, eugenol treatment also increase antioxidant enzymes activity (superoxide dismutase and glutathione peroxidase), while generated a decrease of lipid peroxidation and pro-inflammatory cytokines (TNF-α and IL-1) in brain tissue of rats with induced dementia.

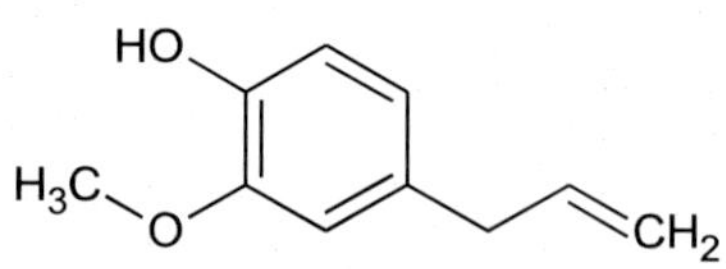

(1)

Thymoquinone (2) belongs to the secondary metabolites family of quinones, isolated from the volatile oil *Nigella sativa* seeds with supported biological activities such as antioxidant, anti-inflammatory, anti-apoptosis, and anti-cancer. To test the potential of this compound in relation to Alzheimer's disease an *in vitro* assay was carried out using cultured human induced pluripotent stem cell-derived cholinergic neurons and neurotoxicity was induced with $A\beta_{42}$ peptide. Authors observed that the treatment with thymoquinone at concentration of 100 nM prevented apoptosis process; in addition, this quinone restored glutathione levels in the cells and inhibited the ROS production and synaptic toxicity produced by $A\beta_{42}$ peptide (Alhibshi et al., 2019).

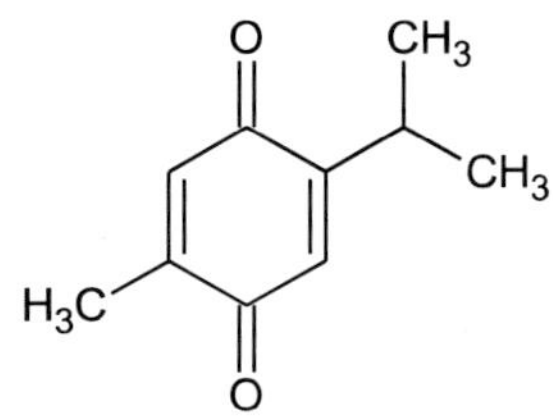

(2)

Icariin (3), is a prenylated flavonoid considered as the major secondary metabolite contained in the Herba Epimedii, a traditional Chinese herbal medicine. This compound has many supported biological activities such as anti-inflammatory, antioxidant, antidepressant and aphrodisiac. Icariin, and its hepatic metabolites, have demonstrated a beneficial effect in pre-clinical models in rodents of dementia and memory loss induced by aluminum chloride, as well in dementia induced by $A\beta_{25-35}$ and $A\beta_{42}$ peptide injection, counter-acting the deposition of this peptide and the formation of amyloid plaques in the rodents brain through an increase in $A\beta_{42}$ clearance and also up-regulating antioxidant enzymes activities, which provoked a decrease in lipid and protein oxidation (Angeloni et al., 2019).

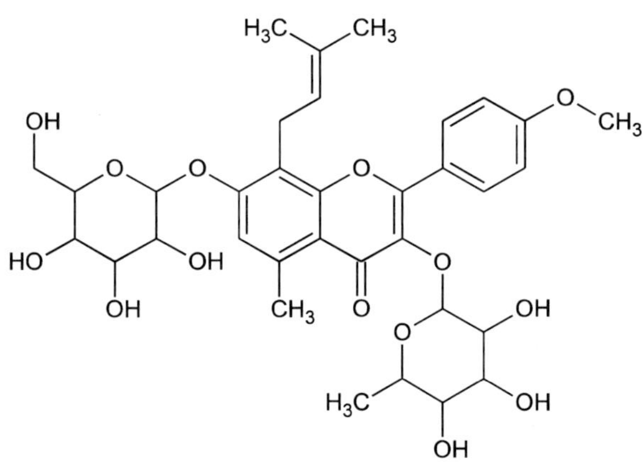

(3)

Hesperidin (4), is a natural glycosylated flavanone contained mostly in citrus fruits, which has demonstrated antioxidant, anti-diabetic and anti-cancer properties, as well anti-acetylcholine esterase potency in pre-clinical model aluminum-induced dementia. Lal et al. (2019), studied the effect that this flavonoid has over learning and memory deficits during LPS-induced neuroinflammation in male Swiss albino mice with treatment doses of 100 and 200 mg/kg administered by intragastric route by 7 days. Results showed that hesperidin treatment significantly improved the learning ability and retention of learned memory in behavioral parameters such as Y maze spontaneous alteration and Morris water maze test in a dose-dependent manner. Moreover, the neuroprotective effect of hesperidin was well supported by histopathological examination of hippocampus zone in the mice with dementia, decreasing severity of cell damage and degree of neuronal cell death compared to LPS-induced dementia control group. Authors suggested that this neuro-protection is due to its antioxidant potency and ability to inhibit acetylcholine esterase activity, as well by its ease of crossing blood brain barrier due to its hydrophobic and polyphenolic nature, a key factor in all of the new molecules evaluated by its possible anti-Alzheimer effect.

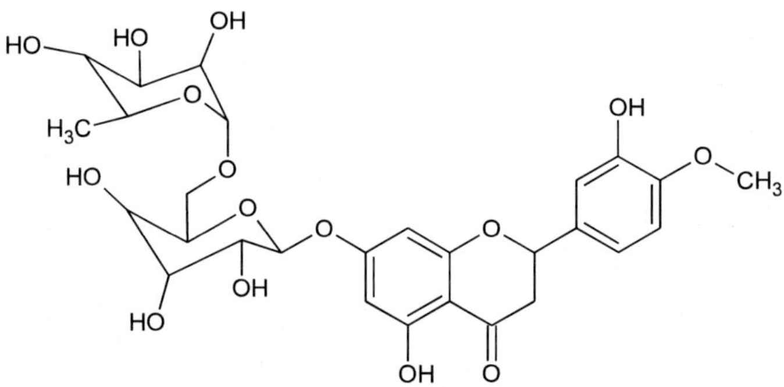

(4)

Rosmarinic acid (5), a caffeic acid ester, is found in many plants and has demonstrated diverse biological activities such as antioxidant and anti-inflammatory, related to Alzheimer's disease it also showed inhibition of acetylcholine esterase enzyme activity in brain tissue of mice with neuro-toxicity induced by scopolamine mostly in the frontal cortex and hippocampus zones, increasing memory, cognitive response and locomotors activity. Also, this metabolite showed a reduction of microglia activation and Aβ_{42} plaques *in vitro* and *in vivo*, increasing the clearance of this peptide. In other pre-clinical murine models it also decrease the levels of pro-inflammatory cytokines in brain tissue of aluminum-induced dementia in mice, through the inhibition of NF-kB factor, as well a decrease of oxidative stress over lipids and proteins increasing antioxidant enzymes activities. Another found neuro-protective effect was observed by this metabolite through the inhibition of caspase-3 activity, key enzymes of apoptosis (Mahboub, 2019).

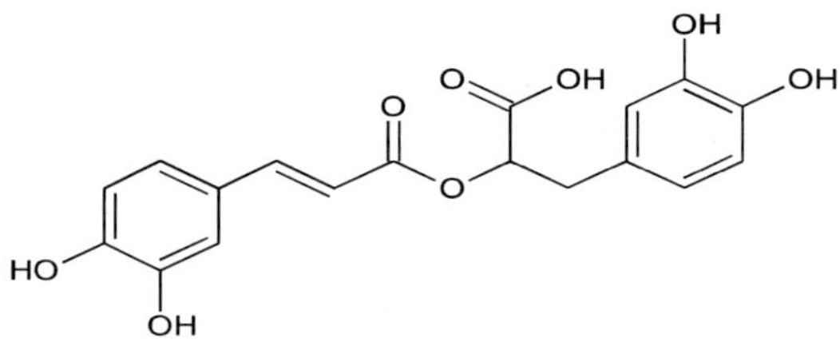

(5)

Bergenin (6), also known as cuscutin, belongs to the carboxylic acids derivatives secondary metabolites family. This natural compound has demonstrated dose-dependent inhibition of both acetylcholine esterase and butyrylcholine esterase *in vitro*, while pre-treatment with bergenin by 14 days in Wistar rats at three doses (20, 40 and 80 mg/kg) administered by intragastric route significantly alleviated amnesia induced by scopolamine in a dose-dependent way. The therapeutic effect of bergenin supplementation for 28 days, at three dose levels, was also evaluated in streptozotocin-induced Alzheimer's model in Wistar rats using Morris water maze and Y maze, where results showed an amelioration of behavioral deficits, inhibit the acetylcholine esterase and butyrylcholine esterase activities in parallel with an increase in reduced glutathione levels in a dose-dependent manner in brain tissue. It also decrease raised $A\beta_{1-42}$ peptides levels and significantly lower levels of p-tau in brain homogenates of rats with neuro-inflammation induced by streptozotocin at dose of 80 mg/kg in a single dose orally (Barai et al., 2018).

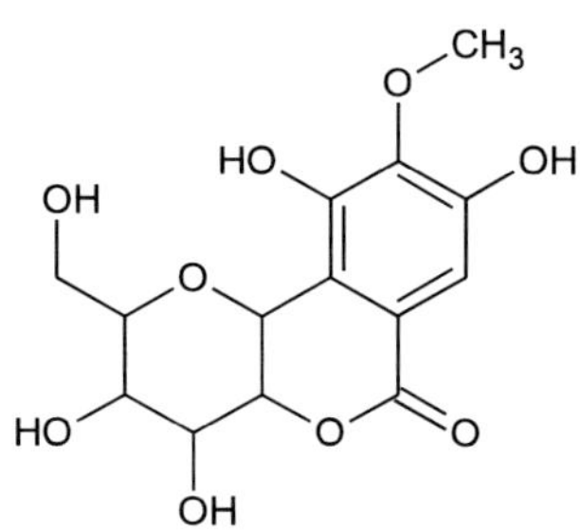

(6)

ε-viniferin, a natural stilbenoid, bio-synthesized in all the woody structures of *Vitis vinifera*, also it's a dehydrodimer of resveratrol a chemical structure which decreases its liver metabolism and also allows it to cross the blood brain barrier. This secondary metabolite has been tested transgenic albino mice (APPswePS1dE9) with predisposition to develops amyloid deposits at 4–6 months, neuro-inflammation and cognitive impairment at 12 months. Mice received weekly intraperitoneal injection of ε-viniferin at 1 and 10 mg/kg. Results showed that this resveratrol derivative induced the disaggregation of $A\beta_{42}$ peptide and inhibited inflammation on murine primary neuronal cultures *in vitro* with a higher efficiency than resveratrol, as well it reduces size and density of amyloid deposits and decreases reactivity of astrocytes and microglia *in vivo* at dose of 10 mg/kg (Caillaud et al., 2019).

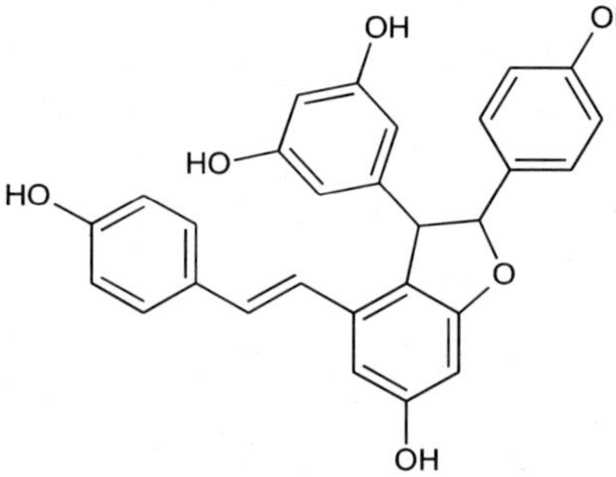

(7)

Pentylcurcumene (8), a terpene isolated from the hydroalcoholic extract from the aerial parts of *Geophila repens*, an Indian medicinal plant used to improve intelligence and memory, has shown anticholinesterase activities *in vitro* with an IC_{50} value of 73.12 ± 0.56 μg/ml for acetylcholine esterase, and 97.65 ± 0.46 μg/ml for butyrylcholine esterase, so this point this terpene as a potential first-line cholinesterase-inhibitor for Alzheimer's treatment (Dash et al., 2019).

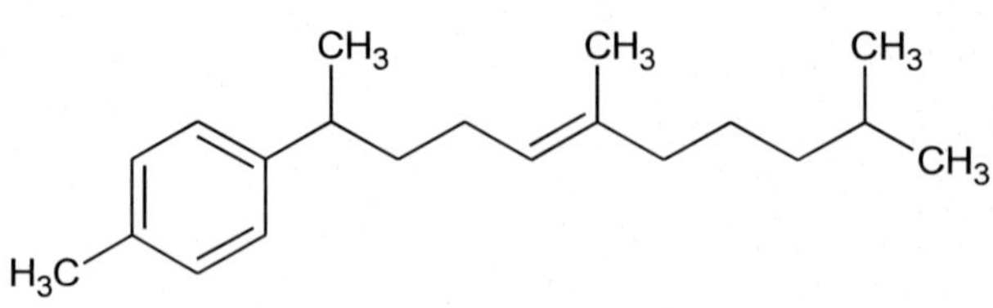

(8)

Isoflavones (9) isolated from soybeans extracts have demonstrated a lot of biological beneficial activities like estrogenic, antioxidant, anti-inflammatory, hypo-cholesterolemic, and anti-cancer in human breast cancer *in vitro*. Essawy et al. (2019), studied its possible beneficial effect against colchicine-induced cognitive dysfunction and oxidative stress in male Wistar rats, where the rich isoflavones fraction was administered by intragastric route at dose 80 mg/kg for 28 days. Results showed that isoflavones treatment before colchicine injection significantly reduced the elevated oxidative stress parameters like lipid peroxidation and restored the reduced antioxidant enzymatic activities (superoxide dismutase and glutathione transferase enzymes). Besides, isoflavones reversed memory impairment in rats subjected to the Morris water maze, the overproduction of β amyloid$_{1-42}$, pro-inflammatory cytokines (TNF-αand IL-1β), and glial fibrillary acidic protein in cortical astrocytes in the brain cortex.

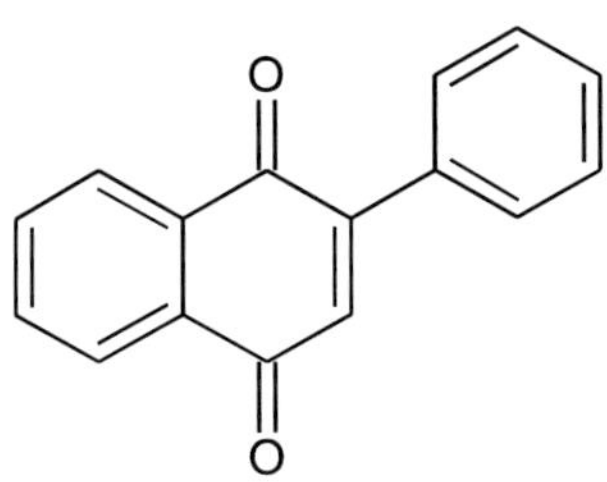

(9)

Trigolline (10), is an alkaloid isolated from *Trigonella foenum-graecum*, has showed several biological scientific supported activities such as has reported to exert hypoglycemic, neuro-protective, antioxidant, anti-apoptotic, anti-inflammatory and memory-improving effects. Fahanik-Babaei et al. (2019), also demonstrated its effect over intra-cerebral Aβ$_{(1-40)}$ injection in rats to emulate Alzheimer's disease consequences in the hippocampal zone, while trigolline was administered orally at dose of 100 mg/kg. Results showed that this alkaloid pre-treatment in Aβ-microinjected rats significantly improves spatial recognition memory in Y maze and performance in novel object recognition task, mitigates hippocampal lipid peroxidation, protein oxidation, and improves mitochondrial membrane potential, reduced glutathione levels, and superoxide dismutase activity in brain tissue. Additionally, trigonelline ameliorated hippocampal levels of glial fibrillary acidic protein, cyclooxygenase 2, and pro-inflammatory cytokines brain levels such as TNF-α and IL-6. Finally, trigonelline pre-treatment prevented loss of hippocampal neurons in Aβ-microinjected group.

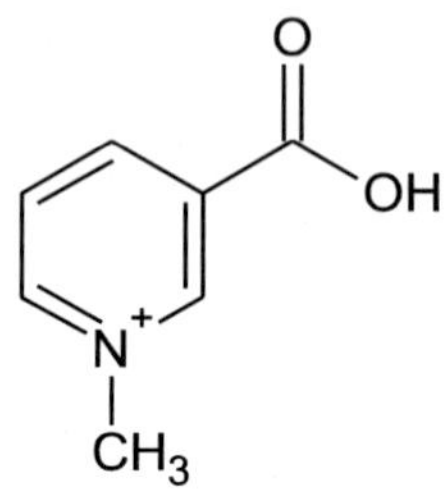

(10)

Aromoline (11), is an isoquinoine alkaloid isolated from *Berberis vulgaris* that has shown inhibitory effect *in vitro* on butyrylcholine esterase with an IC_{50} value of 0.82 ± 0.10 μM, and through docking analysis it was observed that there is a great possibility that this metabolite can cross the brain blood barrier, a crucial step to all anti-Alzheimer agent (Hostalkova et al., 2019).

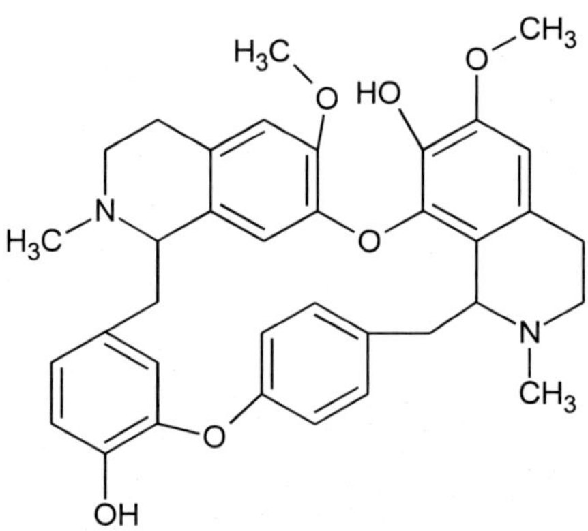

(11)

Kukoamine A (12), an alkaloid isolated from *Lycium chinense* dried root bark, has exhibited anti-inflammatory and antioxidant activities and restore human neuroblastoma cells damaged by peroxide hydrogen. Jiang et al. (2019), also demonstrated that this secondary metabolite had an inhibitory effect over $A\beta_{42}$ aggregation *in vitro* with an IC_{50} value of 11.4 μM.

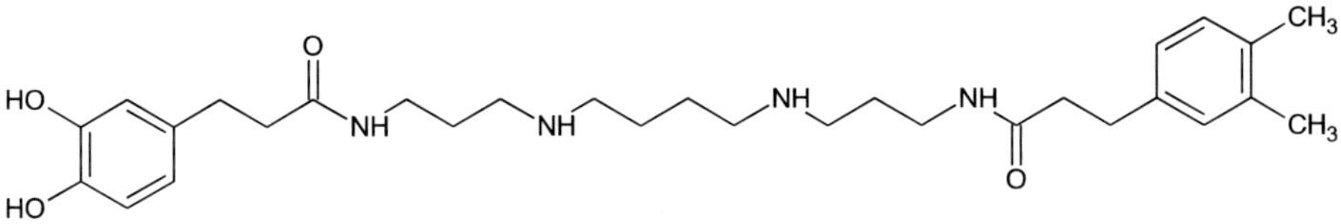

(12)

Umbelliferone (13) and pimpinellin (14) were isolated the dichloromethane fraction of root methanolic extract from *Leiotulus dasyanthus*, and both have shown an important inhibition *in vitro* over butyrylcholine esterase (61.09%) and acetylcholine esterase (66.55%), respectively at 12 μM (Karakaya et al., 2019).

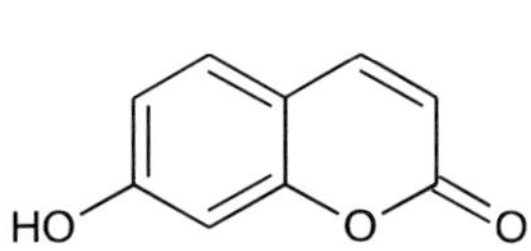

(13)

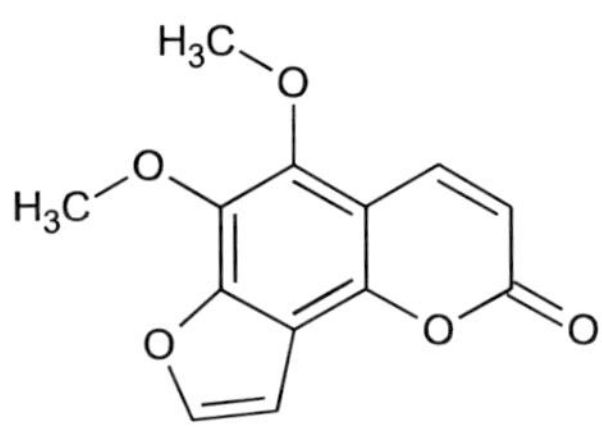

(14)

Abscisic acid (15), is an isoprenoid phytohormone, also produced and accumulated in animal tissues such as mammalian brain, that act as an autocrine and paracrine agent and acts in defensive and inflammatory responses. When this phyto-hormone was injected intra-cerebro-ventriculary at dose of 10 μg/per animal in rats with Alzheimer's condition induced by streptozotocin, authors observed that it significantly prevented the learning and memory impairment in the Morris water maze, and they suggested that PPAR-β/δ receptors and PKA signaling are involved, at least in part in its possible action mechanism (Khorasani et al., 2019).

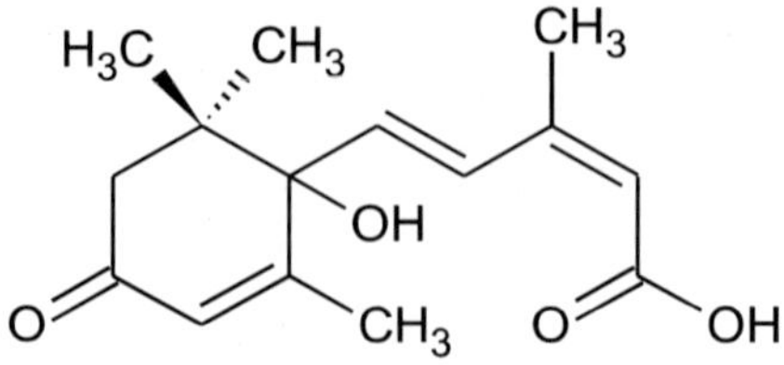

(15)

Cremaphenanthrene F (16), is a biphenanthrenes isolated from the ethanolic extract of the tubers obtained from *Cremastra appendiculata*, which shown a selective inhibition of the butyrylcholine esterase activity *in vitro* with an IC_{50} value of 14.62 ± 2.15 μM, however it did not exert any effect over acetylcholine esterase (Liu et al., 2019a).

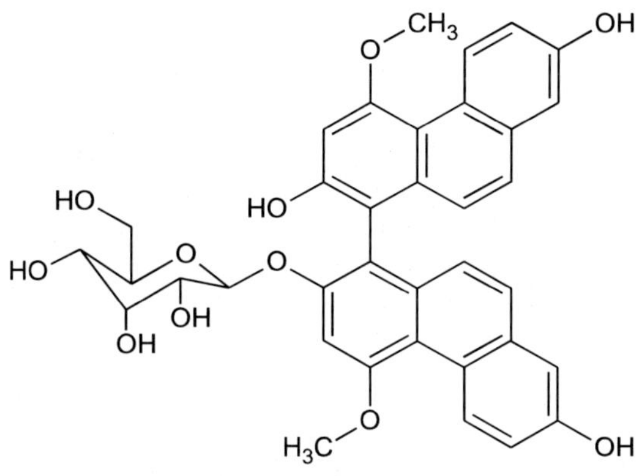

(16)

Puerarin (17), is the major secondary metabolite isolated from the roots of *Pueraria lobata*, which has demonstrated beneficial effects over Alzheimer's disease consequences in pre-clinical studies. This metabolite was administered in amyloid β-peptide-induced Alzheimer in Sprague-Dawley rats at dose of 50, 100 and 200 mg/kg orally for 14 days after the peptide injection. Results showed that puerarin treatment could restrain the acetylcholine esterase activity, restore the memory impairment observed in the Morris water maze, the activities of antioxidant enzymes (superoxide dismutase) and endogenous substances (reduced glutathione) toward normal levels, decrease the expression of inflammatory factors (IL-1β, TNF-α and nitric oxide), lipid peroxidation and apoptosis genes in the brain, especially down-regulated the expressions of cyclooxygenase 2 and caspase-3. The histopathological examination of brain sections and behavioral testing also verified the biochemical observations. All this observed beneficial effects were dose-dependent (Liu et al., 2019b).

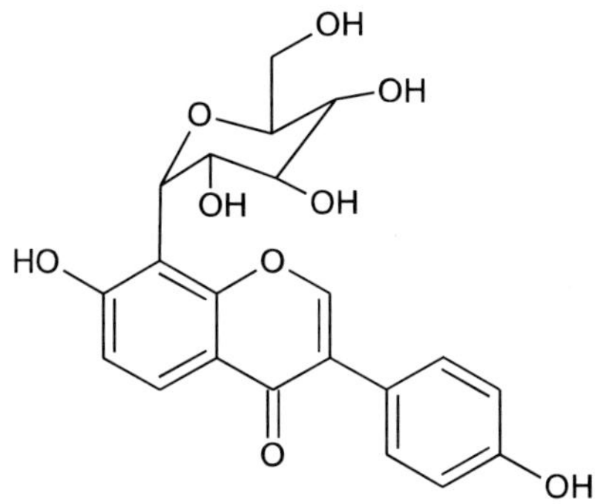

(17)

Resveratrol (18), a well-known polyphenol isolated from plants fruits like grapes, berries and peanuts, has demonstrated to be a potential anti-Alzheimer agent due to its multi-target effect in this disease such as anti-inflammatory and antioxidant actions, reduction of $A\beta_{42}$ production and deposition, reduction of hyper phosphorylation of tau protein, regulation of mi RNA a gene translation, modulation of estrogen-dependent receptors, regulation of cell autophagy and neurotransmissor toxicity, however due to its hydrophilic chemical structure greater doses have to be administer *in vivo* because of its quickly liver metabolism (Cornejo et al., 2019).

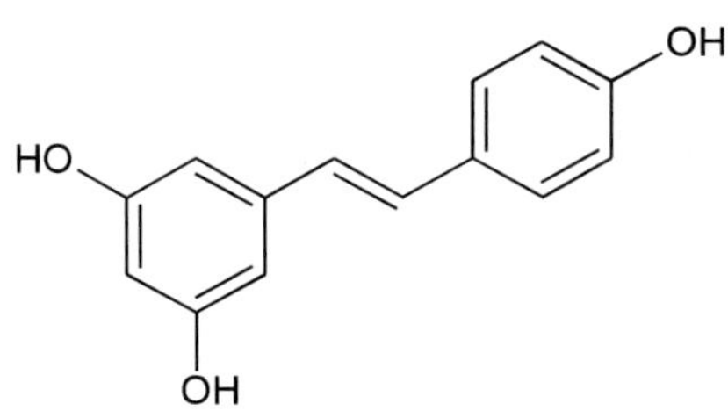

(18)

Epigallocatechin-3-gallate (19) and ferulic acid (20), secondary metabolites both related to the α-secretase pathway in Alzheimer's disease research, were tested both in a pre-clinical model using transgenic mice expressing mutant human amyloid β-protein precursor and presenilin 1 (APP/PS1) to model cerebral amyloidosis which received a mix treatment of both metabolites at dose of 30 mg/kg each orally everyday by 3 months. Results showed that combined treatment reversed cognitive impairment in most tests of learning and memory, including novel object recognition and maze tasks. Moreover, APP/PS1 mice exhibited amelioration of brain parenchymal and cerebral vascular β-amyloid deposits and decreased abundance of amyloid β-proteins compared with either metabolite single treatment. Combined treatment elevated non-amyloidogenic soluble APP-α, and α-secretase candidate and down-regulated amyloidogenic soluble APP-β, β-carboxyl-terminal APP fragment and β-secretase protein expression, providing evidence for a shift toward non-amyloidogenic APP processing. Additional beneficial co-treatment effects included amelioration of neuro-inflammation, oxidative stress, and synaptic toxicity (Mori et al., 2018).

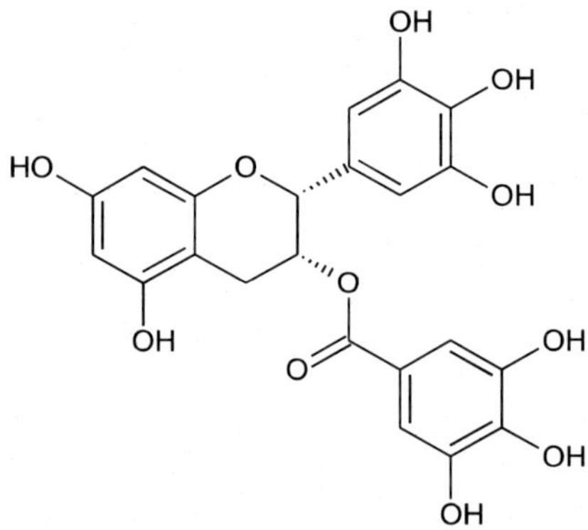

(19)

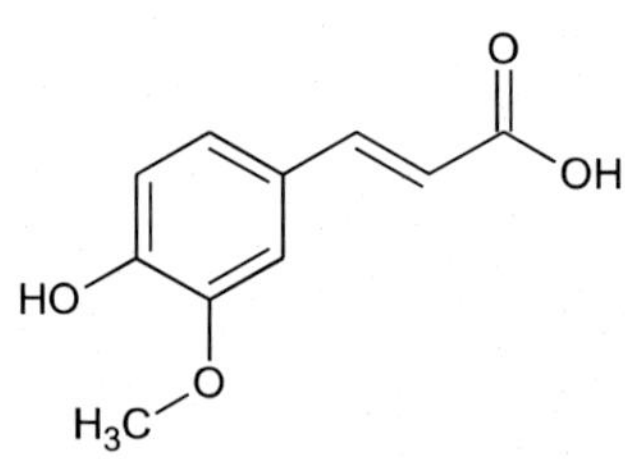

(20)

Betulinic acid (21), carboxylic acid metabolite that was isolated from ethyl acetate extract of *Melaleuca bracteata* leaves, has shown inhibition over acetylcholine esterase in concentration-dependent manner *in vitro* where at 1 mg/ml it exerted an enzyme activity of 50 nM. However, when this metabolite was acetylated this effect was greater, authors suggest that this could be due to in which carbon at position 3 (C-3) was replaced with acetyl group, meanwhile in previous studies, structural modification of triterpenes at C-3 and C-28 improved biological activities, through the interaction or binding to the active sites of this Alzheimer's key enzyme (Osunsanmi et al., 2019).

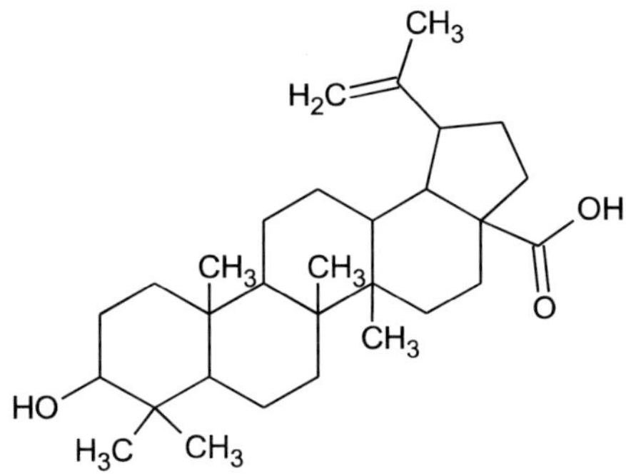

(21)

Cannabidiol (22), is a secondary metabolite isolated from the plant genus *Cannabis spp*, which doesn't have the psycho-active effect but it has been tested for neuro-protection *in vitro* in human MC65 neurons, and researchers found that this metabolite $A\beta_{42}$-induced cytotoxicity with an EC_{50} value of 30 nM, through the removal of intra-neuronal amyloid deposits, and blocking cell death and prevented the cells from accumulating the highly aggregated Aβ, and also it showed ability to stimulate the degradation and removal of preformed, aggregated Aβ from neurons interior (Schubert et al., 2019).

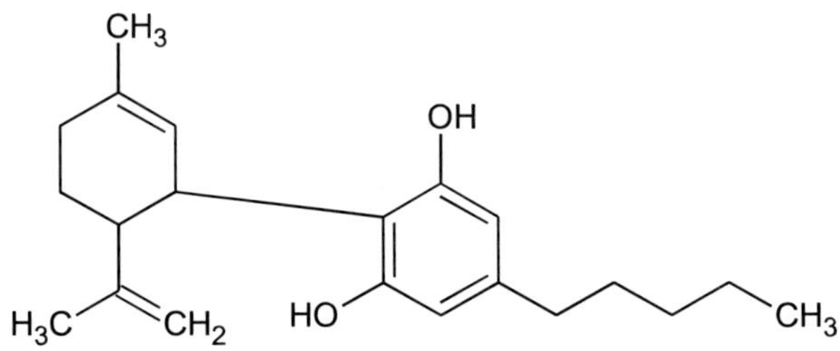

(22)

Berberine (23), is an isoquinoline alkaloid isolated from the stems and roots of various *Berberis* species that has shown multi-target approaches in the Alzheimer's research *in vitro* where is observed that it inhibited acetylcholine esterase activity with an IC_{50} value of 1.85 mM compared to the standard anti-dementia drug tacrine (IC_{50} = 0.12 mM). Also it has effect over Aβ plaque formation restricting the mitogen-activated protein kinase signaling pathway in primary microglia and BV2 cells by inhibiting Aβ-intensified production of interleukin-6 and monocyte chemotactic protein-1. It down-regulates cyclo-oxygenase-2 expression and induces nitric oxide synthase by blocking phosphoinositide 3-kinase/protein kinase β. Due to its ability to cross the brain blood barrier is a potential candidate for *in vivo* studies, for example in Alzheimer's transgenic mouse models berberine ameliorates Aβ pathology, gliosis and cognitive impairment, while intragastric administration of berberine in rabbits decreased hippocampus degeneration, changed behavior. This alkaloid also reduces tau protein phosphorylation, oxidative stress and decrease brain pro-inflammatory cytokines levels (Singh et al., 2019).

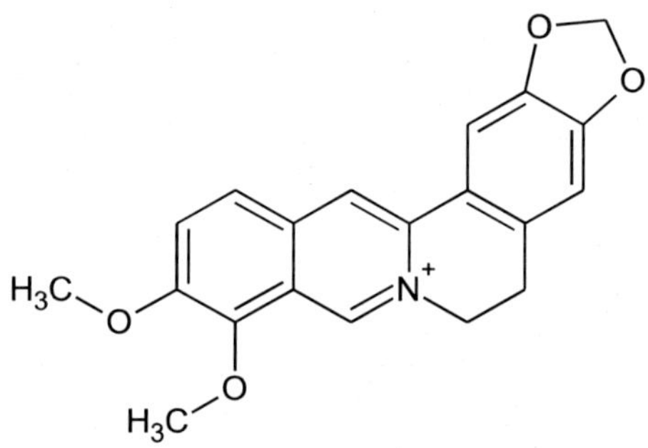

(23)

Amentoflavone (24), a natural isolated bi-flavonoid, has demonstrated to be a potent inhibitor agent of acetylcholine esterase enzyme *in vitro* with an IC_{50} value of 4.8±0.1 μM (Sirimangkalakitti et al., 2019).

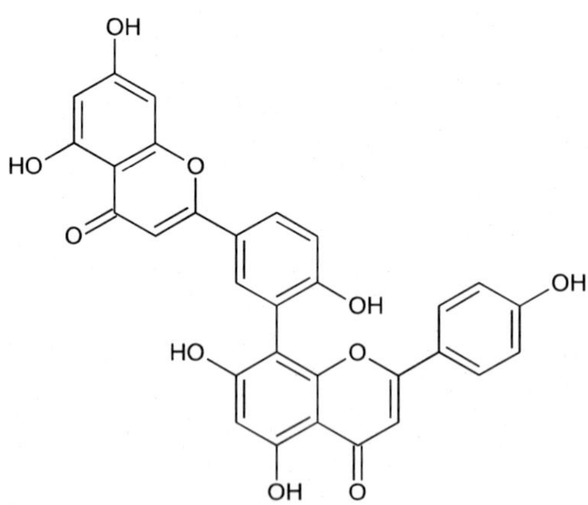

(24)

Tyrosol (25), a phenylethanoid isolated from *Rhodiola rosea*, has demonstrated a significant inhibition of Aβ-induced caspase-3 activation *in vitro*, while when assessed the *in vivo* efficacy of tyrosol by oral administration into Alzheimer's model (5XFAD) transgenic and non-transgenic mice, for both cases this metabolite treatment did not affect body weights of mice, and immune-histochemical analysis of the mice brains revealed that the immune-reactivity of spinophilin, a dendritic synaptic protein, was significantly reduced in three hippocampal sub-regions of Alzheimer affected control group, compared with non-transgenic mice, which was reversed in tyrosol-treated Alzheimer's mice. Also tyrosol treatment prevented the enhancement of 4-hydroxy-2-nonenal immunoreactivity in the hippocampal CA3 region of Alzheimer's mice, being this a lipid peroxidation biomarker in brain tissue. However, it did not have effect over Aβ accumulation, and modestly mitigated spatial memory impairment in transgenic mice (Taniguchi et al., 2019).

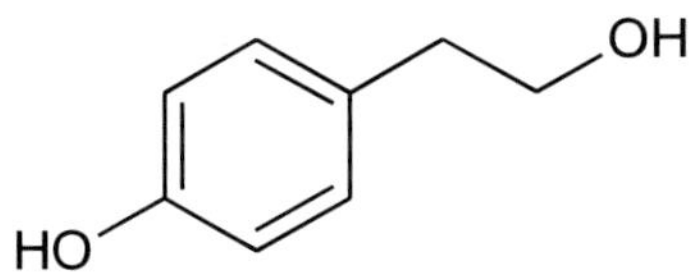

(25)

Tenuifolin (26), is a glycosylated terpene isolated from *Polygala tenuifolia*, a well-known traditional Chinese medicinal plant used to treat dementia. This secondary metabolite has shown a great beneficial inhibitory effect over Alzheimer's pathways *in vitro*. Wang et al. (2019), studied its activity over SH-SY5Y neuroblastoma cells culture, and results showed that tenuifolin prevents $A\beta_{25-35}$-induced inflammation and decreases $A\beta_{1-40}$ and $A\beta_{1-42}$ levels by decreasing BACE1 in SH-SY5Y cells. Moreover, this terpene decreases the mRNA levels of BACE1 but has no impact on the gene expressions of amyloid precursor proteins (APP). 3-MA, the most widely used auto-phagy inhibitor, reverses the effects of tenuifolin in $A\beta_{25-35}$-induced SH-SY5Y cells. The association between tenuifolin and autophagy was further investigated by examining the levels of autophagy markers LC3 II and Beclin 1, as well as the protein levels of mTOR, AMPK, and ULK1. The results showed that tenuifolin increases LC3 II, Beclin 1, and mTOR, inhibits the degradation of AMPK, and increases the expression of ULK1. This suggests that tenuifolin protects against $A\beta_{25-35}$-induced cellular inflammation in an Alzheimer's cell assay through the regulation of autophagy, which, in part, is mediated by the activation of the AMPK/mTOR/ULK1 pathway.

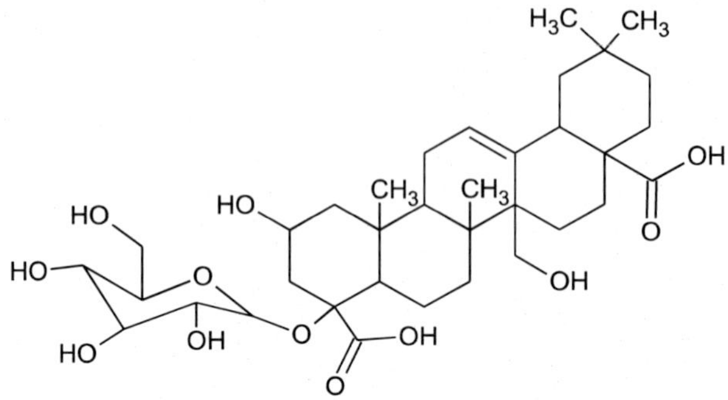

(26)

Lignans (27), isolated from *Schisandra chinensis* rattan stems, were evaluated by $A\beta_{1\text{-}42}$-induced primary microglia cell model *in vitro*. The results have shown that these metabolites could reduce the levels of pro-inflammatory cytokines, including IL-1β, TNF-α, and NO. Moreover, these lignans suppressed the phosphorylations of NF-κB and IκBα as well as p38, JNK and ERK proteins in $A\beta_{1\text{-}42}$-induced microglia cells. These metabolites could attenuate microglia cells from neuro-inflammation by activating the NF-κB/MAPK signaling pathway (Yang et al., 2018).

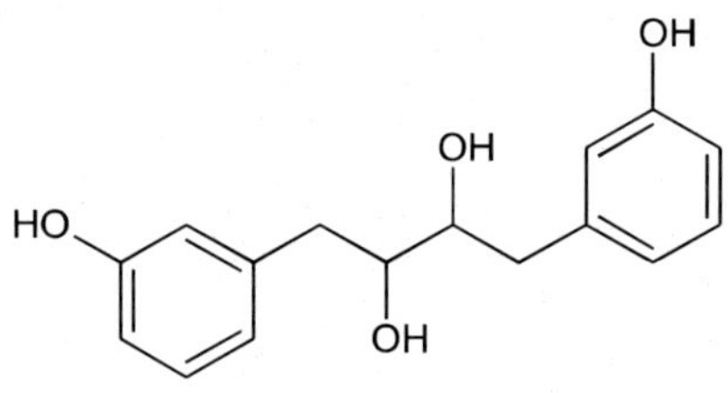

(27)

Osthole (28), chemical compound which is a derivative of coumarin and could be isolated from medicinal plants such as *Cnidium monnieri*; it has been demonstrated in human neuroblastoma (SH-SY5Y) *in vitro* assay, and later in APP/PS1 double transfected mice in a C57BL/6 background (which can effectively simulate the pathological features of Alzheimer's patients mostly those induction mechanisms related to $A\beta_{42}$ aggregation), the effect that this metabolite could exert over this neurodegenerative disease. After this time osthole was given by intragastric administration at dose of 20 mg/kg twice daily for 8 weeks, and the Morris water maze was carried out to evaluate memory *in vivo*, while for the *in vitro* technique apoptotic cells were evaluated by flow cytometry, and finally the expression of tau protein was detected through Western Blot. Results showed that osthole could significantly improve learning and memory dysfunction, ameliorate the histology structure of damaged neural cells in hippocampal area. Moreover, we also found that osthole could decrease tau protein phosphorylation as well as inhibit cells apoptosis. To explore the underlying mechanism, we used LY294002 to block PI3K/Akt/GSK-3β signaling pathway, the results from Western blot showed that the expression of related proteins in PI3K signaling pathway were decreased with LY294002 treated. This metabolite could decrease phosphorylated tau protein levels via activation of PI3K/Akt/ GSK-3β signaling pathway (Yao et al., 2019).

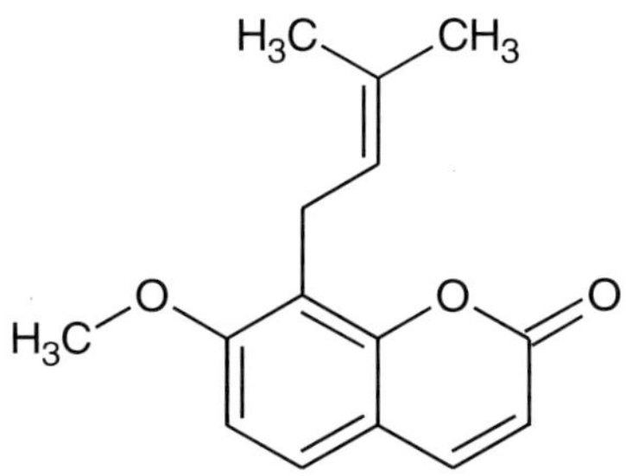

(28)

DISCUSSION

The study of the anti-Alzheimer's effect that compounds isolated from natural sources, mainly medicinal plants, has increased in recent years due to the great need to discover and test new therapies; however, most of the studies have only been carried out *in vitro* or at a pre-clinical stage, and from those only almost 21% pass to the clinical phase, since in humans it has been observed that these compounds exerted a low biological activity, due to poor absorption or bio-activation of reactive metabolites by hepatic metabolism, coupled with that various extracts of medicinal plants have showed to have toxic effect or generate adverse side effects over liver and kidneys (Andrade et al., 2019; Habtemariam, 2019).

From previous results, we observed that many of the main studies conducted on the anti-Alzheimer's effect of medicinal plants, and their isolated secondary metabolites, focus on the *in vitro* inhibition of the enzymes acetyl and butyrylcholine esterase activities, followed by the anti-inflammatory effect over the diverse immunological pathways related to this neuro-degenerative disease, as well the study of this natural compounds over $A\beta_{42}$ clearance and antioxidant effect during experimental Alzheimer *in vivo*.

Then we found the study of medicinal plants extracts effect over acetyl and butyrylcholine esterase activities *in vivo*, and $A\beta_{42}$ clearance and plaque's disaggregation *in vitro* in neuroblastome cell culture, followed by anti-inflammatory effect *in vitro* and microglial activation *in vivo*; continue with those studies related to the amelioration of apoptosis response, as well inactivation of microglial both *in vitro* and p-tau phosphorylation inhibition *in vivo*. Then we have the measure of the antioxidant potency *in vitro* of the natural compounds, and finally p-tau phosphorylation inhibition *in vitro*.

Also we observed that almost all the studied extracts were polar ones (ethanolic, methanolic and hydroalcoholic), which mainly contain secondary metabolites of a very hydrophilic nature, but also those with amphiphilic characteristics (hydro- and lipophilic nature), being this last property one of the most important due to that all the anti-Alzheimer's molecules must overcome a first primary step: to get through the brain blood barrier (where the lipophilic part of the molecule is important) (Hostalkova et al., 2019; Singh et al., 2019), and then when the molecule reach to the brain tissue, the neuro-protective effect could be exerted by the hydrophilic part of the molecule (such as anti-oxidant and anti-inflammatory effect).

Our search results showed that in the context of anti-Alzheimer's activity from isolated natural compounds from medicinal plants, the most analyzed secondary metabolites both *in vitro* and *in vivo* studies were flavonoids > alkaloids > terpenes > carboxylic acids > coumarines and their chemical derivatives.

Another important step to overcome is that the molecules have to exert a great bioavailability in the organism, with a longer half-life in the body which allows it to be in adequate concentrations in both blood and brain tissue. To achieve this goal, researchers have to alter the original chemical structure of these secondary metabolites for example, Osunsanmi et al. (2019) found the importance of the triterpenes betulinic acid over Alzheimer's disease, and they observed that after an acetylation process, the resultant product showed a greater biological activity compared to the original molecule. Also Caillaud et al. (2019), observed that ε-viniferin, showed a greater chemical structural complexity than resveratrol, which decrease its hepatic metabolism and bio-transformation, increasing its half-life in the body as well its therapeutic effect over Alzheimer's development in lower doses compared to resveratrol, which although it has demonstrated a great neuro-protective potential, through the inhibition of several Alzheimer's developmental pathways *in vitro*; when the study was carried out *in vivo,* large and repeated doses of this metabolite were required to reach its effective concentration in blood, since its biotransformation and elimination of the body is faster, due to its very hydrophilic nature and little complexity in its chemical structure (Cornejo et al., 2019).

For flavonoids, researchers suggested that their therapeutic effect over Alzheimer's disease, is due to their multiple neuro-protective actions within the brain, such as protection of neurons from neurotoxins, suppression of neuro-inflammation and thus improve memory, learning and cognitive function through theirs antioxidant and anti-inflammatory potency, mostly by inhibiting directly ROS, or inactivating its production sources in the organism, thanks to the large number of functional groups such as hydroxyl and aromatic rings that have in their chemical structure, which serve as donors of protons to stabilize free radicals (Singh and Hembrom, 2018); also through the reduction of the exacerbation of inflammatory process, since a large number of pro-inflammatory markers are expressed thanks to the translocation to the cell nucleus of NF-kB, and this is activated by the action of free radicals (Jha et al., 2019).

However, the large number of hydroxyl groups in their chemical structure are also what limits their passage through the brain blood barrier, due to its increased hydrophilic profile which accelerates and facilitates its biotransformation and elimination, thus reducing its half-life in the body, requiring very large doses, as well chemical structure modification with lipophilic groups to increase their absorption, so they could reach brain tissue. On the other hand, unlike polyphenolic compounds, those of a non-polar nature such as terpenes, need to be added with hydrophilic groups to facilitate their absorption at the gastric and intestinal level, and that can reach the bloodstream until they reach the brain tissue (Deshpande et al., 2019).

Despite this, there are secondary metabolites, naturally biosynthesized, which can reach the brain because they have functional groups that facilitate their absorption and passage through membranes, such as the nitro and amino groups of the alkaloids; however, despite the great potential of these metabolites on the development of Alzheimer's disease, toxicological studies should be carried out to establish the effective and lethal doses of the alkaloids before moving on to a clinical phase study (Deshpande et al., 2019).

Conclusion

The study of medicinal plants, even today, offers possible pharmacological agents for treatments of chronic degenerative diseases such as Alzheimer, in the search for new therapies with greater therapeutic effect, and lower toxic effects than conventional current therapies. However, the greatest limitation that still exists in this matter is to transpose the results obtained in the pre-clinical phase into the clinical phase, which implies time and investment funds, which is why bio-directed studies, and changes in the chemical structure of metabolites, are viable tools that allow us to facilitate research. It was also concluded that those natural compounds that have amphipathic characteristics, and a small molecular weight, are the most viable candidates to continue their studied in clinical stages, such as modified alkaloids and flavonoids, which exert a therapeutic multi-effect at various levels of Alzheimer's disease, mainly in the inhibition of enzymes key like acetyl and butyrylcholine esterase.

References

Alhibshi, A. H., A. Odawara, and I. Suzuki. "Neuroprotective Efficacy of Thymoquinone against Amyloid Beta-Induced Neurotoxicity in Human Induced Pluripotent Stem Cell-Derived Cholinergic Neurons." *Biochemistry and Biophysics Reports* 17 (2019/03/01/ 2019): 122-26.

Andrade, Stephanie, J. Maria Ramalho, A. Joana Loureiro, and D. Maria Pereira. "Natural Compounds for Alzheimer's Disease Therapy: A Systematic Review of Preclinical and Clinical Studies." *International Journal of Molecular Sciences* 20, no. 9 (2019).

Angeloni, Cristina, Maria Cristina Barbalace, and Silvana Hrelia. "Icariin and Its Metabolites as Potential Protective Phytochemicals against Alzheimer's Disease." *Frontiers in Pharmacology* 10 (2019): 271.

Aranda, Mónica, and Alejandro Calabria. "Impacto Económico-Social De La Enfermedad De Alzheimer." [Economic-Social Impact of Alzheimer's Disease]. *Neurología Argentina* 11, no. 1 (2019/01/01/ 2019): 19-26.

Arredondo, Armando, and Raul Aviles. "Costs and Epidemiological Changes of Chronic Diseases: Implications and Challenges for Health Systems." [In eng]. *PloS one* 10, no. 3 (2015): e0118611-e11.

Barai, Priyal, Nisith Raval, Sanjeev Acharya, Ankit Borisa, Hardik Bhatt, and Niyati Acharya. "Neuroprotective Effects of Bergenin in Alzheimer's

Disease: Investigation through Molecular Docking, *in Vitro* and *in Vivo* Studies." *Behavioural Brain Research* 356 (2019/01/01/ 2019): 18-40.

Brito-Aguilar, Rafael. "Dementia around the World and the Latin America and Mexican Scenarios." *Journal of Alzheimer's Disease* 71, no. 1 (2019): 1-5.

Caillaud, Martial, Jérôme Guillard, Damien Richard, Serge Milin, Damien Chassaing, Marc Paccalin, Guylène Page, and Agnès Rioux Bilan. "Trans E Viniferin Decreases Amyloid Deposits and Inflammation in a Mouse Transgenic Alzheimer Model." *PLOS ONE* 14, no. 2 (2019): e0212663.

Castillo Bautista, C.M., Torres Tapia, L.W., Rangel Méndez, J.A., PerazaSánchez, S.R., Cortés, D., Velasco, I., MooPuc, R.E. "Neuroprotective Effect of Mayan Medicinal Plant Extracts against Glutamate-Induced Toxicity." *Journal of Natural Medicines* 73, no. 3 (2019): 672-78.

Chen, Nai-Ching, Chih-Kuang Liang, Chun-Hao Yin, Yu-Te Lin, Ching-Chih Lee, and Chien-Liang Chen. "Effects of Socioeconomic Status on Alzheimer Disease Mortality in Taiwan." *The American Journal of Geriatric Psychiatry* (2019/06/24/ 2019).

Cornejo, L., Varela, A., Ruiz, A. "Resveratrol as a Possible Multitarget Drug for Alzheimer's Disease." *MOL2NET, International Conference Series on Multidisciplinary Sciences* 4 (2019): 1-4.

Cummings, J.L., Tong, G., Ballard, C. "Treatment Combinations for Alzheimer's Disease: Current and Future Pharmacotherapy Options." *Journal of Alzheimer's Disease* 67, no. 3 (2019): 779-94.

Cummings, Jeffrey, Garam Lee, Aaron Ritter, and Kate Zhong. "Alzheimer's Disease Drug Development Pipeline: 2018." *Alzheimer's & Dementia: Translational Research & Clinical Interventions* 4 (2018): 195-214.

Dash, Umesh Chandra, Satish Kanhar, Anshuman Dixit, Jagnehswar Dandapat, and Atish Kumar Sahoo. "Isolation, Identification, and Quantification of Pentylcurcumene from *Geophila Repens*: A New Class of Cholinesterase Inhibitor for Alzheimer's Disease." *Bioorganic Chemistry* 88 (2019/07/01/ 2019): 102947.

Deshpande, Prajakta, Neha Gogia, and Amit Singh. "Exploring the Efficacy of Natural Products in Alleviating Alzheimer's Disease." *Neural Regeneration Research* 14, no. 8 (August 1, 2019 2019): 1321-29.

DeTure, Michael A., and Dennis W. Dickson. "The Neuropathological Diagnosis of Alzheimer's Disease." *Molecular Neurodegeneration* 14, no. 1 (2019/08/02 2019): 32.

dos Santos Picanço, L.C., F. Ozela Priscilla, Brito Maiara de Fatima de Brito, A. Pinheiro Abraao, C. Padilha Elias, S. Braga Francinaldo, Silva Carlos

Henrique Tomich de Paula da, et al. "Alzheimer's Disease: A Review from the Pathophysiology to Diagnosis, New Perspectives for Pharmacological Treatment." *Current Medicinal Chemistry* 25, no. 26 (2018): 3141-59.

Escher, C.M., Sannemann, L., Jessen, F. "Stress and Alzheimer's Disease." *Journal of Neural Transmission* 126, no. 9 (2019): 1155–61.

Essawy, A.E., Abdou, H.M., Ibrahim, H.M., Bouthahab, N.M. "Soybean Isoflavone Ameliorates Cognitive Impairment, Neuroinflammation, and Amyloid Β Accumulation in a Rat Model of Alzheimer's Disease." *Environmental Science and Pollution Research* 26, no. 25 (2019): 26060–70.

Fahanik-Babaei, J., Baluchnejadmojarad, T., Nikbakht, F., Roghani, M. "Trigonelline Protects Hippocampus against Intracerebral $A\beta_{(1-40)}$ as a Model of Alzheimer's Disease in the Rat: Insights into Underlying Mechanisms." *Metabolic Brain Disease* 34, no. 1 (2019): 191-201.

Femminella, Grazia Daniela, Tony Thayanandan, Valeria Calsolaro, Klara Komici, Giuseppe Rengo, Graziamaria Corbi, and Nicola Ferrara. "Imaging and Molecular Mechanisms of Alzheimer's Disease: A Review." [In eng]. *International journal of molecular sciences* 19, no. 12 (2018): 3702.

Folch, J., M. Ettcheto, D. Petrov, S. Abad, I. Pedrós, M. Marin, J. Olloquequi, and A. Camins. "Una Revisión De Los Avances En La Terapéutica De La Enfermedad De Alzheimer: Estrategia Frente a La Proteína Β-Amiloide." [A Review of Advances in Alzheimer's Therapeutics: Strategy Against Frente-Amyloid Protein]. *Neurología* 33, no. 1 (2018/01/01/ 2018): 47-58.

Frozza, Rudimar L., Mychael V. Lourenco, and Fernanda G. De Felice. "Challenges for Alzheimer's Disease Therapy: Insights from Novel Mechanisms Beyond Memory Defects." [In English]. *Frontiers in Neuroscience* 12, no. 37 (2018-February-06 2018).

Graham, W. Vallen, Alessandra Bonito-Oliva, and Thomas P. Sakmar. "Update on Alzheimer's Disease Therapy and Prevention Strategies." *Annual Review of Medicine* 68, no. 1 (2017/01/14 2017): 413-30.

Gutiérrez-Rebolledo, Gabriel Alfonso, Leticia Garduño-Siciliano, Rosa Virginia García-Rodríguez, Mariana Zuleima Pérez-González, María Isabel Chávez, Moustapha Bah, Georgina Alicia Siordia-Reyes, Germán Alberto Chamorro-Cevallos, and María Adelina Jiménez-Arellanes. "Anti-Inflammatory and Toxicological Evaluation of *Moussonia Deppeana* (Schldl. & Cham) Hanst and Verbascoside as a Main Active Metabolite." *Journal of Ethnopharmacology* 187 (2016/07/01/ 2016): 269-80.

Gutiérrez-Robledo, L.M., Arrieta-Cruz, I. "Dementia in Mexico: The Need for a National Alzheimer's Plan." *Gaceta Médica de México* 151, no. 5 (2015): 667-73.

Habtemariam, Solomon. "Natural Products in Alzheimer's Disease Therapy: Would Old Therapeutic Approaches Fix the Broken Promise of Modern Medicines?" [In eng]. *Molecules (Basel, Switzerland)* 24, no. 8 (2019): 1519.

Hajat, Cother, and Emma Stein. "The Global Burden of Multiple Chronic Conditions: A Narrative Review." *Preventive Medicine Reports* 12 (2018/12/01/ 2018): 284-93.

Herrera-Ruiz, M., M. A. Santillán-Urquiza, O. Romero-Cerecero, A. Zamilpa, E. Jiménez-Ferrer, and J. Tortoriello. "Antidepressant-Like Effect of *Bauhinia Blakeana* Dunn in a Neuroinflammation Model in Mice." *Medical Principles and Practice* (2019): 1-8.

Hostalkova, Anna, Jana Marikova, Lubomir Opletal, Jan Korabecny, Daniela Hulcova, Jiri Kunes, Lucie Novakova, et al. "Isoquinoline Alkaloids from *Berberis Vulgaris* as Potential Lead Compounds for the Treatment of Alzheimer's Disease." *Journal of Natural Products* 82, no. 2 (2019/02/22 2019): 239-48.

Jha, Niraj Kumar, Saurabh Kumar Jha, Rohan Kar, Parma Nand, Kumari Swati, and Vineet Kumar Goswami. "Nuclear Factor-Kappa B as a Therapeutic Target for Alzheimer's Disease." *Journal of Neurochemistry* 150, no. 2 (2019/07/01 2019): 113-37.

Jiang, G., Takase, M., Aihara, Y., Shigemori, H. "Inhibitory Activities of Kukoamines a and B from Lycii Cortex on Amyloid Aggregation Related to Alzheimer's Disease and Type 2 Diabetes." *Journal of Natural Medicines* (2019).

Karakaya, Songul, Mehmet Koca, Oksana Sytar, and Hayri Duman. "The Natural Phenolic Compounds and Their Antioxidant and Anticholinesterase Potential of Herb *Leiotulus Dasyanthus* (K. Koch) Pimenov & Ostr." *Natural Product Research* 18 (2019): 1-3.

Khorasani, Ali, Mehdi Abbasnejad, and Saeed Esmaeili-Mahani. "Phytohormone Abscisic Acid Ameliorates Cognitive Impairments in Streptozotocin-Induced Rat Model of Alzheimer's Disease through Pparβ/Δ and Pka Signaling." *International Journal of Neuroscience* 129, no. 11 (2019/11/02 2019): 1053-65.

Kim, Namkwon, Cindy Cruz Martínez, Dae Sik Jang, Jong Kil Lee, and Myung Sook Oh. "Anti-Neuroinflammatory Effect of *Iresine Celosia* on

Lipopolysaccharide-Stimulated Microglial Cells and Mouse." *Biomedicine & Pharmacotherapy* 111 (2019/03/01/ 2019): 1359-66.

Kubínová, R., M. Gazdová, Z. Hanáková, S. Jurkaninová, S. Dall'Acqua, J. Cvačka, and O. Humpa. "New Diterpenoid Glucoside and Flavonoids from *Plectranthus Scutellarioides* (L.) R. Br." *South African Journal of Botany* 120 (2019/01/01/ 2019): 286-90.

Lal, M., Rai, P., Bainwad, M., Shaikh, A., Juvekar, A.R., Gurvashi, M., Gawali, N. "Neuroprotective Effect of Hesperidin in Lipopolysaccharide Induced Memory Impairment Model of Alzheimer's Disease." *World Journal of Pharmaceutical Research* 8, no. 7 (2019): 1494-513.

Lancet, The, Spencer L. James, Degu Abate, Kalkidan Hassen Abate, Solomon M. Abay, Cristiana Abbafati, Nooshin Abbasi, et al. "Global, Regional, and National Incidence, Prevalence, and Years Lived with Disability for 354 Diseases and Injuries for 195 Countries and Territories, 1990–2017: A Systematic Analysis for the Global Burden of Disease Study 2017." *The Lancet* 392, no. 10159 (2018/11/10/ 2018): 1789-858.

Liu, Liang, Qi-Meng Yin, Qian Gao, Jun Li, Yong Jiang, and Peng-Fei Tu. "New Biphenanthrenes with Butyrylcholinesterase Inhibitory Activitiy from *Cremastra Appendiculata*." *Natural Product Research* (2019a): 1-7.

Liu, Song, Xiao-Lu Cao, Guang-Qi Liu, Tong Zhou, Xi-Liang Yang, and Bing-Xin Ma. "The *in Silico* and *in Vivo* Evaluation of Puerarin against Alzheimer's Disease." *Food & Function* 10, no. 2 (2019b): 799-813.

Lou Diana, M.M., Yadav, K., Bhutia, G.T., Owoalade, S.A. "Review on Aetiology, Diagnosis and Treatment of Alzheimer's Disease." *Journal of Drug Delivery & Therapeutics* 9, no. 3 (2019): 626-33.

Mahboubi, Mohaddese. "*Melissa Officinalis* and Rosmarinic Acid in Management of Memory Functions and Alzheimer Disease." *Asian Pacific Journal of Tropical Biomedicine* 9, no. 2 (February 1, 2019 2019): 47-52.

Mancarz, Graziele Francine Franco, Laressa Carolina Laba, Elaine Cristina Pinto da Silva, Maria Rosa Machado Prado, Lauro Mera de Souza, Daiany de Souza, Tomoe Nakashima, and Rosiane Guetter Mello. "*Liquidambar Styraciflua* L.: A New Potential Source for Therapeutic Uses." *Journal of Pharmaceutical and Biomedical Analysis* 174 (2019/09/10/ 2019): 422-31.

Marabotti, Claudio, Paolo Piaggi, Paolo Scarsi, Elio Venturini, Romina Cecchi, and Alessandro Pingitore. "Mortality for Chronic-Degenerative Diseases in Tuscany: Ecological Study Comparing Neighboring Areas with Substantial Differences in Environmental Pollution." *International Journal of Occupational Medicine and Environmental Health* 30, no. 4 (2017 2017): 641-53.

Morán-Santibañez, Karla, H. Abimael Vasquez, Armando Varela-Ramirez, Veronica Henderson, Janae Sweeney, Valerie Odero-Marah, Karine Fenelon, and Rachid Skouta. "*Larrea Tridentata* Extract Mitigates Oxidative Stress-Induced Cytotoxicity in Human Neuroblastoma Sh-Sy5y Cells." *Antioxidants* 8, no. 10 (2019): 427-46.

Mori, T., Koyama, N., Tan, J., Segawa, T., Maeda, M., Town, T. "Combined Treatment with the Phenolics (−)-Epigallocatechin-3-Gallate and Ferulic Acid Improves Cognition and Reduces Alzheimer-Like Pathology in Mice." *Journal of Biological Chemistry* 294 (2018): 2714-31.

Osunsanmi, F.O., Zharare, G.E., Mosa, R.A., Ikhile, M.I., Shode, F.O., Opoku, A.R. "Anti-Oxidant, Anti-Inflammatory and Antiacetylcholinesterase Activity of Betulinic Acid and 3β-Acetoxybetulinic Acid from *Melaleuca Bracteata* 'Revolution Gold'." *Tropical Journal of Pharmaceutical Research* 18, no. 2 (2019): 303-09.

Pedraza-Alva, Gustavo, Cristina E. Ramírez-Serrano, Fernando Pedraza, Rosario del Carmen Flores-Vallejo, María Luisa Villarreal, and Leonor Pérez-Martínez. "From Traditional Remedies to Cutting-Edge Medicine: Using Ancient Mesoamerican Knowledge to Address Complex Disorders Relevant to Psychoneuroimmunology." *Brain, Behavior, and Immunity* 79 (2019/07/01/ 2019): 3-5.

Ramírez-Serrano, Cristina E., Enrique Jiménez-Ferrer, Maribel Herrera-Ruiz, Alejandro Zamilpa, Gabriela Vargas-Villa, Ricardo Jair Ramírez-Carreto, Anahí Chavarría, et al. "A *Malva Parviflora´*S Fraction Prevents the Deleterious Effects Resulting from Neuroinflammation." *Biomedicine & Pharmacotherapy* 118 (2019/10/01/ 2019): 109349.

Schubert, D., Kepchia, D., Liang, Z., Dargusch, R., Goldberg, J., Maher, P. "Efficacy of Cannabinoids in a Pre-Clinical Drug-Screening Platform for Alzheimer's Disease." *Molecular Neurobiology* 56, no. 11 (2019): 7719-30.

Secretary, Mexican Health. "*Dirección General De Epidemiología: Anuario De Morbilidad 1984-2017, Sistema Único De Información Y Vigilancia Epidemiológica (Suive).*" [*General Directorate of Epidemiology: Yearbook of Morbidity 1984-2017, Unique Information System and Epidemiological Surveillance*]. Mexico: Mexican Health Secretary, 2018.

Shakir, M.A. "The Effect of *Aloe Vera* Extract on Acetylcholinesterase and Monoamine Oxidase." *Al-Mustansiriyah Journal of Science* 29, no. 4 (2018): 1-5.

Sherzai, D., Sherzai, A. "Preventing Alzheimer's: Our Most Urgent Health Care Priority." *American Journal of Lifestyle Medicine* 13, no. 5 (2019): 451-61.

Singh, A.K., Singh Santosh Kumar, K. Nandi Manmath, Mishra Gaurav, Maurya Anand, Rai Arati, Rai Gopal Kumar, et al. "Berberine: A Plant-Derived Alkaloid with Therapeutic Potential to Combat Alzheimer's Disease." *Central Nervous System Agents in Medicinal Chemistry* 19 (2019): 1-17.

Singh, D., and Hembrom, S. "Neuroprotective Effect of Flavonoids: A Systematic Review." *International Journal of Aging Research* 1 (2018): 28-45.

Sirimangkalakitti, Natchanun, Lia Dewi Juliawaty, Euis H. Hakim, Irpan Waliana, Naoki Saito, Kiyotaka Koyama, and Kaoru Kinoshita. "Naturally Occurring Biflavonoids with Amyloid Β Aggregation Inhibitory Activity for Development of Anti-Alzheimer Agents." *Bioorganic & Medicinal Chemistry Letters* 29, no. 15 (2019/08/01/ 2019): 1994-97.

Takeda, Shuko. "Progression of Alzheimer's Disease, Tau Propagation, and Its Modifiable Risk Factors." *Neuroscience Research* 141 (2019/04/01/ 2019): 36-42.

Taniguchi, K., Yamamoto, F., Arai, T., Yang, J., Sakai, Y., Itoh, M., Mamada, N., Sekiguchi, M., Yamada, D., Saitoh, A., Kametanig, F., Tamaoka, A., Araki, Y.M., Wada, K., Mizusawa, H., Araki, W. "Tyrosol Reduces Amyloid-Β Oligomer Neurotoxicity and Alleviates Synaptic, Oxidative, and Cognitive Disturbances in Alzheimer's Disease Model Mice." *Journal of Alzheimer's Disease* 70, no. 3 (2019): 937-52.

Valencia-González, Damaris, Rocío Ramírez-Santos, and Gilberto Isaac Acosta-Castillo. "Prevalence of Dementia in a General Hospital in Mexico City." *Alzheimer's & Dementia: The Journal of the Alzheimer's Association* 13, no. 7 (2017): P840.

Vázquez-García, M., Poser, G.L.V., Apel, M., Tlatilpa, R.C., Mendoza-Ruiz, A., Villarreal, M.L., Henriques, A.T., Taketa, A.C. "Anticholinesterase Activity and Identification of Huperzine a in Three Mexican Lycopods: *Huperzia Cuernavacensis, Huperzia Dichotoma* and *Huperzia Linifolia* (Lycopodiaceae)." *Pakistan Journal of Pharmaceutical Sciences* 30 (2017): 235-39.

Wang, Jun, Ben J. Gu, Colin L. Masters, and Yan-Jiang Wang. "A Systemic View of Alzheimer Disease — Insights from Amyloid-Β Metabolism Beyond the Brain." *Nature Reviews Neurology* 13, no. 10 (09/29/online 2017): 612-23.

Wang, Lin, Guifang Jin, Hehan Yu, Qiao Li, and Hong Yang. "Protective Effect of Tenuifolin against Alzheimer's Disease." *Neuroscience Letters* 705 (2019/07/13/ 2019): 195-201.

Weller, J, and A Budson. "Current Understanding of Alzheimer's Disease Diagnosis and Treatment." *F1000Research* 7, no. 1161 (2018).

Wu, S., Rodriguez, F., Jin, H., Vega, W.A. *Chapter 4: Latino and Alzheimer's: Social Determinants and Personal Factors Contributing to Disease Risk.* Contextualizing Health and Aging in the Americas. Edited by Angel J. Vega W., Gutiérrez Robledo L., Markides K. Switzerland: Springer, Cham, 2018. doi:10.1007/978-3-030-00584-9_4.

Yang, Bingyou, Wei Han, Hua Han, Yan Liu, Wei Guan, and Haixue Kuang. "Lignans from *Schisandra Chinensis* Rattan Stems Suppresses Primary $A\beta_{1-42}$-Induced Microglia Activation Via Nf-Kb/Mapk Signaling Pathway." *Natural Product Research* 33, no. 18 (2019/09/17 2019): 2726-29.

Yao, Yingjia, Yameng Wang, Liang Kong, Yuqing Chen, and Jingxian Yang. "Osthole Decreases Tau Protein Phosphorylation Via Pi3k/Akt/Gsk-3β Signaling Pathway in Alzheimer's Disease." *Life Sciences* 217 (2019/01/15/ 2019): 16-24.

Zhao, Y., Wang, D., Bais, S., Wang, H. "Modulation of Pro-Inflammatory Mediators by Eugenol in $Alcl_3$ Induced Dementia in Rats." *International Journal of Pharmacology* 15 (2019): 457-64.

In: Medicinal Plants …
Editors: A. Cardador Martínez et al.
ISBN: 978-1-53618-061-9

Chapter 5

CANCER OF INFECTIOUS ORIGIN AND NUTRITION

Andrea Orellana-Manzano[1,2,*], PhD, Diana Maldonado[1,2] and María José Vizcaíno[1,2]
[1]ESPOL Polytechnic University, Escuela Superior Politécnica del Litoral, ESPOL, Facultad de Ciencias de la Vida (FCV), Guayaquil, Ecuador
[2]ESPOL Polytechnic University, Escuela Superior Politécnica del Litoral, ESPOL, Laboratoty for Biomedical Research, Facultad de Ciencias de la Vida (FCV), Guayaquil, Ecuador

ABSTRACT

It is essential to emphasize the role of nutrition in the treatment of cancer and nutritional therapy to help patients maintain a healthy weight, strength, and reduce the effects of treatment. It is necessary for promote the consumption of fruits and vegetables, according to the literature review, which to prevent cancer.

For this chapter, we performed a literature search of PubMed®/ ScienceDirect on March 15, 2019, using the following search items "Infectious diseases and cancer," "cancer of infectious origin." The authors (AOM, DM) screened titles and abstracts for relevance. Articles that did not include an abstract or full-text available in English or Spanish and

[*] Corresponding Author's Email: akorella@espol.edu.ec.

original articles were excluded. The remaining publications that included information on infectious diseases and cancer were analyzed in-depth. After this literature research, sixteen scientific studies were selected and compared according to the WHO statistics in cancer.

Keywords: cancer, infectious diseases, *Helicobacter pylori, Human papillomavirus, Hepatitis virus*

INTRODUCTION

Cancer is the second cause of death worldwide. Around 9.6 million deaths are evidenced in 2018, of which 70% occur in low and middle resource countries (Bray et al. 2018). Because of the late presentation of the disease, diagnosis, and treatment are inaccessible due to its high costs (WHO 2018).

The number of cancer cases will grow as the population adopts lifestyle behaviors that increase cancer risk. Mainly due to physical inactivity, excess body weight, low consumption of fruits and vegetables, tobacco consumption, and alcohol (Torre et al. 2016). Moreover, predictions suggest that by 2030, 30 million people will die of cancer each year (Lancet 2018). The World health organization-defined incidence as the number of cases that occur in a specific period and geographic area, so in cancer, there is evidenced as a rate of 100,000 people per year. According to this, Australia has the highest incidence of cancer worldwide (4.68 million cases), followed by New Zeland (4.68 million cases, Ireland with 3.73 million cases, Hungary 3.88 million cases, United States of America with 3.52 million cases (WHO 2018) which still has a high prevalence. In the South America region, the estimated age-standardized incidence rates (World) in 2018, all cancers, both sexes, all ages, Uruguay has a higher incidence of cancer with 2.63 million cases, following by Argentina, Brazil and Chile with 2.18, 2.17, 1.95 million cases (Antoni et al., 2016), respectively.

Carcinogenic infections are an important cause of cancer; in 2008, it was estimated that 16% of cancer cases are attributable to infections (Siegel, Miller, and Jemal 2019). There have been classified 11 infectious agents as carcinogens, according to the International Agency for Research on Cancer (IARC) (International agency for Research of Cancer, 2019).

Helicobacter pylori, hepatitis B virus (HBV), hepatitis C virus (HCV), human papillomavirus (HPV), Human Herpesvirus type 8 (HHV-8), lymphotropic virus type 1, *Clonorhis sinensis, Schistosoma haematobium*, Epstein-Barr virus (EBV), *Opisthorchis viverrini*, and HIV type 1 (Plummer et al. 2016). However, the human immunodeficiency virus (HIV) increases the risk of cancer when combined with other infectious agents (de Martel et al. 2015, Romesser et al. 2012). Additionally, four of this infectious agents, are the cause of the majority of cancer cases worldwide, as reported in the IARC: *H. pylori* (35.8% = 770,000 cases), *Human papillomavirus* (29.3% = 630,000 cases), Hepatitis Virus B (19.1% = 410,000 cases), Hepatitis C virus (7.9% = 170,000 cases), other agents (7.9% = 170,000 cases) (Lancet 2018).

According to studies carried out on stem cells, the risk of cancer increases when an agent acts directly on the DNA (America Cancer Society & Society, 2011; Garcion et al., 2009; Themeli et al., 2013; Wykes & Lewin, 2018).

This infectious agent could cause mutations or modifications in the number of its replications (Garcion et al., 2009; Hollstein et al., 2017; Phillips, 2018). It is known that some contagious agents can generate an increase in cell proliferation in a prolonged time. The extended exposition could cause necrosis, mitogenesis, and blockage of cell differentiation capacity, and increase the risk of carcinogenesis in infectious processes (Buonaguro, Lewis, and Pelicci 2006).

Nowadays, the purpose is to prevent chronic diseases such as cancer and avoid the progression of it. There are several epidemiological research indicating the need to establish a regular diet to prevent it (Paul et al. 2015, Song, Garrett, and Chan 2015, Moynihan and Petersen 2004). On the other hand, studies are showing that an imbalanced diet could promote the next steps of carcinogenesis (Chan, Estaki, and Gibson 2013). Fat could enhance carcinogenesis by contributing to the formation of peroxides and other reactive forms of oxygen, which lead to DNA damage, and there are no specific pathways that lead to (Neuhouser et al. 2004). A high-fat diet increased the excretion of sterol metabolites in the gut, which in turn may promote tumorigenesis in the colonic epithelium (Martinez et al. 2013, Pierre et al. 2006, Poesen et al. 2014). Also, certain fatty acids in diet could be incorporated into cell membranes, possibly produce changes in cell behavior that are associated with cancer promotion (Marian 2010).

METHODS

Literature Review

We performed database searches in ScienceDirect, PubMed, and google scholar for any cancer infectious diseases with time limitation 20 years "1999-2019." We used specific words for the searches, including "Infectious diseases and cancer," "cancer of Infectious origin" we focused only on "originals articles" and only in which the main focus is human. After the literature search, the references from the studies were merged, obtaining a total of 875 articles, we used another filter "human," "free full text" and all the rest of the references were excluded. We did perform an abstract reading focusing the articles leaving a total of sixteen scientific studies of cancer of infectious origin focusing on gastric, prostate, hepatocellular, cervical cancer.

RESULTS

Table 1 shows the results of the literature searching about "cancer of infectious diseases origin." The sixteen papers selected into five cancer types were reduced according to the WHO incidences of cancer infectious diseases origin. According to WHO, there are mainly four pathogens that affect most of the worldwide cancer population. *Helicobacter pylori*, *Human papillomavirus*, *Hepatitis virus B, and C, that could lead to gastric, cervical, and hepatocellular cancer.*

Gastric Cancer (GC) and *H. pylori*

Gastric cancer is the 6th incidence of cancer cause worldwide in 2018, with 5.7% of cases, and one of the leading causes of this cancer is the chronic infection of *H. pylori*. *H. pylori* infection causes superficial gastritis that produces atrophy, a pre-cancerous condition. In 1994, the International Agency for Research on Cancer of the World Health Organization included *H. pylori* as a carcinogenic biological agent for humans (category 1) based on epidemiological evidence that associated it with gastric cancer (Ishaq and Nunn 2015).

This bacteria is one of the most studies bacteria worldwide (Daugule and Rowland 2008, Goh et al. 2011), and the prevalence change according to the region, geography, ethnicity, age, and socioeconomic factors (Gomez et al. 2004, de Martel and Parsonnet 2006). *H. pylori* is a microaerophile microorganism that lives in human gastric mucosa. It has a spiral form and could adopt coccoid form in cellular systems or when it is committed to unfavorable growing systems (Bauer and Meyer 2011), and the main transmission is oral-oral or fecal-oral (Goh et al. 2011). This bacterium, once established in the

Table 1. Cancer of infectious diseases origin

Paper	Cancer type	Pathogen	Mechanism of carcinogenesis	Study population	N	Country	Prevalence WHO	Reference
The prevalence of EBV and CMV DNA in epithelial ovarian cancer	Epithelial ovarian cancer	Epstein-Barr Virus (EBV) cytomegalovirus (CMV)	CMV contains several oncoproteins with the potential to cause immunological evasion and affect the progression of the human cell cycle and angiogenesis.	Adult women with epithelial ovarian cancer (55-64 years)	198	Denmark	NA*	(Ingerslev et al. 2019)
Gastric cancer risk estimate in patients with chronic gastritis associated with *H. pylori* infection in a clinical setting	Gastric cancer	*Helicobacter pylori*	The bacterium *Helicobacter pylori* generate chronic inflammation leading to gastritis, ulcers-peptic disease, gastric cancer, and primary gastric lymphoma. Carcinogenesis begins with a process of chronic gastritis, followed by glandular atrophy, intestinal metaplasia, dysplasia, and finally, adenocarcinoma.	Male and female patients (77% women) with an average age of 38.6 ± 13.1.	111	Venezuela	6.7% (1,589,752 cases)	(Arismendi-Morillo et al. 2013)
Progression of chronic atrophic gastritis associated with *H pylori* infection increases the risk of gastric cancer	Gastric cancer	*Helicobacter pylori*	*H. pylori* cause of chronic atrophic gastritis (CAG), as shown in rodent models. The current model for stomach carcinogenesis begins with gastritis, proceeds to CAG, then to intestinal metaplasia, dysplasia, and, finally, carcinoma.	males, from 40 to 59 years of age	5706	Japan	6.7% (1,589,752 cases)	(Ohata et al. 2004)

Table 1. (Continued)

Paper	Cancer type	Pathogen	Mechanism of carcinogenesis	Study population	N	Country	Prevalence WHO	Reference
Mycoplasma genitalium Infection and Chronic Inflammation in Human Prostate Cancer: Detection Using Prostatectomy and Needle Biopsy Specimens	Prostate cancer	*Mycoplasma genitalium*	*M.genitalium* is capable of inducing tumorigenesis not only indirectly through a local chronic progressive inflammatory response, but also directly through bacterial protein products such as p37 that exert oncogenic effects.	Men with prostate cancer	133	Japan	15.73% (3,724,658 cases)	(Miyake, Ohnishi, Hori, Nakano, Nakano, Yano, Ohnishi, Owari, Morizawa, Itami, et al. 2019)
A prospective cohort study to evaluate immunosuppressive cytokines as predictors of viral persistence and progression to a pre-malignant lesion in the cervix in women infected with HR-HPV: study protocol	Cervical cancer	Human papillomavirus (HPV)	The progression of CC has been associated with an undesirable change of Th1 to Th2 cytokine type induced by two epitopes derived from HPV E7 and an increase in the expression of IL-10.	Women with positive human papillomavirus (30 years or older)	200	Mexico	6.22% (1,474,265 cases)	(Torres-Poveda et al. 2018)

Paper	Cancer type	Pathogen	Mechanism of carcinogenesis	Study population	N	Country	Prevalence WHO	Reference
Serum IL-6 levels and the risk for hepatocarcinogenesis in chronic hepatitis C patients: An analysis based on gender differences	Carcinoma hepatocellular	Hepatitis C virus	Serum IL-6 levels are elevated in patients with chronic inflammation of the liver, including alcoholic hepatitis, hepatitis B, HCV infections, and steatohepatitis. In chronic hepatitis, IL-6, produced mainly by activated Kupffer cells, intensifies local inflammatory responses, and induces the compensatory proliferation of hepatocytes, facilitating the malignant transformation of hepatocytes.	One hundred fifty men and 180 women with a median age of 60 years (interquartile range, 52-65).	330	Japan	2.85% (675,210 cases)	(Nakagawa et al. 2009)
Study of the liver in HBV-related hepatocellular carcinoma: Stereology shows quantitative differences in liver structure	Hepatocellular carcinoma	*Hepatitis B virus (HBV) and Hepatitis C virus (HCV)*	In the infectious process of the chronic mixed infection of HBV + HBV, signs such as hepatocyte modification and the destruction of cytoplasmic organelles occur. Functional deterioration and degeneration of the liver structure leading to the risk of hepatocellular carcinoma.	40 cases had HBV infection (28 men and 12 women, median = 58 years), 41 patients with HCC (32 men and nine women, median = 56 years), and 40 patients with HBV + HCC (29 men and 11 women, median = 59 years)	121	Iran	2.85% (675,210 cases)	(Moudi, Heidari, and Mahmoudzadeh-Sagheb 2018)

Table 1. (Continued)

Paper	Cancer type	Pathogen	Mechanism of carcinogenesis	Study population	N	Country	Prevalence WHO	Reference
"Risk of cervical dysplasia among human papillomavirus-infected women in Korea: a multicenter prospective study.	Cervical cancer	*Human papillomavirus* (HPV)	Chronic infection leads to inflammation and can progress from precursor lesions (if left untreated) even after several years. This precancerous stage, is complicated to detect due to the absence of symptoms in the infected individual.	Women between 20 to 60 years old	1027	Korea	6.22% (1,474,265 cases)	(Park et al. 2019)
Urinary microbiota in patients with prostate cancer and benign prostatic hyperplasia	Prostate cancer	Bacteroidetes bacteria, Alphaproteobacteria, Firmicutes bacteria, Lachnospiraceae, Propionicimonas, and Sphingomonas	Gram-negative enteric bacteria are frequently associated with urinary tract infections that can cause chronic bacterial prostatitis. Bacterial-induced chronic bacterial prostatitis may improve proinflammatory responses that may contribute to prostate cancer.	Male patients included in the study were younger than 75 years old and were diagnosed with BPH or prostate cancer	34	China	15.73% (3,724,658 cases)	(Yu et al. 2015)
Helicobacter pylori Infection and the Development of Gastric Cancer	Gastric cancer	*Helicobacter pylori*	*H. pylori* infection is associated with the development of gastric cancer of both intestinal and diffuse types. Patients with severe atrophy may generate intestinal metaplasia and gastritis with a predominance of the corpus.	Japanese patients who had duodenal ulcers, gastric ulcers, gastric hyperplasia, or non-ulcer dyspepsia. (869 men and 657 women)	1526	Japan	6.7% (1,589,752 cases)	(Uemura et al. 2001)

Paper	Cancer type	Pathogen	Mechanism of carcinogenesis	Study population	N	Country	Prevalence WHO	Reference
Analysis of *cagA* in *Helicobacter pylori* strains from Colombian populations with contrasting gastric cancer risk reveals a biomarker for disease severity	Gastric cancer	*Helicobacter pylori*	CagA interacts with multiple components of the host cell and causes numerous alterations in cell signaling and morphology.	males between the ages of 39 and 60 years with dyspeptic symptoms	36	Colombia	6.7% (1,589,752 cases)	(Loh et al. 2011)

gastric mucosa, generates a chronic inflammatory process triggering multiple clinical manifestations such as gastritis, ulcers, and adenocarcinoma (Orellana-Manzano et al. 2016, Bauerfeind et al. 1997, Goh et al. 2011). Many factors can affect the prevalence of the infection, such as overpopulation, nonhygienic system, and no public water (O'Ryan et al. 2013). Several studies indicate that the prevalence of the disease in adults is between 60-79%, and it depends on the socio-economic, sanitary, educational levels of the study population (Ortega et al. 2010, Khedmat et al. 2013, Sepúlveda et al. 2012).

As we mentioned before, *H. pylori* infection plays a crucial role in gastric carcinogenesis, but also exerts oncogenic effects on gastric mucosa through a complex interaction between bacterial virulence factors (McGee and Mobley 2000, Delahay and Rugge 2012) and host inflammatory responses (Niwa et al. 2010). The most studied virulence factors are CagA (cytotoxin-associated gene A antigen) and VacA (vacuolating cytotoxin). Cag A is injected into the gastric cell by bacterial type IV secretion system; after its entry is phosphorylated by tyrosine kinases, interacting with cellular proteins, acting in signal transduction pathways, inducing changes in the cytoskeleton, disruption of cell-cell junctions, stimulating the growth factor signaling and increasing cell proliferation (Backert, Tegtmeyer, and Selbach 2010). VacA induces the formation of vacuoles in eukaryotic cells and stimulates apoptosis in epithelial cells (Yamaoka 2010). This way, *H. pylori* infection modifies host gene expression patterns involved in defense mechanisms, inflammatory and immunological response, cell proliferation, and apoptosis, generating gastric damage (Obayashi et al. 2016). Recently, new mechanisms have been described involving the regulation of miRNA expression in precancerous lesions, gastric cancer, and inflammatory processes induced by *H. pylori* (Cadamuro et al. 2014).

There are several studies in which determined gastric cancer biomarkers. In children, there are biomarkers related to gene expression in gastric cancer, such as CXCL13, LCN2, MUC5AC, PIMP2, REG3A, SLC5A8, β-catenin, and variation on the methylation such as CALCA, CDH1, CRABP1, DAPK1, GATA-4, GRING2B, HIC1, THBS1, TIMP3, TWIST1. Studies including mucosa samples of infected, compared to non-infected children, have reported increased expression of CXCL13, LC N2, PIMP2, REG3A, β-catenin (Ikuse et al. 2012, Villarreal-Calderon et al. 2014, Obayashi et al. 2016). There were decreased expression levels of MUC5AC (Park et al. 2015) and SCL5A8 (Orellana-Manzano et al. 2016, O'Ryan et al. 2015) among infected children to non-infected children. SLC5A8 has also been reported in blood samples of *H pylori*-infected, apparently healthy children compared to non-infected age-matched controls (Orellana-Manzano et al. 2016). LCN2 and CXCL13 genes were involved in the inflammatory and cancer process. There were reported genes related to the cell cycle (TGFA, CDT1, NUSAP1, BTG3) and apoptosis, programmed cell death (C3ORF38, GZMH, TIAM 1, IFNG, HIPK2) not shown (Chen et al. 2015, O'Ryan et al. 2015). In a study in Mexican children with gastritis, there were six genes (CDX2, EpB4, MMP3, MIF, p53, and E-cadherin) with differential expression in infected versus non-infected children at histological level (Villarreal-Calderon et al. 2014).

The epigenetic modifications have been on the sciences hot spot during the last ten years, and there are many associations between *H. pylori* infection and this modification (Hanada and Graham 2014, Valenzuela et al. 2015). It has been known that H. pylori persistent infection-induced chronic inflammation and epigenetics modification can produce gastric cancer in the future (Matsusaka et al. 2014, Nardone et al. 2007, Valenzuela et al. 2015, Hanada and Graham 2014). This several molecular changes generated for *H. pylori* persistent infection-induced this different epigenetic changes, including DNA methylation and histone modifications, which are one of the causes for tumor progression, and cancer development (Shin et al. 2013, Shimazu et al. 2015, Hur et al. 2010, Xia et al. 2008, Valenzuela et al. 2015).

H. pylori generate epigenetics changes in the adult population (Wang et al. 2014, Shin et al. 2010, Shimazu et al. 2015), creating a pathogenic mechanism to cancer development. It has been proved that there are tumoral suppressor genes that can be hypermethylated and silenced in gastric cancer, such as CDKN2A, CDH|, MKH1, and RUNX3. This information could lead to an epigenetic mechanism originated by *H. pylori* chronic infection (Ushijima and Hattori 2012). There is also another mechanism to modify the gene expression during the pathogenicity of *H. pylori* infection, miRNA. The miRNA is a small non-coding molecule of RNA, which regulate the post-transcriptional gene expression negatively, principally to RNA degradation, and translational repression (Bartel 2004). A miRNA can be able to control of several mRNA molecules, and their deregulation could affect several cell signaling pathways. This miRNA mechanism can contribute to the inflammatory progression of cancer (Ranjha and Paul 2013). *H. pylori* could affect miRNAs expression at the gastric mucosa (Matsushima et al. 2011), and these can regulate the inflammatory process through its action on mRNAs of pro- and anti-inflammatory cytokines (Cadamuro et al. 2014). Together these miRNAs can participate in the pathological process triggered by *H. pylori* in the gastric mucosa and influence the inflammatory response of the host against the infectious process (Rossi et al. 2016).

Several studies indicated the influence of the diet in the *H. pylori* infections, and some components possess the activity such as cranberry (Gotteland et al. 2008), broccoli (Yanaka et al. 2009), virgin oil (Castro et al. 2012). Also, the sociocultural practice could influence the food choice in Peninsular Malaysia, such as the consumption of tea and locally produced foods, "pegaga" and "budu" are associated with *H. pylori* protection (Lee et al. 2012). Xia et al. (2016) determinate in a cross-sectional study that a high carbohydrate diet is associated with *H. pylori* infection, and the high intake of animal offal, fish, seafood is related to a reduction in *H. pylori* infection. These results were obtained with a prevalence of 1, 65 (1.27-2.17), OR (95%CI).

Cervix Cancer (GC) and Human Papillomavirus

Cervical cancer originates in cells that line the cervix (Crosbie et al. 2013). Epidemiological studies have shown that high-risk human papillomavirus (HPV) is the main etiological factor for cervical cancer that is caused by a persistent infection of the virus (Zur Hausen 2002, Torres-Poveda et al. 2018). HPV types sixteen and eighteen are responsible for approximately 70% of all cases of cervical cancer worldwide. The HPV oncogenes that are expressed in these cells are involved in their transformation and immortalization and are necessary for the progression towards malignancy (Álvarez Aldana, Sepúlveda Arias, and Siller López 2012). Crosbie et al. (2013) demonstrated that the virus exclusively infects the epithelium and produces new viral particles only in fully mature epithelial cells and that human HPV interrupts the standard control of the cell cycle, promoting cell division uncontrolled and the accumulation of genetic damage.

Worldwide, the incidence of HPV is 3.2% (569,847 /18'078.957 cases) of all types of cancer. According to the continents, Asia presents 55.3% (315,346), Africa 10.7% (119 284), Europe 10.7% (61,072), Latin America and the Caribbean 9.9% (56,187) North America 2.7% (15,502), and Oceania 0.47% (2,456). Regarding mortality, HPV represents 1.54% (311,365/9,555,027 deaths), being the fourth cause of death related to cancer.

Hepatitis Viruses and Hepatocellular Carcinoma

Hepatocellular carcinoma (HCC) is the primary neoplasia malignancy of the liver, and it develops in patients who have cirrhosis caused by the hepatitis

B virus (HBV) or hepatitis C virus (HCV) (Poustchi et al. 2011, Forner et al. 2014, Balogh et al. 2016).

The mechanisms by which hepatitis viruses induce hepatic carcinogenesis remains a subject of investigation. Di Bisceglie (2009) discusses that this difference can be related to the fact that HBV is a DNA virus. The DNA virus is integrated into the chromosomes of infected hepatocytes, the integration of viral genetic material that occurs in a critical location within the cellular genome, and produces the HBVx protein that can play a crucial regulatory role in the development of HCC.

In contrast, HCV is an RNA virus that replicates in the cytoplasm and does not integrate into the DNA of the host (Kew 1998).

Worldwide, the incidence of HCC is 4.7% (841,080 / 18'078.957 cases) of all types of cancer. According to the continents, Asia presents 72.5% (609,596), Europe 9.8% (82,466), Africa 7.7% (64,779), North America 5% (41,851), Latin America and the Caribbean 4.6% (38,400) and Oceania 0.47% (3,988). Regarding mortality, HCC represents 8.2% (781,631 / 9,555,027 deaths), being the fourth cause of death related to cancer. A study showed that mean ages of diagnosis with HCC vary by continent; in Asia, it is between 55 to 59 years, in Europe and North America it was 63 to 65 years, and in the other continents, the highest incidence of HCC is among individuals aged 75 or older (El-Serag 2012).

Prostate Cancer and Other Pathogens

Prostate cancer develops when the cells of the prostate gland start to grow uncontrollably. This type of cancer is common in men because this gland is only found in the male sex. Generally, all prostate cancers are adenocarcinomas.

Worldwide, the incidence of prostate cancer is 7.1% (1'276.106 /18'078.957 cases) of all types of cancer. According to the continents, Europe presents 35.2% (449,761), Asia 23.3% (297,215), North America 18.4% (234,278), Latin America and the Caribbean 14.9% (190,385), Africa 6.3% (80,971) and Oceania 1.8% (23,496). Regarding mortality, prostate cancer represents 3.8% (358,989 / 9,555,027 deaths), being the eighth cause of death related to cancer.

Recent epidemiological, genetic, and molecular studies suggest that infection and inflammation initiate prostate cancer (Klein and Silverman 2008, Omabe and Ezeani 2011). Infectious agents can directly induce tumorigenesis through viral or bacterial protein products that have oncogenic effects (Namiki et al. 2009).

Some studies suggest the possible role of *Mycoplasma genitalium* and *Mycoplasma hominis* in the development of prostate cancer (Zarei, Rezania, and Mousavi 2013). Miyake, Ohnishi, Hori, Nakano, Nakano, Yano, Ohnishi, Owari, Morizawa and Itami (2019) examined surgical and biopsy samples from 45 patients with prostate cancer against *Mycoplasma genitalium*, using the polymerase chain reaction and examined the severity of intraprostatic inflammation. In the analysis, the *Mycoplasma genitalium* infection rate was significantly different between the prostate cancer cohort and the benign prostatic hyperplasia cohorts ($p = 0.03$). Likewise, Barykova et al. (2011) investigated the possible participation of *M. Hominis* infection in prostate cancer by detecting biopsies of two groups of men who underwent a diagnosis. In the results, *M. Hominis* was detected by standard PCR in 15% of 125 patients in the first group and by quantitative real-time PCR in 37.4% of 123 men in the second group.

Nutrition in Cancer

Malnutrition, anorexia, and weight loss are high incidence problems in oncology; more than half of people with cancer lose weight, and more than a third lose more than 5% of their healthy weight (Skipworth et al. 2007). These effects are due to inadequate food intake, decreased physical activity, and catabolic disorders. In this sense, nutritional therapy, which includes evaluation and early diagnosis, nutritional support, and pharmacological treatments, plays an essential role in the quality of life of the cancer patient (Gomez et al. 2004).

The assessment of nutritional status should be an interdisciplinary work, instituted at the time of diagnosis, re-evaluated, and followed throughout the treatment and recovery (Arends et al. 2017). In the oncological patient, the subjective global assessment (VGS) is necessary since it allows us to have a global vision of the digestive and metabolic symptoms that occur in patients who have the disease. The VGS method classifies patients into:

A. Well-nourished (weight unchanged or increased and absence of edema)
B. Moderately malnourished or with suspected malnutrition (weight loss ≥5% in previous weeks, or average, but with edema/ascites)
C. Severe malnutrition (weight loss of ≥10%).

The VGS scale includes the clinical history that incorporates recent changes in weight, alterations in intake, food intolerances, drugs that interfere with appetite, and persistent gastrointestinal symptoms for two weeks. Another component is the physical examination, whose objective is to detect signs and symptoms of fatty compartment deficit and the presence of edema or ascites (Cáceres Lavernia et al. 2016). Likewise, there are other necessary tools for the evaluation of the oncogenic patient, such as the questionnaires of activities of daily living (ADL), the criteria of frequent toxicity (CTF), and the index in the scale of performance of Karnofsky (ERK).

Nutritional support has as main objectives to prevent or reverse malnutrition and favor compliance with oncological therapies and improve the quality of life of the patient (Lobbe 2008).

In oncology, nutritional support considers the factors linked to the patient and his illness, categorizing them according to their aggressiveness and complexity. According to these parameters, adequate nutritional support is indicated (Cáceres Lavernia et al. 2016).

- Oral feeding: The patient must cover 75% of their caloric-protein requirement. In these cases, the use of nutritional supplements should be one more tool to achieve an adequate income of macro and micronutrients, but they only complement the food intake.
- Enteral nutrition: Indicated in patients who cannot meet their caloric-protein requirements orally, as long as there is an adequate gastrointestinal function.
- Oral, parenteral nutrition, supplementation: It is indicated only when there is an absolute impossibility or contraindication to using the digestive tract (Lobbe 2008).

The European Society of Enteral and Parenteral Nutrition (ESPEN) recommends that the total energy expenditure of cancer patients if it is not measured individually, is assumed to be like healthy subjects and generally ranges from 25 to 30 kcal/kg/ day (Arends et al. 2017). Besides, the American Society for Parenteral and Enteral Nutrition (ASPEN) recommends to patients with obesity a caloric intake of 21 to 25 kcal/kg / day, and to patients with slight hypermetabolism who need to gain weight or are anabolic an intake of 30 at 35 kcal / kg / day (Grant 2013). Regarding proteins, ESPEN recommends that proteins be greater than 1 g /kg/day and, if possible, up to 1.5 g /kg/day.

The management of fluids in cancer care should ensure that hydration and electrolyte balance is adequate so it can prevent hypovolemia and dehydration. A recommendation is 1ml of liquid for each kcal of the calculated energy needs (Malone and Hamilton 2013).

There are ten key points that people with cancer must take into Account to ensure enough, balanced, and safe food is:

- Distribute food into four or five times a day.
- Eat five servings of fruits and vegetables a day.
- Ensure daily protein intake.
- Ensure the necessary energy that the body needs.
- Consume dairy daily.
- Maintain proper hydration.
- Always use virgin olive oil.
- Prioritize simple preparations and cooking with little fat.
- Limit the consumption of alcohol and reduce the consumption of foods rich in added sugars, saturated fats, or salt.
- Eat accompanied.

Diet therapy aims to agree with the symptoms that the oncological patient presents. Sometimes it is necessary to apply strategies to modify the dietary intake, and it depends on a specific problem for the consumer and the nutritional status of the person.

When the patient presents anorexia, it is necessary to take advantage of the time of day where is more appetite for foods with higher energy and protein content. At the same time, it is essential to enrich the diet to have a more significant contribution of nutrients. Add to:

- Soups and purees: chicken, cheese, milk, and egg.
- Salads: pasta, rice, vegetables. Other dishes that allow mayonnaise cheese, tuna, egg, nuts, and ham.
- Milk: cocoa powder or honey.
- Yogurt: fruits, honey, nuts, cereals.

In a patient with nausea and vomiting, it is necessary to make frequent meals and little volume. Likewise, it is needed to consume soft and low-fat foods such as white meats (Brown et al. 2001).

In constipation, it is necessary to drink many liquids and take a lot of foods rich in fiber such as cereals and whole grains, vegetables, nuts, among others. Likewise, it is advisable to reduce astringent foods such as quince, banana, tea, wine (Brown et al. 2001).

DISCUSSION AND CONCLUSION

This paper is showing the relevance of several pathogens in the carcinogenesis process. In the results section, Table 1 references the important pathogen to generate cancer is *H. pylori*, with a 35,8% (770,000 cases) of cancer prevalence worldwide. This pathogen one has established in the gastric epithelial tissue generates chronic inflammation and metabolic changes to origin in longterm carcinogenesis. As we mentioned before, this several molecular changes caused for *H. pylori* persistent infection could induce different metabolic changes, including DNA methylation and histone modifications, tumoral suppressor genes that can be hypermethylated and silenced in gastric cancer, such as CDKN2A, CDH|, MKH1, and RUNX3 (Hur et al. 2010, Shimazu et al. 2015, Shin et al. 2013, Valenzuela et al. 2015, Xia et al. 2016); miRNA as a gene expression control during *H. pylori* pathogenicity (Bartel 2004). This regulation mechanism can contribute to the inflammatory progression of cancer (Ranjha and Paul 2013).

The second relevant pathogen associated with cancer is *Human papillomavirus,* which generates cervix cancer, with 29.3% (630,000 cases) of cancer prevalence worldwide. As *H. pylori*, this pathogen causes cancer by persistent infection of HPV. The metabolic changes during these processes are related to the transformation and immortalization of the epithelium cells (Álvarez Aldana, Sepúlveda Arias, and Siller López 2012), such as interrupts the standard control of the cell cycle, cell division, and genetic damages (Crosbie et al. 2013). Other mechanisms influence cervical cancer risks, such as folate deficiency (Ziegler, Weinstein, and Fears 2002), DNA methylation, riboflavin interaction, and genotype (Powers 2005). *Ziegler, R et al.* 2002 in the large multiethnic community-based-case-control study of invasive cervical cancer in U.S. demonstrated the moderate risk of folate measures in serum and homocysteine is an indicator of inadequate metabolism (Ziegler, Weinstein, and Fears 2002). An efficient one-carbon metabolism requires folate, vitamins, and multiple enzymes. In one-carbon metabolism, homocysteine accepts a methyl group from 5-methyltetrahydrofolate for methionine in a vitamin B-12-dependent reaction (Selhub 1999). This homocysteine is degraded by transsulfuration to cystathionine in a vitamin B-6-dependent reaction (Selhub 1999, Jacques et al. 2001).

In summary, elevated homocysteine could be a possible biomarker of inefficient one-carbon metabolism caused by folate deficiency, vitamin B12, vitamin B6, and riboflavin (Ziegler, Weinstein, and Fears 2002) and additionally causes gene expression changes (Lievers et al. 2001). These metabolic changes could influence the DNA/RNA synthesis, DNA repairs, and DNA/RNA methylation (Choi and Mason 2000). The association with Folate, nutrition, and DNA stability is in the pyrimidine synthesis, in which are involved several enzymes such as methylenetetrahydrofolate reductase (MTHFR) (Powers 2005). This enzyme transformed the 5,10-methylene THF into 5-Me THF, and this product is a substrate into the homocysteine-methionine process to the DNA methylation.

It has been described that DNA hypomethylation is associated with cervical dysplasia and cervical cancer (Kim et al. 1994; Fowler et al. 1998). Additionally, the hypomethylation maybe also a biomarker of this cervical cancer progression, in which serum folate and cervical tissue were inversely associated (Fowler et al. 1998). Another study determines the relevance of this folate metabolic signaling, which involved a polymorphism of the methylenetetrahydrofolate reductase (MTHFR) (Powers 2005), and the MTHFR C677T.. This polymorphism appears to interact with the folate and riboflavin in modulating cancer risk (Lambropoulos et al. 2003). There may be an association between the polymorphism, folate metabolism, and cervical cancer, but there are no consensus results.

Rudlowski et al. (2003) indicated the relation between GLUT1 gene expression and malignant transformation to cervical cancer. They showed that cervical tumor cells respond to enhanced glucose utilization by GLUT1 mRNA overexpression. This overexpression can suggest an early event in cervical neoplasia.

There are dietary patterns that could represent a risk factor for cervical neoplasia (Seo et al. 2016) and could have a synergy with the dominance of *A. vaginae* in the cervical microbiota. The semi-wester diet characterized by higher intake of bread, dairy products, eggs, and soft drinks and relatively higher fat intake ratio is the dietary pattern associated with this cancer (Ford and Capewell 2013), with an odds ratio [OR] 3.44, 95% confidence interval [CI] 1.11–10.7, $p = 0.03$ (Seo et al. 2016). This association with the imbalance of nutrients or lack of fiber, vitamins could determinate the progression of cancer (Oh et al. 2013).

The third and fourth pathogens are Hepatitis Virus B (19.1% = 410,000 cases), Hepatitis C virus (7.9% = 170,000 cases) of cancer prevalence worldwide, and can cause the hepatocellular carcinoma. The molecular mechanisms associated with both viruses and carcinogenesis remain a subject of investigation. The chronical infection and inflammatory processes address the carcinogenesis pathway. There could be a progression with non-cirrhotic livers, fibrosis response, oxidative stress, DNA damage generating liver cancer (Tu, Bühler, and Bartenschlager 2017). The HBV replication occurs with hepatocytes causing the normal processes of infection in the liver, but the DAN integration is a unique way that HBV is reported to drive HCC. The DNA virus integration into the host cell genome leads to mutagenesis, chromosomal instability, and activation of tumor-associated genes. In the HCV infection, there are metabolic reprogramming of the infect cells; this virus leads to hepatosteatosis, increasing the triglyceride deposition in the hepatocytes (Pekow et al. 2007). HCV generates long-term stress response, oxidative stress via ROS and NADPH production, creating an alteration of cell survival, mitosis, and differentiation pathways (Smirnova et al. 2016, Bartenschlager and Vogt 2013). HCV virus can directly interact with the block of tumor suppressor genes such as the retinoblastoma tumour suppressor protein (Rb) (Munakata et al. 2005, Nakagawa et al. 2009), the epidermal growth factor receptor (EGFR) (Zona et al. 2013), the DEAD-box RNA helicase (DDX3) (Chao et al. 2006), p53 (Otsuka et al. 2000, Lan et al. 2002) and microRNA (miR)-122 (Luna et al. 2015).

In summary, this pathogen reviewed in this chapter has one common factor, namely, that they create chronic inflammation, modifying the metabolic patterns to generate long-term carcinogenesis. Other associated pathogens should increase interest in these cancer association, and their relation with nutrition.

ACKNOWLEDGMENTS

The authors would like to thank to Corporación Ecuatoriana para el Desarrollo de la Investigación y Academia - CEDIA for the financial support given to the present re-search, development, and innovation work through its CEPRA program, especially for the "Análisis molecular de *Helicobacter pylori* (genes de patogenicidad y ancestría) en biopsias gástricas de pacientes de la Sierra y Oriente Ecuatorianos." CEDIA-CEPRA XI molecular analysis and ESPOL FCV-27-2017 supported this work.

REFERENCES

Álvarez Aldana, Adalucy, Juan Carlos Sepúlveda Arias, and Fernando Siller López. 2012. "Carcinogénesis inducida por el virus del papiloma humano. [Human Papilloma Virus-Induced Carcinogenesis]." *Investigaciones Andina* 14 (24):438-456.

America Cancer Society, A., & Society, A. C. (2011). *Cancer Facts & Figures* 2011. American Cancer Society, 1(1), 1–68. https://doi.org/10.3322/caac.20121.

Antoni, S., Soerjomataram, I., Møller, B., Bray, F., & Ferlay, J. (2016). Évaluation des méthodes GLOBOCAN pour établir des estimations nationales de l'incidence du cancer. [Evaluation of GLOBOCAN methods for establishing national cancer incidence estimates]. *Bulletin of the World Health Organization*, 94(3), 174–184. https://doi.org/10.2471/BLT.15.164384.

Arends, Jann, Patrick Bachmann, Vickie Baracos, Nicole Barthelemy, Hartmut Bertz, Federico Bozzetti, Ken Fearon, Elisabeth Hütterer, Elizabeth Isenring, and Stein Kaasa. 2017. "ESPEN guidelines on nutrition in cancer patients." *Clinical Nutrition* 36 (1):11-48. doi: 10.1016/j.clnu.2016.07.015.

Arismendi-Morillo, G., I. Hernandez, E. Mengual, N. Abreu, N. Molero, A. Fuenmayor, G. Romero, and M. Lizarzabal. 2013. "Estimación de riesgo de cáncer gástrico en pacientes con gastritis crónica asociada a la infección por *Helicobacter pylori* en un escenario clínico. [Gastric cancer risk estimate in patients with chronic gastritis associated with *Helicobacter pylori* infection in a clinical setting]." *Revista de Gastroenterología de México* 78 (3):135-43. doi: 10.1016/j.rgmx.2013.01.004.

Backert, Steffen, Nicole Tegtmeyer, and Matthias Selbach. 2010. "The versatility of *Helicobacter pylori* CagA effector protein functions: The master key hypothesis." *Helicobacter* 15 (3):163-176. doi: 10.1111/j.1523-5378.2010.00759.x.

Balogh, Julius, Emad H. Asham David Victor III, Sherilyn Gordon Burroughs, Maha Boktour, Ashish Saharia, Xian Li, R. Mark Ghobrial, and Howard P. Monsour Jr. 2016. "Hepatocellular carcinoma: a review." *Journal of Hepatocellular Carcinoma* 3:41.

Bartel, David P., 2004. "MicroRNAs: genomics, biogenesis, mechanism, and function." *Cell* 116 (2):281-297. DOI: 10.1016/S0092-8674(04)00045-5.

Bartenschlager, Ralf, and P. K. Vogt. 2013. *Hepatitis C virus: from molecular virology to antiviral therapy*: Springer.

Barykova, Yulia A., Denis Yu Logunov, Maxim M. Shmarov, Andrei Z. Vinarov, Dmitry N. Fiev, Natalia A. Vinarova, Irina V. Rakovskaya, Patricia Stanhope Baker, Inna Shyshynova, and Andrew J. Stephenson. 2011. "Association of Mycoplasma hominis infection with prostate cancer." *Oncotarget* 2 (4):289. doi: 10.18632/oncotarget.256.

Bauer, Bianca, and Thomas F. Meyer. 2011. "The Human Gastric Pathogen *Helicobacter pylori* and Its Association with Gastric Cancer and Ulcer Disease." *Ulcers* 2011. doi: 10.1155/2011/340157.

Bauerfeind, P., R. Garner, B. E. Dunn, and H. L. Mobley. 1997. "Synthesis and activity of *Helicobacter pylori* urease and catalase at low pH." *Gut* 40 (1):25-30. doi: 10.1136/gut.40.1.25.

Bray, F., J. Ferlay, I. Soerjomataram, R. L. Siegel, L. A. Torre, and A. Jemal. 2018. "Global cancer statistics 2018: GLOBOCAN estimates of incidence and mortality worldwide for 36 cancers in 185 countries." *CA: A Cancer Journal for Clinicians* 68 (6):394-424. doi: 10.3322/caac.21492.

Brown, Jean, Tim Byers, Kevin Thompson, Barbara Eldridge, Colleen Doyle, and Alexis M Williams. 2001. "Nutrition during and after cancer treatment: A guide* for informed choices by cancer survivors." *CA: A Cancer Journal for Clinicians* 51 (3):153-181.

Buonaguro, Franco M., George K. Lewis, and Piergiuseppe Pelicci. 2006. "Introducing infectious agents and cancer." *Infectious agents and cancer* 1 (1):1-1. doi: 10.1186/1750-9378-1-1.

Cáceres Lavernia, Haslen, Elia Neninger Vinageras, Yanet Menéndez Alfonso, and Jesús Barreto Penié. 2016. "Intervención nutricional en el paciente con cáncer. [Nutritional Intervention in Cancer Patient]." *Revista Cubana de Medicina* 55 (1):0-0.

Cadamuro, Aline Cristina Targa, Ana Flávia Teixeira Rossi, Nathália Maciel Maniezzo, and Ana Elizabete Silva. 2014. "*Helicobacter pylori* infection: host immune response, implications on gene expression and microRNAs." *World Journal of Gastroenterology: WJG* 20 (6):1424. doi: 10.3748/wjg.v20.i6.1424.

Castro, Manuel, Concepción Romero, Antonio de Castro, Julio Vargas, Eduardo Medina, Raquel Millan, and Manuel Brenes. 2012. "Assessment of *Helicobacter pylori* eradication by virgin olive oil." *Helicobacter* 17 (4):305-311. doi: 10.1111/j.1523-5378.2012.00949.x.

Crosbie, Emma J., Mark H. Einstein, Silvia Franceschi, and Henry C. Kitchener. 2013. "Human papillomavirus and cervical cancer." *The Lancet* 382 (9895):889-899. doi: 10.1016/S0140-6736(13)60022-7.

Chan, Y. K., M. Estaki, and D. L. Gibson. 2013. "Clinical consequences of diet-induced dysbiosis." *Annals of Nutrition and Metabolism* 63 28-40. doi: 10.1159/000354902.

Chao, Chi-Hong, Chun-Ming Chen, Pei-Lin Cheng, Jing-Wen Shih, Ann-Ping Tsou, and Yan-Hwa Wu Lee. 2006. "DDX3, a DEAD box RNA helicase with tumor growth–suppressive property and transcriptional regulation activity of the p21waf1/cip1 promoter, is a candidate tumor suppressor." *Cancer Research* 66 (13):6579-6588. doi: 10.1158/0008-5472.CAN-05-2415.

Chen, Liangdong, Deqiang Zhuo, Jiakuan Chen, and Hongyin Yuan. 2015. "Screening feature genes of lung carcinoma with DNA microarray analysis." *International Journal of Clinical and Experimental Medicine* 8 (8):12161.

Choi, Sang-Woon, and Joel B Mason. 2000. "Folate and carcinogenesis: an integrated scheme." *The Journal of nutrition* 130 (2):129-132. doi: 10.1093/jn/130.2.129.

Daugule, I., and M. Rowland. 2008. "*Helicobacter pylori* infection in children." *Helicobacter* 13 Suppl 1:41-6. doi: 10.1111/j.1523-5378.2008.00632.x.

de Martel, C., and J. Parsonnet. 2006. "*Helicobacter pylori* infection and gender: a meta-analysis of population-based prevalence surveys." *Digestive Diseases and Sciences* 51 (12):2292-301. doi: 10.1007/s10620-006-9210-5.

de Martel, C., M. S. Shiels, S. Franceschi, E. P. Simard, J. Vignat, H. I. Hall, E. A. Engels, and M. Plummer. 2015. "Cancers attributable to infections among adults with HIV in the United States." *Aids* 29 (16):2173-81. doi: 10.1097/qad.0000000000000808.

Delahay, R. M., and M. Rugge. 2012. "Pathogenesis of *Helicobacter pylori* infection." *Helicobacter* 17 Suppl 1:9-15. doi: 10.1111/j.1523-5378.2012.00976.x.

Di Bisceglie, Adrian M. 2009. "Hepatitis B and hepatocellular carcinoma." *Hepatology* 49 (S5):S56-S60. doi: 10.1002/hep.22962.

El-Serag, Hashem B. 2012. "Epidemiology of viral hepatitis and hepatocellular carcinoma." *Gastroenterology* 142 (6):1264-1273. e1. doi: 10.1053/j.gastro.2011.12.061.

Ford, Earl S., and Simon Capewell. 2013. "Trends in total and low-density lipoprotein cholesterol among US adults: contributions of changes in dietary fat intake and use of cholesterol-lowering medications." *PloS one* 8 (5):e65228. doi: 10.1371/journal.pone.0065228.

Forner, Alejandro, Marine Gilabert, Jordi Bruix, and Jean-Luc Raoul. 2014. "Treatment of intermediate-stage hepatocellular carcinoma." *Nature Reviews Clinical Oncology* 11 (9):525.

Garcion, E., Naveilhan, P., Berger, F., & Wion, D. (2009). Cancer stem cells: Beyond Koch's postulates. In *Cancer Letters* (Vol. 278, Issue 1, pp. 3–8). https://doi.org/10.1016/j.canlet.2008.09.006.

Goh, K. L., W. K. Chan, S. Shiota, and Y. Yamaoka. 2011. "Epidemiology of *Helicobacter pylori* infection and public health implications." *Helicobacter* 16 Suppl 1:1-9. doi: 10.1111/j.1523-5378.2011.00874.x.

Gomez, N. A., A. Salvador, P. E. Vargas, J. A. Zapatier, and J. Alvarez. 2004. "Seroprevalence of *Helicobacter pylori* among the child population of Ecuador." *Revista de Gastroenterología del Peru* 24 (3):230-3.

Gotteland, Martin, Monica Andrews, Marcela Toledo, Loreto Muñoz, Paola Caceres, Alyerina Anziani, Emma Wittig, Hernan Speisky, and Gabriela Salazar. 2008. "Modulation of *Helicobacter pylori* colonization with cranberry juice and *Lactobacillus johnsonii* La1 in children." *Nutrition* 24 (5):421-426. doi: 10.1016/j.nut.2008.01.007.

Hanada, Katsuhiro, and David Y. Graham. 2014. "*Helicobacter pylori* and the molecular pathogenesis of intestinal-type gastric carcinoma." *Expert Review of Anticancer Therapy* 14 (8):947-954. doi: 10.1586/14737140.2014.911092.

Hollstein, M., Alexandrov, L. B., Wild, C. P., Ardin, M., & Zavadil, J. (2017). Base changes in tumour DNA have the power to reveal the causes and evolution of cancer. In *Oncogene* (Vol. 36, Issue 2, pp. 158–167). Nature Publishing Group. https://doi.org/10.1038/onc.2016.192.

Hur, Keun, Tohru Niwa, Takeshi Toyoda, Tetsuya Tsukamoto, Masae Tatematsu, Han-Kwang Yang, and Toshikazu Ushijima. 2010. "Insufficient role of cell proliferation in aberrant DNA methylation induction and involvement of specific types of inflammation." *Carcinogenesis* 32 (1):35-41. doi: 10.1093/carcin/bgq219.

Ikuse, Tamaki, Yoshikazu Ohtsuka, Takahiro Kudo, Kenji Hosoi, Naho Obayashi, Keisuke Jimbo, Yo Aoyagi, Tohru Fujii, Satoru Nagata, and Toshiaki Shimizu. 2012. "Microarray analysis of gastric mucosa among children with *Helicobacter pylori* infection." *Pediatrics International* 54 (3):319-324. doi: 10.1111/j.1442-200X.2012.03573.x.

Ingerslev, Kasper, Estrid Høgdall, Wojciech Skovrider-Ruminski, Tine Henrichsen Schnack, Marianne Lidang, Claus Høgdall, and Jan Blaakaer. 2019. "The prevalence of EBV and CMV DNA in epithelial ovarian cancer." *Infectious Agents and Cancer* 14 (1):7. doi: 10.1186/s13027-019-0223-z.

International agency for Research of Cancer. (2019). *Cancers Attributable to Infections*.

Ishaq, Sauid, and Lois Nunn. 2015. "*Helicobacter pylori* and gastric cancer: a state of the art review." *Gastroenterology and Hepatology from Bed to Bench* 8 (Suppl 1):S6-S14.

Jacques, Paul F., Andrew G. Bostom, Peter W. F. Wilson, Sharron Rich, Irwin H. Rosenberg, and Jacob Selhub. 2001. "Determinants of plasma total homocysteine concentration in the Framingham Offspring cohort." *The American Journal of Clinical Nutrition* 73 (3):613-621. doi: 10.1093/ajcn/73.3.613.

Kew, M. C. 1998. "Hepatitis viruses and hepatocellular carcinoma." *Research in Virology* 149 (5):257-262. doi: 10.1016/S0923-2516(99)89003-7.

Khedmat, Hossein, Reza Karbasi-Afshar, Shahram Agah, and Saeed Taheri. 2013. "*Helicobacter pylori* Infection in the general population: A Middle Eastern perspective." *Caspian Journal of Internal Medicine* 4 (4):745-753.

Klein, Eric A., and Robert Silverman. 2008. "Inflammation, infection, and prostate cancer." *Current Opinion in Urology* 18 (3):315-319. doi: 10.1097/MOU.0b013e3282f9b3b7.

Lambropoulos, A. F., T. Agorastos, Z. J. Foka, S. Chrisafi, T. C. Constantinidis, J. Bontis, and A. Kotsis. 2003. "Methylenetetrahydrofolate reductase polymorphism C677T is not associated to the risk of cervical dysplasia." *Cancer Letters* 191 (2):187-191. doi: 10.1016/S0304-3835(02)00675-4.

Lan, Keng-Hsin, Meei-Ling Sheu, Shinn-Jang Hwang, Sang-Hue Yen, Shiow-Yi Chen, Jaw-Ching Wu, Yuan-Jan Wang, Naoya Kato, Masao Omata, and Full-Young Chang. 2002. "HCV NS5A interacts with p53 and inhibits p53-mediated apoptosis." *Oncogene* 21 (31):4801. doi: 10.1038/sj.onc.1205589.

Lancet. 2018. "GLOBOCAN 2018: counting the toll of cancer." *Lancet* 392 (10152):985. doi: 10.1016/s0140-6736(18)32252-9.

Lee, Yeong Yeh, Ahmad Wazi Ismail, Nazri Mustaffa, Kamarul Imran Musa, Noorizan Abdul Majid, Keng Ee Choo, S. Mahendra Raj, Mohammad H. Derakhshan, Hoda M. Malaty, and David Y. Graham. 2012. "Sociocultural and dietary practices among Malay subjects in the north-eastern region of Peninsular Malaysia: a region of low prevalence of *Helicobacter pylori* infection." *Helicobacter* 17 (1):54-61. doi: 10.1111/j.1523-5378.2011.00917.x.

Lobbe, V. 2008. "Inflammatory Process-Immunity." In *Clinic and Therapeutics in Adult Nutrition*, 449–463.

Loh, J. T., C. L. Shaffer, M. B. Piazuelo, L. E. Bravo, M. S. McClain, P. Correa, and T. L. Cover. 2011. "Analysis of cagA in Helicobacter pylori strains from Colombian populations with contrasting gastric cancer risk reveals a biomarker for disease severity." *Cancer Epidemiology, Biomarkers and Prevention* 20 (10):2237-49. doi: 10.1158/1055-9965.epi-11-0548.

Luna, J. M., T. K. Scheel, T. Danino, K. S. Shaw, A. Mele, J. J. Fak, E. Nishiuchi, C. N. Takacs, M. T. Catanese, Y. P. de Jong, I. M. Jacobson, C. M. Rice, and R. B. Darnell. 2015. "Hepatitis C virus RNA functionally sequesters miR-122." *Cell* 160 (6):1099-110. doi: 10.1016/j.cell.2015.02.025.

Malone, Ainsley, and Cynthia Hamilton. 2013. "The Academy of Nutrition and Dietetics/the American Society for Parenteral and Enteral Nutrition consensus malnutrition characteristics: application in practice." *Nutrition in Clinical Practice* 28 (6):639-650. doi: 10.1177/0884533613508435.

Marian, Mary. 2010. "Introduction to the nutritional management of oncology patients." *Clinical Nutrition for Oncology Patients*:1.

Martinez, I., D. J. Perdicaro, A. W. Brown, S. Hammons, T. J. Carden, T. P. Carr, K. M. Eskridge, and J. Walter. 2013. "Diet-induced alterations of host cholesterol metabolism are likely to affect the gut microbiota composition in hamsters." *Applied and Environmental Microbiology* 79 (2):516-24. doi: 10.1128/aem.03046-12.

Matsusaka, Keisuke, Sayaka Funata, Masashi Fukayama, and Atsushi Kaneda. 2014. "DNA methylation in gastric cancer, related to *Helicobacter pylori* and Epstein-Barr virus." *World Journal of Gastroenterology: WJG* 20 (14):3916. doi: 10.3748/wjg.v20.i14.3916.

Matsushima, Kayoko, Hajime Isomoto, Naoki Inoue, Toshiyuki Nakayama, Tomayoshi Hayashi, Masaaki Nakayama, Kazuhiko Nakao, Toshiya Hirayama, and Shigeru Kohno. 2011. "MicroRNA signatures in *Helicobacter pylo*ri-infected gastric mucosa." *International Journal of Cancer* 128 (2):361-370. doi: 10.1002/ijc.25348.

McGee, David J., and Harry L. T. Mobley. 2000. "Pathogenesis of *Helicobacter pylori* infection." *Current Opinion in Gastroenterology* 16 (1):24-31.

Miyake, M., K. Ohnishi, S. Hori, A. Nakano, R. Nakano, H. Yano, S. Ohnishi, T. Owari, Y. Morizawa, Y. Itami, Y. Nakai, T. Inoue, S. Anai, K. Torimoto, N. Tanaka, T. Fujii, H. Furuya, C. J. Rosser, and K. Fujimoto. 2019. "*Mycoplasma genitalium* Infection and Chronic Inflammation in Human Prostate Cancer: Detection Using Prostatectomy and Needle Biopsy Specimens." *Cells* 8 (3). doi: 10.3390/cells8030212.

Miyake, Makito, Kenta Ohnishi, Shunta Hori, Akiyo Nakano, Ryuichi Nakano, Hisakazu Yano, Sayuri Ohnishi, Takuya Owari, Yosuke Morizawa, and Yoshitaka Itami. 2019. "*Mycoplasma genitalium* infection and chronic inflammation in human prostate cancer: detection using prostatectomy and needle biopsy specimens." *Cells* 8 (3):212. doi: 10.3390/cells8030212.

Moudi, Bita, Zahra Heidari, and Hamidreza Mahmoudzadeh-Sagheb. 2018. "Study of liver in HBV-related hepatocellular carcinoma: Stereology shows quantitative differences in liver structure." *European Journal of Histochemistry* 62 (3):2950. doi: 10.4081/ejh.2018.2950.

Moynihan, P., and P. E. Petersen. 2004. "Diet, nutrition and the prevention of dental diseases." *Public Health and Nutrition* 7 (1a):201-26.

Munakata, Tsubasa, Mitsuyasu Nakamura, Yuqiong Liang, Kui Li, and Stanley M Lemon. 2005. "Down-regulation of the retinoblastoma tumor suppressor by the hepatitis C virus NS5B RNA-dependent RNA polymerase." *Proceedings of the National Academy of Sciences* 102 (50):18159-18164. doi: 10.1073/pnas.0505605102.

Nakagawa, H., S. Maeda, H. Yoshida, R. Tateishi, R. Masuzaki, T. Ohki, Y. Hayakawa, H. Kinoshita, M. Yamakado, N. Kato, S. Shiina, and M. Omata. 2009. "Serum IL-6 levels and the risk for hepatocarcinogenesis in chronic hepatitis C patients: an analysis based on gender differences." *International Journal of Cancer* 125 (10):2264-9. doi: 10.1002/ijc.24720.

Namiki, Kazunori, Steve Goodison, Stacy Porvasnik, Robert W Allan, Kenneth A Iczkowski, Cydney Urbanek, Leticia Reyes, Noboru Sakamoto, and Charles J Rosser. 2009. "Persistent exposure to Mycoplasma induces malignant transformation of human prostate cells." *PloS one* 4 (9):e6872. doi: 10.1371/journal.pone.0006872.

Nardone, Gerardo, Debora Compare, Patrizia De Colibus, Germana De Nucci, and Alba Rocco. 2007. "*Helicobacter pylori* and epigenetic mechanisms underlying gastric carcinogenesis." *Digestive Diseases* 25 (3):225-229. doi: 10.1159/000103890.

Neuhouser, Marian L., Beti Thompson, Gloria D. Coronado, and Cam C. Solomon. 2004. "Higher fat intake and lower fruit and vegetables intakes are associated with greater acculturation among mexicans living in Washington State." *Journal of the American Dietetic Association* 104 (1):51-57. doi: 10.1016/j.jada.2003.10.015.

Niwa, Tohru, Tetsuya Tsukamoto, Takeshi Toyoda, Akiko Mori, Harunari Tanaka, Takao Maekita, Masao Ichinose, Masae Tatematsu, and Toshikazu Ushijima. 2010. "Inflammatory Processes Triggered by <em> Helicobacter pylori</em> Infection Cause Aberrant DNA

Methylation in Gastric Epithelial Cells." *Cancer Research*:0008-5472.CAN-09-2755. doi: 10.1158/0008-5472.CAN-09-2755.

O'Ryan, M. L., M. Rabello, H. Cortes, Y. Lucero, A. Pena, and J. P. Torres. 2013. "Dynamics of Helicobacter pylori detection in stools during the first 5 years of life in Chile, a rapidly developing country." *Pediatr Infectious Disease Journal* 32 (2):99-103. doi: 10.1097/INF.0b013e318278b929.

O'Ryan, Miguel L, Yalda Lucero, Marcela Rabello, Nora Mamani, Ana María Salinas, Alfredo Peña, Juan Pablo Torres-Torreti, Asunción Mejías, Octavio Ramilo, and Nicolas Suarez. 2015. "Persistent and transient *Helicobacter pylori* infections in early childhood." *Clinical Infectious Diseases* 61 (2):211-218. doi: 10.1093/cid/civ256.

Obayashi, Naho, Yoshikazu Ohtsuka, Kenji Hosoi, Tamaki Ikuse, Keisuke Jimbo, Yo Aoyagi, Tohru Fujii, Takahiro Kudo, Daisuke Asaoka, and Mariko Hojo. 2016. "Comparison of gene expression between pediatric and adult gastric mucosa with *Helicobacter pylori* infection." *Helicobacter* 21 (2):114-123. doi: 10.1111/hel.12245.

Oh, Hea Young, Mi Kyung Kim, Myoungsook Lee, and Young Ok Kim. 2013. "Macronutrient composition and sodium intake of diet are associated with risk of metabolic syndrome and hypertension in Korean women." *PloS one* 8 (10):e78088. doi: 10.1371/journal.pone.0078088.

Ohata, H., S. Kitauchi, N. Yoshimura, K. Mugitani, M. Iwane, H. Nakamura, A. Yoshikawa, K. Yanaoka, K. Arii, H. Tamai, Y. Shimizu, T. Takeshita, O. Mohara, and M. Ichinose. 2004. "Progression of chronic atrophic gastritis associated with *Helicobacter pylori* infection increases risk of gastric cancer." *International Journal of Cancer* 109 (1):138-43. doi: 10.1002/ijc. 11680.

Omabe, Maxwell, and Martin Ezeani. 2011. "Infection, inflammation and prostate carcinogenesis." *Infection, Genetics and Evolution* 11 (6):1195-1198. doi: 10.1016/j.meegid.2011.03.002.

Orellana-Manzano, A., M. G. O'Ryan, A. J. Lagomarcino, S. George, M. S. Munoz, N. Mamani, C. A. Serrano, P. R. Harris, O. Ramilo, A. Mejias, J. P. Torres, Y. Lucero, and A. F. Quest. 2016. "*Helicobacter pylori* Infection Is Associated with Decreased Expression of SLC5A8, a Cancer Suppressor Gene, in Young Children." *Frontiers in Cellular and Infection Microbiology* 6:121. doi: 10.3389/fcimb.2016.00121.

Ortega, J. P., A. Espino, B. A. Calvo, P. Verdugo, M. Pruyas, E. Nilsen, L. Villarroel, O. Padilla, A. Riquelme, and A. Rollan. 2010. "Infección por *Helicobacter pylori* en pacientes sintomáticos con patología gastroduodenal benigna. Análisis de 5.664 pacientes. [*Helicobacter pylori* infection in symptomatic patients with benign gastroduodenal diseases: analysis of 5.664 cases]." *Revista Medica de Chile* 138 (5):529-35. doi: /S0034-98872010000500001.

Otsuka, Motoyuki, Naoya Kato, Keng-Hsin Lan, Hideo Yoshida, Jun Kato, Tadashi Goto, Yasushi Shiratori, and Masao Omata. 2000. "Hepatitis C virus core protein enhances p53 function through augmentation of DNA binding affinity and transcriptional ability." *Journal of Biological Chemistry* 275 (44):34122-34130. doi: 10.1074/jbc.M000578200.

Park, Ji Sook, Jung-Sook Yeom, Ji-Hyun Seo, Jae-Young Lim, Chan-Hoo Park, Hyang-Ok Woo, Hee-Shang Youn, Jin-Su Jun, Ji-Hoe Park, and Gyung-Hyuck Ko. 2015. "Immunohistochemical Expressions of MUC 2, MUC 5 AC, and MUC 6 in Normal, *Helicobacter pylori* Infected and Metaplastic Gastric Mucosa of Children and Adolescents." *Helicobacter* 20 (4):260-268. doi: 10.1111/hel.12198.

Park, Y., T. J. Kim, C. S. Hwang, C. H. Cho, D. H. Jeong, S. J. Seong, J. K. Lee, S. Hur, M. K. Kee, J. Seong, and M. Ki. 2019. "Risk of cervical dysplasia among human papillomavirus-infected women in Korea: a multicenter prospective study." *Journal of Gynecologic Oncology* 30 (3):e50. doi: 10.3802/jgo.2019.30.e50.

Paul, B., S. Barnes, W. Demark-Wahnefried, C. Morrow, C. Salvador, C. Skibola, and T. O. Tollefsbol. 2015. "Influences of diet and the gut microbiome on epigenetic modulation in cancer and other diseases." *Clinical Epigenetics* 7:112. doi: 10.1186/s13148-015-0144-7.

Pekow, Joel R., Atul K. Bhan, Hui Zheng, and Raymond T. Chung. 2007. "Hepatic steatosis is associated with increased frequency of hepatocellular carcinoma in patients with hepatitis C-related cirrhosis." *Cancer* 109 (12):2490-2496. doi: 10.1002/cncr.22701.

Phillips, D. H. (2018). Mutational spectra and mutational signatures: Insights into cancer aetiology and mechanisms of DNA damage and repair. In *DNA Repair* (Vol. 71, pp. 6–11). Elsevier B.V. https://doi.org/10.1016/j.dnarep.2018.08.003.

Pierre, F., G. Peiro, S. Tache, A. J. Cross, S. A. Bingham, N. Gasc, G. Gottardi, D. E. Corpet, and F. Gueraud. 2006. "New marker of colon cancer risk associated with heme intake: 1,4-dihydroxynonane mercapturic acid." *Cancer Epidemiology, Biomarkers & Prevention* 15 (11):2274-9. doi: 10.1158/1055-9965.Epi-06-0085.

Plummer, M., C. de Martel, J. Vignat, J. Ferlay, F. Bray, and S. Franceschi. 2016. "Global burden of cancers attributable to infections in 2012: a synthetic analysis." *Lancet Global Health* 4 (9):e609-16. doi: 10.1016/s2214-109x(16)30143-7.

Poesen, Ruben, Karen Windey, Rosalinde Masereeuw, Petra Broek, Pieter Evenepoel, Bjorn Meijers, and Kristin Verbeke. 2014. "*influence of a high protein diet on the human metabolome.*" 51st ERA-EDTA Congress. Amsterdam Netherlands.

Poustchi, Hossein, Geoffrey C. Farrell, Simone I. Strasser, Alice U. Lee, Geoffrey W. McCaughan, and Jacob George. 2011. "Feasibility of conducting a randomized control trial for liver cancer screening: is a randomized controlled trial for liver cancer screening feasible or still needed?" *Hepatology* 54 (6):1998-2004. doi: 10.1016/S0140-6736(18)30010-2.

Powers, Hilary J. 2005. "Interaction among folate, riboflavin, genotype, and cancer, with reference to colorectal and cervical cancer." *The Journal of Nutrition* 135 (12):2960S-2966S. doi: 10.1093/jn/135.12.2960s.

Ranjha, R., and J. Paul. 2013. "Micro-RNAs in inflammatory diseases and as a link between inflammation and cancer." *Inflammation Research* 62 (4):343-355. doi: 10.1007/s00011-013-0600-9.

Romesser, P. B., J. C. Romanyshyn, K. D. Schupak, J. Setton, N. Riaz, S. L. Wolden, D. Y. Gelblum, E. J. Sherman, D. Kraus, and N. Y. Lee. 2012. "Percutaneous endoscopic gastrostomy in oropharyngeal cancer patients treated with intensity-modulated radiotherapy with concurrent chemotherapy." *Cancer* 118 (24):6072-8. doi: 10.1002/cncr.27633.

Rossi, Ana Flávia Teixeira, Aline Cristina Targa Cadamuro, Joice Matos Biselli-Périco, Kátia Ramos Moreira Leite, Fábio Eduardo Severino, Patricia P Reis, José Antonio Cordeiro, and Ana Elizabete Silva. 2016. "Interaction between inflammatory mediators and miRNAs in Helicobacter pylori infection." *Cellular Microbiology* 18 (10):1444-1458. doi: 10.1111/cmi.12587.

Rudlowski, Christian, Albert J. Becker, Willibald Schroder, Werner Rath, Reinhard Büttner, and Markus Moser. 2003. "GLUT1 messenger RNA and protein induction relates to the malignant transformation of cervical cancer." *American Journal of Clinical Pathology* 120 (5):691-698. doi: 10.1309/4KYNQM5862JW2GD7.

Selhub, Jacob. 1999. "Homocysteine metabolism." *Annual Review of Nutrition* 19 (1):217-246. doi: 10.1146/annurev.nutr.19.1.217.

Seo, Sang-Soo, Hea Young Oh, Jae-Kwan Lee, Ji-Sook Kong, Dong Ock Lee, and Mi Kyung Kim. 2016. "Combined effect of diet and cervical microbiome on the risk of cervical intraepithelial neoplasia." *Clinical Nutrition* 35 (6):1434-1441. doi: 10.1016/j.clnu.2016.03.019.

Sepúlveda, Ester, Jessica Moreno, María L Spencer, Sandra Quilodrán, Ursula Brethauer, Carlos Briceño, and Apolinaria García. 2012. "Comparación de *Helicobacter pylori* en cavidad oral y mucosa gástrica de acuerdo a genotipo de virulencia (cagA y vacAm 1). [Comparison of *Helicobacter pylori* in oral cavity and gastric mucosa according to virulence genotype (CagA and VacA m 1)]." *Revista Chilena de Infectología* 29:278-283.

Shimazu, Taichi, Kiyoshi Asada, Hadrien Charvat, Chika Kusano, Yosuke Otake, Yasuo Kakugawa, Hidenobu Watanabe, Takuji Gotoda, Toshikazu Ushijima, and Shoichiro Tsugane. 2015. "Association of gastric cancer risk factors with DNA methylation levels in gastric mucosa of healthy Japanese: a cross-sectional study." *Carcinogenesis* 36 (11):1291-1298. doi: 10.1093/carcin/bgv125.

Shin, Cheol Min, Nayoung Kim, Younmu Jung, Ji Hyun Park, Gyeong Hoon Kang, Joo Sung Kim, Hyun Chae Jung, and In Sung Song. 2010. "Role of *Helicobacter pylori* infection in aberrant DNA methylation along multistep gastric carcinogenesis." *Cancer Science* 101 (6):1337-1346. doi: 10.1111/j.1349-7006.2010.01535.x.

Shin, Cheol Min, Nayoung Kim, Hye Seung Lee, Ji Hyun Park, Soyeon Ahn, Gyeong Hoon Kang, Jung Mogg Kim, Joo Sung Kim, Dong Ho Lee, and Hyun Chae Jung. 2013. "Changes in aberrant DNA methylation after Helicobacter pylori eradication: a long-term follow-up study." *International Journal of Cancer* 133 (9):2034-2042. doi: 10.1002/ijc. 28219.

Siegel, R. L., K. D. Miller, and A. Jemal. 2019. "Cancer statistics, 2019." *CA: A Cancer Journal for Clinicians* 69 (1):7-34. doi: 10.3322/caac.21551.

Skipworth, Richard J. E., Grant D. Stewart, Cornelis H. C. Dejong, Tom Preston, and Kenneth CH Fearon. 2007. "Pathophysiology of cancer cachexia: much more than host–tumour interaction?" *Clinical Nutrition* 26 (6):667-676. doi: 10.1016/j.clnu.2007.03.011.

Smirnova, Olga A., Olga N. Ivanova, Birke Bartosch, Vladimir T. Valuev-Elliston, Furkat Mukhtarov, Sergey N. Kochetkov, and Alexander V. Ivanov. 2016. "Hepatitis C virus NS5A protein triggers oxidative stress by inducing NADPH oxidases 1 and 4 and cytochrome P450 2E1." *Oxidative Medicine and Cellular Longevity* 2016. doi: 10.1155/2016/8341937.

Song, Mingyang, Wendy S. Garrett, and Andrew T. Chan. 2015. "Nutrients, Foods, and Colorectal Cancer Prevention." *Gastroenterology* 148 (6):1244-1260.e16. doi: 10.1053/j.gastro.2014.12.035.

Themeli, M., Kloss, C. C., Ciriello, G., Fedorov, V. D., Perna, F., Gonen, M., & Sadelain, M. (2013). Generation of tumor-targeted human T lymphocytes from induced pluripotent stem cells for cancer therapy. *Nature Biotechnology*, 31(10), 928–933. https://doi.org/10.1038/nbt.2678.

Torre, L. A., R. L. Siegel, E. M. Ward, and A. Jemal. 2016. "Global Cancer Incidence and Mortality Rates and Trends--An Update." *Cancer Epidemiol Biomarkers Prev* 25 (1):16-27. doi: 10.1158/1055-9965.Epi-15-0578.

Torres-Poveda, K., M. Bahena-Roman, K. Delgado-Romero, and V. Madrid-Marina. 2018. "A prospective cohort study to evaluate immunosuppressive cytokines as predictors of viral persistence and progression to pre-malignant lesion in the cervix in women infected with HR-HPV: study protocol." *BMC Infectious Diseases* 18 (1):582. doi: 10.1186/s12879-018-3490-1.

Tu, Thomas, Sandra Bühler, and Ralf Bartenschlager. 2017. "Chronic viral hepatitis and its association with liver cancer." *Biological Chemistry* 398 (8):817-837. doi: 10.1515/hsz-2017-0118.

Uemura, N., S. Okamoto, S. Yamamoto, N. Matsumura, S. Yamaguchi, M. Yamakido, K. Taniyama, N. Sasaki, and R. J. Schlemper. 2001. "*Helicobacter pylori* infection and the development of gastric cancer." *New England Journal of Medicine* 345 (11):784-9. doi: 10.1056/NEJMoa 001999.

Ushijima, Toshikazu, and Naoko Hattori. 2012. "Molecular pathways: Involvement of *Helicobacter pylori*–triggered inflammation in the formation of an epigenetic field defect, and its usefulness as cancer risk and exposure markers." *Clinical Cancer Research* 18 (4):923-929. doi: 10.1158/1078-0432.CCR-11-2011.

Valenzuela, Manuel A., Jimena Canales, Alejandro H. Corvalán, and Andrew F. G. Quest. 2015. "*Helicobacter pylori*-induced inflammation and epigenetic changes during gastric carcinogenesis." *World Journal of Gastroenterology* 21 (45):12742. doi: 10.3748/wjg.v21.i45.12742.

Villarreal-Calderon, Rodolfo, Arturo Luévano-González, Mariana Aragón-Flores, Hongtu Zhu, Ying Yuan, Qun Xiang, Benjamin Yan, Kathryn Anne Stoll, Janet V. Cross, and Kenneth A. Iczkowski. 2014. "Antral atrophy, intestinal metaplasia, and preneoplastic markers in Mexican children with *Helicobacter pylori*–positive and *Helicobacter pylori*–negative gastritis." *Annals of Diagnostic Pathology* 18 (3):129-135. doi: 10.1016/j.anndiagpath.2014.02.003.

Wang, Fei, Wenbo Meng, Bingyuan Wang, and Liang Qiao. 2014. "*Helicobacter pylori*-induced gastric inflammation and gastric cancer." *Cancer Letters* 345 (2):196-202. doi: 10.1016/j.canlet.2013.08.016.

WHO. 2018. "*Cancer Today.*" World Health Organization, accessed April 29, 2018. https://gco.iarc.fr/today/data-sources-methods.

Wykes, M. N., & Lewin, S. R. (2018). Immune checkpoint blockade in infectious diseases. In *Nature Reviews Immunology* (Vol. 18, Issue 2, pp. 91–104). Nature Publishing Group. https://doi.org/10.1038/nri.2017.112.

Xia, Guoqing, Regine Schneider-Stock, Antje Diestel, Caroline Habold, Sabine Krueger, Albert Roessner, Michael Naumann, and Uwe Lendeckel. 2008. "*Helicobacter pylori* regulates p21WAF1 by histone H4 acetylation." *Biochemical and biophysical research communications* 369 (2):526-531. doi: 10.1016/j.bbrc.2008.02.073.

Xia, Yang, Ge Meng, Qing Zhang, Li Liu, Hongmei Wu, Hongbin Shi, Xue Bao, Qian Su, Yeqing Gu, and Liyun Fang. 2016. "Dietary patterns are associated with *Helicobacter pylori* infection in Chinese adults: a cross-sectional study." *Scientific Reports* 6:32334.

Yamaoka, Yoshio. 2010. "Mechanisms of disease: *Helicobacter pylori* virulence factors." *Nature reviews Gastroenterology & hepatology* 7 (11):629. doi: 10.1038/nrgastro.2010.154.

Yanaka, Akinori, Jed W. Fahey, Atsushi Fukumoto, Mari Nakayama, Souta Inoue, Songhua Zhang, Masafumi Tauchi, Hideo Suzuki, Ichinosuke Hyodo, and Masayuki Yamamoto. 2009. "Dietary sulforaphane-rich broccoli sprouts reduce colonization and attenuate gastritis in *Helicobacter pylori*–infected mice and humans." *Cancer Prevention Research* 2 (4):353-360. doi: 10.1158/1940-6207.CAPR-08-0192.

Yu, Haining, Hongzhou Meng, Feng Zhou, Xiaofeng Ni, Shengrong Shen, and Undurti N. Das. 2015. "Urinary microbiota in patients with prostate cancer and benign prostatic hyperplasia." *Archives of Medical Science: AMS* 11 (2):385-394. doi: 10.5114/aoms.2015.50970.

Zarei, Omid, Simin Rezania, and Atefeh Mousavi. 2013. "Mycoplasma genitalium and cancer: a brief review." *Asian Pacific Journal of Cancer Prevention* 14 (6):3425-3428. doi: 10.7314/apjcp.2013.14.6.3425.

Ziegler, Regina G., Stephanie J. Weinstein, and Thomas R. Fears. 2002. "Nutritional and genetic inefficiencies in one-carbon metabolism and cervical cancer risk." *The Journal of nutrition* 132 (8):2345S-2349S.

Zona, Laetitia, Joachim Lupberger, Nazha Sidahmed-Adrar, Christine Thumann, Helen J. Harris, Amy Barnes, Jonathan Florentin, Rajiv G. Tawar, Fei Xiao, and Marine Turek. 2013. "HRas signal transduction promotes hepatitis C virus cell entry by triggering assembly of the host tetraspanin receptor complex." *Cell Host & Microbe* 13 (3):302-313. doi: 10.1016/j.chom.2013.02.006.

Zur Hausen, Harald. 2002. "Papillomaviruses and cancer: from basic studies to clinical application." *Nature Reviews Cancer* 2 (5):342. doi: 10.1038/nrc798.

In: Medicinal Plants …
Editors: A. Cardador Martínez et al.
ISBN: 978-1-53618-061-9

Chapter 6

MORINGA OLEIFERA AND ITS MULTIPLE BENEFITS FOR HUMAN HEALTH

Sara Aviles-Gaxiola[1], Luis A. Cabanillas-Bojórquez[1], Gabriela Vázquez-Olivo[1], Leticia X. López-Martínez[2], Erick P. Gutiérrez-Grijalva[2] and J. Basilio Heredia[1,*]

[1]Centro de Investigación en Alimentación y Desarrollo, A. C. Coordinación Culiacán, Sinaloa, México

[2]Cátedras CONACYT - Centro de Investigación en Alimentación y Desarrollo, A. C. Coordinación Culiacán, Sinaloa, México

ABSTRACT

Moringa oleifera Lam (Moringaceae), known as "drumstick tree" or "horseradish tree" is a highly valued medicinal plant native to India and already distributed in tropical countries worldwide. All parts of the *Moringa oleifera* tree are suitable both for human and animal intake, being exceptionally nutritious. The consumption and usage of this plant have been increasing over the years, so much that nowadays, it is used as a food supplement and herbal medicine, being sold in urban consumption centers around the world. The most studied parts of *Moringa oleifera* tree are leaves and seeds, either as extracts or as flours. These have shown to be effective against several conditions, including cancer, obesity, diabetes, hypercholesterolemia, Parkinson, and Alzheimer's disease, among others.

[*] Corresponding Author's Email: jbheredia@ciad.mx.

Phytochemicals with nutraceutical properties, such as polyphenols, carotenoids, glucosinolates, alkaloids, and phytosterols, are responsible for the observed effects. The present study focuses on describing the phytochemical profile found in all parts of the *Moringa oleifera* tree and the role they play as preventive and curative agents in high prevalence diseases.

Keywords: *Moringa oleifera,* phytochemicals, polyphenols, carotenoids, alkaloids, cancer, diabetes, obesity

INTRODUCTION

Taxonomy

Moringa oleifera Lam is a tree species belonging to *Moringaceae,* within the order Brassicales (Table 1) (Bennett et al. 2003). *M. oleifera* is a wild plant widely distributed in nature. It is mainly found in countries with tropical and subtropical climates (Fahey 2005, Vongsak et al. 2013). This tree can grow in different and complicated conditions such as hot, drylands and humid tropics. Also, it is resistant to droughts and poor soils (Mbikay 2012, Anwar et al. 2007). Its structure, varying in height, can reach up to 10 m. *M. oleifera* has feathery leaves of intense green color with an extension of up to 60 cm. Also, its flowers are constituted of five petals of variant colors, going from white to a creamy yellow. These flowers give off a very characteristic smell. As for their reproductive morphology, they are bisexuals, producing both eggs and sperms (Paul and Didia 2012, Liu et al. 2018).

M. oleifera flowering usually occurs from April to June, which is linked to climatic conditions, because the flowering is favored in seasonal temperatures with constant rainfall (Santiago and Neto 2017).

The tree possesses a whitish corky bark and 3-sided hanging pods (Gupta et al. 2018). As for the fruits, after three years of tree planting, they can reach up to 1000 grains per pod. Regarding the color of the plant, depending on the environment, it varies from green to deciduous (Liu et al. 2018).

Table 1. Botanical description of *Moringa oleifera* (Muhammad, Asmawi, and Khan 2016)

Taxonomic subdivisions	Description
Kingdom	Plantae
Subkingdom	Tracheobionta
Supervision	Spermatophyta
Division	Magnoliophyta
Class	Magnoliopsida
Subclass	Dilleniidae
Order	Brassicales
Family	Moringaceae
Genus	*Moringa*
Species	*Moringa oleifera*

Due to their phytochemical profiles (polyphenols, tannins, phytosterols, carotenoids, glucosinolates, isothiocyanates, saponins, alkaloids, among others), all *M. oleifera* anatomical parts (barks, flowers, leaves, pods, roots, and seeds) have been studied either as a whole or as selective extracts for the treatment of several diseases.

Origin

M. oleifera is an angiosperm plant that belongs to the Moringaceae family. It is native to sub-Himalayan tracts of Northern India. This family is made up of only 13 species (Table 2) (Olson, 2002). Among the 13 species, *M. oleifera,* also known as "the miracle plant" or "the tree of life," has been by far the most studied one, and its leaves and seeds have been chemically characterized and studied for at least the last 30 years (Faizi et al. 1992). *Moringa stenopetala*, *Moringa concanensis*, and *Moringa peregrina* have also been studied, although to a much lesser extent. As for the others, they are only distributed in Madagascar and Africa, whereby they have been less studied (Rani et al. 2018).

This tree has been given different names according to the region of the world where it is located. Besides moringa, these names include the drumstick tree, horseradish tree, and ben oil tree or benzoil tree. The synonyms to moringa are given in Table 3.

M. oleifera has been of great interest throughout history due to its many therapeutic applications since little or no adverse effects have been associated with its consumption. For instance, Ayurveda, an Indian tradition, has claims that *M. oleifera* leaves can prevent and treat more than 300 ailments (Ganguly

2013). Moreover, its seeds oil has been used as part of the formulation of a variety of cosmetic and fragrance industries. Nowadays, its oil is being studied as lubricants in machinery and for biodiesel production (Boukandoul, Casal, and Zaidi 2018).

Table 2. Moringa species and their origin of cultivation (Boukandoul, Casal, and Zaidi 2018, Leone et al. 2015)

Species	Origin
M. arborea Verdc.	Kenya
M. borziana Mattei	Somalia and Kenia
M. concanensis Nimmo	Sub-Himalayan tracts of Northern India
M. drouhardii Jum.	Madagascar
M. hildebrandtii Engl.	Madagascar
M. longituba Engl.	Kenya, Ethiopia, and Somalia
M. oleifera Lam.	Sub-Himalayan tracts of Northern India
M. ovalifolia Dinter & Berger	Namibia and Angola
M. peregrine (Forssk.) Fiori	Red sea and Horn of Africa
M. pygmaea Verdc.	Somalia
M. rivae Chiov.	Kenya and Ethiopia
M. ruspoliana Engl.	Ethiopia
M. stenopetala (Bak. f.) Cuf.	Kenya and Ethiopia

Table 3. Names by which the *Moringa oleifera* tree is known around the world (Rani et al. 2018)

Language	Name
English	Drumstick tree, Horseradish tree
Spanish	Moringa, Angela, Ben
Chinese	La ken
French	Morungue
Latin	*Moringa oleifera*
Arabian	Rawag
Hindi	Sainjna,Saguna
Gujarati	Suragavo
Malayalam	Murinna, Sigru
Tamil	Mulaga, Munaga
Unani	Sahajan
Ayurvedic	Akshiva, Haritashaaka

Production, Commercialization, and Consumption

As previously mentioned, *M. oleifera* is native to sub-Himalayan tracts of Northern India. Nevertheless, it has been subsequently distributed more widely in Africa, India, Ethiopia, The Philippines, and the Sudan, where this plant is the one contributing the most to herbal sale income (Leone et al. 2016).

Since *M. oleifera* tree is capable of growing in any tropical climate, nowadays is also found in tropical Asia, Latin America, The Caribbean, Florida, and the Pacific Islands, among other countries (Figure 1).

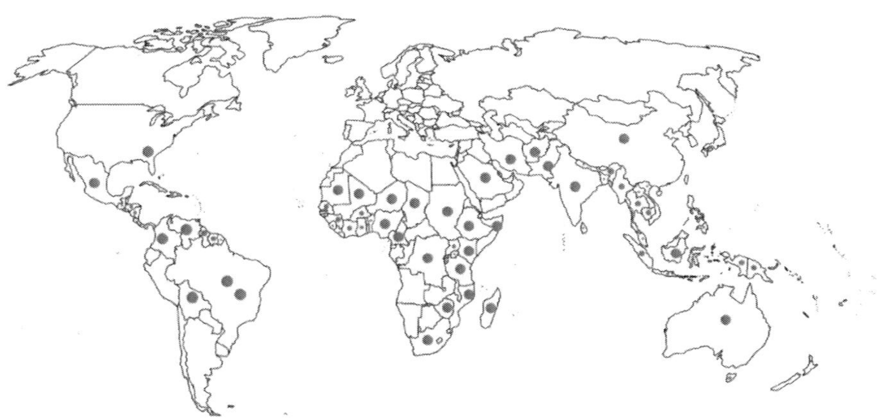

Figure 1. *Moringa oleifera* worldwide presence (green dots indicate in which countries are the tree distributed).

For *M. oleifera* to grow optimally, it requires a temperature between 18 and 28°C, a loose-textured soil with a pH going from 4.5 to 8, an altitude up to 600 m above sea level and an annual rainfall between 760 and 2500 mm (Leone et al. 2015). As for the above, *M. oleifera* is resistant to drought but not to excess rain, so it is not recommended for it to be grown in the rainy season (Meza-Carranco et al. 2016).

The seeds are 1 cm in diameter with coloration going from brown to black and a semi-permeable hull constituted of 3 papery wings. As a whole, the average weight is 0.3 g/seed. Seeds germinate ten days after sowing, and under optimal conditions, they can reach a height of up to 5 m in the first year and up to 10 m as an adult tree. Each tree can produce up to 25,000 seeds each year. It is recommended for the crop to be harvested at 85-90 days after sowing since harvesting earlier usually leads to a thin and weak stem. The pests that affect the plants immediately after germination are ants (*Formica* spp.), mainly atta (*Atta cephalotes*) and small mocis moth (*Mocis latipes*).

India is the *M. oleifera* largest producer with a yield of 1.2 tons per year. Adhara Pradesh, Karnataka, and Tamil Nadu are the major growers of *M. oleifera* trees in this country where 156.6, 102.8, and 74.09 km^2 are devoted to their production, respectively (Ravani et al. 2017).

All parts of the *M. oleifera* tree bark, pods, leaves, nuts, seeds, tubers, roots, and flowers are used for different purposes, and they are suitable both for human and animal consumption showing to be exceptionally nutritious. Egyptians were among the first civilizations taking advantage of *M. oleifera* tree health benefits using the oil obtained from their seeds to produce balms for skincare, perfumes, and lubricants (Barakat and Ghazal 2016). Nowadays, it is known that *M. oleifera* seed oil is rich in oleic acid, tocopherols, and sterols, so it is also used as cooking oil substituting others such as olive and also it is applied as a fertilizer (Gopalakrishnan et al. 2016).

While *Moringa oleifera* has been part of traditional food and medicine in South Asia and Africa for thousands of years, in many countries of America this plant was mainly used as an ornamental until recent, that its production had a boom due to different discoveries, for example, their anti-cancer chemoprotective properties (Olson and Alvarado-Cárdenas 2016). Those discoveries have caused that variants of unpleasant taste to disappear a long time ago in their native countries and recently in America.

Nowadays, in many countries, seeds are eaten either green, toasted, powdered, infused for tea, or even used to make curries (Wadhwa 2013). The tree trunk is whitish-gray, thick, and rough. It is wounded to produce gums. The gum is initially white, but it changes to a reddish-brown or brownish-black when exposed to air and light. The tree wood is used as fuel for bonfires in native countries, and sometimes for building. In India, *M. oleifera* wood is also used for the production of newsprint, textiles, and cellophane.

The flower, 10-25 cm long fragrant, bisexual and yellowish-white, is used for water purification and for infusions known to have hypocholesterolemic properties. They are also edible, and its flavor is compared to that of mushrooms (Arise et al. 2014). As for the leaves, green hairless bipinnate, or tripinnate, they were used as forage and lately, due to its high protein content, as a food source. In developing countries, *M. oleifera* leaves are offered to children and also to breastfeeding mothers for increasing milk production (Olson and Alvarado-Cárdenas 2016). Although the root is less consumed because of the presence of alkaloids, it is used ground as a condiment with a very particular hot flavor. *M.*

oleifera root infusions are also known to have beneficial effects over heart complaints, dyspepsia, and eye conditions (Ferreira et al. 2008).

The consumption and usage of all parts of the tree has been increasing so much (Table 4) they are being used as food supplement and herbal medicine, and even sold at urban consumption centers around the world, as well as incorporated into different dishes such as soups, and different pastry products (Oyeyinka and Oyeyinka 2018). *M. oleifera* has been included as part of various commercial products formulations, and it has been found that it improves some organoleptic properties as well as increases product shelf life, oxidative stability as well as nutritional value (Falowo et al. 2018). In developing countries such as Ghana, *M. oleifera* leaves flour have been introduced in different dishes on schools to children of 4 to 13 years, improving macronutrients and micronutrients intake, specially β-carotene, Zn, Mn, and Fe, being accepted by the children after the sensory test (Glover-Amengor et al. 2017). *M. oleifera* leaf powder has also been included in complementary foods for infants aged 8 to 12 months, mainly as part of a cereal-legume blend. The use of leaf powder is an effort to combat malnutrition, improving blood retinol concentrations (Dewey, Yang, and Boy 2009). It has also been incorporated in yogurt in Mwanza, Tanzania, with flavors of locally-grown fruit purees, aiming to increase the nutritional value and health benefits of the product (Hekmat et al. 2015). Soup powders have been supplemented with *M. oleifera* leaf, raising vitamin C, protein, and fiber content, which is highly acceptable, even by six months children (Farzana et al. 2017). Recently wound dressing formulations containing *M. oleifera* leaf extracts have been developed (3% W/V), its phenolic compounds (vicenin-2, chlorogenic acid, gallic acid, quercetin, kaempferol, rosmarinic acid, and rutin) promotes dermal fibroblast and human keratinocytes cell proliferation and migration properties (Chin et al. 2018).

Table 4. Old and recent uses of the different parts of the *Moringa oleifera* tree

Tree part	Uses	References
Leave	Scholar snacks, baby food, yogurt, forage, juice, infusions, and balms	(Wadhwa 2013, Gopalakrishnan et al. 2016)
Seeds	Balm, perfume, lubricant, cooking oil and fertilizer	(Barakat and Ghazal 2016)
Flower	Water purification, infusions and as mushroom substitute	(Arise et al. 2014)
Pod	Natural preservative, water purification, the main ingredient in soups and pastry	(Arise et al. 2014)
Root	Infusions and as a condiment	(Alves de Almeida et al. 2017, Ferreira et al. 2008)

Despite the above, the commercialization and production of *M. oleifera* products are still very informal, making it difficult to get reliable information about its production volumes and prices. With the recent recognition of *M. oleifera* nutritional, pharmacokinetic, and industrial properties, there is a growing interest in promoting its cultivation worldwide (Palada et al. 2014).

Physicochemical Profile

M. oleifera tree contains both high concentrations of vitamins and phytochemicals, which make it an excellent alternative to alleviate some noncommunicable diseases. The whole tree is a storehouse of valuable phytochemicals and nutrients (Tables 5 and 6). For instance, the leaves, the most characterized and studied part of the tree, is rich in minerals and vitamins. Also, they are rich in phytochemicals such as tannins, flavonoids, alkaloids, and saponins (Gopalakrishna et al. 2016).

M. oleifera has a high content of compounds containing rhamnose, and it is rich in phytochemicals known as glucosinolates and isothiocyanates (Fahey 2005). Because of this characteristics, *M. oleifera* is considered as the miracle tree, since each part of the plant serves for many purposes, including their use in both food and pharmaceutical industries (Moyo et al. 2011). Also, for its high protein content, *M. oleifera* has been considered as an option to treat malnutrition problems around the world. The main amino acids contained in its protein are leucine (492.2-650 mg/100 g), valine (374.5-540 mg/100 g), isoleucine (299.6-440 mg/100 g), threonine (117.7-390 mg/100 g) and arginine (360 to 406.6 mg/100 g) (Yameogo et al. 2011, Amabye, 2015). Also, *M. oleifera* leaves are a low-calorie food that has been considered to be used in obese people's diets to supply nutrient demand (Gopalakrishnan et al. 2016). As part of their protein profile, there is a serine protease considered as an anti-nutrient, trypsin inhibitor. Trypsin inhibitor forms complexes by strongly inhibiting the activity of the pancreatic enzymes chymotrypsin and trypsin, so proteins are not properly digested, and amino acids are not released to be absorbed (Avilés-Gaxiola, Chuck-Hernández, and Serna Saldivar 2018). The activity of trypsin inhibitor in *M. oleifera* leaves of 1.45 units/mg. It is much lower than those of other high protein food sources, for example, legumes like soybean, which has a trypsin inhibitor activity of 107.22 units/mg (Teixeira et al. 2014). *M. oleifera* trypsin inhibitor is an 18.2 kDa polypeptide which acts against the *Aedes aegypti* larvae, egg, and pupae (Pontual et al. 2014). Its activity in the tree flowers is about 0.18 U/mg. As for *M. oleifera* seeds, trypsin inhibitor activity is about 2.3 units/mg. Every part of the tree also has high vitamin and mineral content. Among the main minerals are calcium, potassium, zinc, magnesium, iron, and copper (Table 7).

Table 5. Phytochemical content of extracts from the tissues of *Moringa oleifera* tree obtained with different solvents

Extraction solvent	Tree fraction	Phytochemicals	References
Water	-Leaves -Root -Flower	-Myricetin, quercetin, and kaempferol -4(a-L-Rhamnosyloxy)benzyl isothio- cyanate -Phtalic acid diesters	(Matshediso, Cukrowska, and Chimuka 2015, Eilert, Wolters, and Nahrstedt 1981, Anand et al. 2016)
Ethanol	-Roots -Leaves -Seed	- Aurantiamide acetate and 1,3-dibenzyl urea -Crypto-chlorogenic acid, isoquercetin, and astragalin. - *O*-ethyl-4-(α-l-rhamnosyloxy)benzyl carbamate, , 4(α-l-rhamnosyloxy)-benzyl isothiocyanate, niazimicin, niazirin, β-sitosterol, glycerol-1-(9-octadecanoate), 3-*O*-(6′-*O*-oleoyl-β-d-glucopyranosyl)-β-sitosterol, and β-sitosterol-3-*O*-β-d-glucopyranoside	(Sashidhara et al. 2009, Vongsak, Sithisarn, and Gritsanapan 2013)
Methanol	-Leaves - Flowers	-Galic acid, chlorogenic acid, ellagic acid, ferulic acid, kaempferol, quercetin and rutin -Ethyl olate, quinic acid, cis-9-hexadecanal, palmitic acid, gamma-sitosterol and stigmasterol	(Verma et al. 2009, Inbathamizh and Padmini 2012)
Hydro-methanolic	-Leaves	-Quercetin, kaempferol, glucosides and glucoside malonates	(Coppin et al. 2013)
Hydro-ethanol	-Stem bark -Leaves -Pods	-Azulene, quinoline, ethyl ester, cis-13-octadecenoic acid, methyl ester, dodecane, eicosane 2, isopropyl myristate, stigmasterol, hexadecanoic acid, methyl ester, lupeol, hexadecane, n-hexadecanoic acid, benzoic acid, dodecane, heptadecane, and β-sitosterol - kaempferol, quercetin, multiflorin-B, and apigenin -Niaziridin	(Vasanth et al. 2015, Karthivashan et al. 2013, Shanker et al. 2007)
Butanol	-Oil seed	- 3,5,7,3′,4′,5′-hexahydroxyflavone (myricetin)	(Lalas and Tsaknis 2002)
Petroleum ether	-Seed	-Palmitic acid, stearic acid, oleic acid, docosanoic acid	(Abdulkarim et al. 2005)

Table 6. Nutritional composition of *Moringa oleifera* tree

Fraction	Moisture (%)	Crude protein (%)	Fats (%)	Crude fiber (%)	Ash (%)	Total carbohydrate (%)	Bibliography
Dry leaves	4.86-8.1	26.2-27.6	12.5-16.9	15.7-20.0	8.2-16.0	35.7-43.3	(Yameogo et al. 2011, Amabye, 2015)
Dry pods	8.1-8.33	18.4-19.81	1.9-16.9	24.43-39.2	5.49-6.7	10.4-34.81	(Abdulkadir, Zawawi, and Jahan 2016, Gidamis et al. 2003)
Dry seeds	7.0-10.60	18.86 - 31.4	13.35-36.7	5.03-7.3	4.77 - 6.2	18.4-53.36	(Ijarotimi, Adeoti, and Ariyo 2013, Leone et al. 2016)
Dry Root	6.06-8.6	12.25-16.87	2.66-10.88	13.80-45.43	3.37-13.40	14.92-51.83	(Mgbemena and Obodo 2016, Verma and Nigam 2014)
Dry flower	5.8-7.92	25.16-18.92	1.57-2.91	7.55-32.45	6.01-9.68	28.12-53.67	(Sánchez-Machado et al. 2010, Arise et al. 2014)

Table 7. Mineral profile of *Moringa oleifera* tree part (Dhakar et al. 2011, Naik et al. 2018, Kumssa et al. 2017, Fakankun, Babayemi, and Utiaruk 2013)

Mineral (mg)	Pods (per 100 g)	Leaves fresh weight (per 100 g)	Flower fresh weight (per 100 g)	Seeds (per 100 g)	Root wood (per 100 g)
Calcium	30	440	32.34	125	170
Magnesium	24	24	-	310	6.5
Phosphorous	110	70	19.66	-	-
Potassium	24	24	671	-	500
Copper	3.1	1.1	-	0.402	15
Iron	5.3	0.7	48.11	4.98	-
Oxalic acid	10	101	-	-	-
Sulfur	137	137	-	-	-

PHYTOCHEMICALS

Vitamins

Vitamins are organic substances essential for metabolic processes. They are present in different food sources, including plants. Inadequate vitamin intake can cause a variety of diseases (Mozafar, 2018). For example, scurvy and blindness. The first one is caused by a vitamin C deficit, while the other is promoted by vitamin A low consumption. Their prevalence is higher in developing countries.

Among *M. oleifera* excellent nutritional properties, it is its high content of vitamins A, C, and E (Vergara-Jimenez, Almatrafi, and Fernandez 2017). Furthermore, *M. oleifera* leaves fresh and dried vitamin A content is four and ten times higher, respectively, when compared to carrots. As for vitamin C, is concentration is seven-fold higher when compared to the one of orange. Dry *M. oleifera* leaves contain 41.17 mg/g of vitamin C (Ademiluyi et al. 2018). Additionally, it has been reported that dry *M. oleifera* leaves contain 0.5 g/kg of Vitamin E (Zeng et al. 2019) and 13.4 mg/100g α-carotene (Barichella et al. 2018). α and β carotene are known to be vitamin A precursors (Nagarajan et al. 2017).

The different ways in which *M. oleifera* leaves are processed, affect their nutrient content, including vitamin levels. For instance, cooked and oven-dried *M. oleifera* leaves lose 32 and 74% of its vitamin C content, respectively (Sahay, Yadav, and Srinivasamurthy 2017). However, this process enhances the availability of β–carotene (Saha and Sen, 2019).

As for *M. oleifera* pods, they are also excellent sources of vitamin C, containing 145 μg/100 g. For these, consuming the pods and leaves of this tree has been related to an improved immunity system.

Regarding the other anatomical parts of *M. oleifera* tree, its vitamin profile has not yet been reported. For example, it is known that their seeds are high in both vitamin A and E content, nevertheless the exact content is not known. As for other moringa species such as *Moringa peregrina,* their seeds have high amounts of vitamin C (14 mg/100 g) and vitamin A (24.8 mg/100 g) (Asghari, Palizban, and Bakhshaei 2015).

Polyphenols

Polyphenols are secondary metabolites occurring mostly in vegetables, cereals, and fruits. These compounds are related to defense systems against unfavorable conditions such as biotic and abiotic factors. Their consumption has been related to the cure and treatment of different diseases such as cancer and diabetes. Moreover, their chemical structure is characterized by the presence of at least a phenol group. More than 8,000 polyphenols have been identified, and each plant has a particular profile. Polyphenols are classified in flavanols, flavanones, flavonols, hydroxycinnamic acids, and anthocyanins (Pandey and Rizvi 2009).

M. oleifera is a rich source of phenolic acids and flavonoids. These polyphenols are known by its many bioactive properties, mainly for its high antioxidant potential. *M. oleifera* leaves bioactive compounds content, including polyphenols, have been reviewed (Leone et al. 2015). From all plant tissues, the leaves have been reported to possess the highest concentration of flavonoids (Amaglo et al. 2010). Besides, leaves contain proanthocyanidins and phenolic acids. The concentration of flavonoids, flavonols, phenols, and proanthocyanidins in leaves was found to be 295.01 quercetin, 120.33 tannic acids, and 32.50 catechin equivalent/g, respectively (Moyo, Oyedemi and Masika 2012).

M. oleifera leaves and seeds are rich in polyphenols, mainly phenolic acids and flavonoids. Naringin and quercetin are the main flavonoids found in *M. oleifera* leaf, and benzoic and salicylic acids are the main phenolic acids (Helmy et al. 2017). The seeds are rich in luteolin, *p*-coumaric acid, gallic acid, caffeic acid, apigenin, quercetin, and rutin (Adedayo et al. 2018). Additionally, *M. oleifera* seeds were reported to contain bound and free phenolics, 4173 and 780 mg/100 g, respectively. The main phenolics present in seeds are catechin, epicatechin, coumaric acid, gallic acid, protocatechuic acid, catechin gallate, and ferulic acid (Pandu, Cherupanalli, and Muthukumar 2018).

Another investigation revelated that leaves and seeds contain ellagic, chlorogenic, gallic acids, kaempferol, isoquercetin, rutin, and quercetin (Oyeleye et al. 2019).

The variation in phenolic content of an *M. oleifera* plant might be due to several factors, such as differences in the maturity stage, climatic conditions, and type of solvent used for their extraction (Hani et al. 2017). The identification of polyphenols reported for *M. oleifera* is summarized in Table 8.

Table 8. Polyphenols reported in the different parts of the *Moringa oleifera* tree

Origin	Part of the plant	Components	Reference
Salem, Tamil Nadu, Southern India	Leaf Root Flower Bark Seed	Coumaric acid, myricetin, quercetin, kaempferol, resveratrol, naringenin, biochanin A, naringin and catechin	(Prabakaran et al. 2018)
Akure metropolis, Nigeria	Leaf	Gallic acid, catechin, chlorogenic acid, caffeic acid, ellagic acid, epicatechin, rutin, quercetin and kaempferol	(Ademiluyi et al. 2018)
Himayatnagar, Hyderabad, Andhra Pradesh, India.	Seed	1H-pyrazol-4-yl-methanol, 1-(2-Methyl-5-nitro-1H-imidazol-1-yl) propan-2-ol, Benzoyl-β-d-glucoside, 13-Hydroperoxy octadecadienoic acid, 1,4-Naphthoquinone, Luteolin-6-c-glucoside, 4-O-(6-Vanillyl1)-β-d-glucopyranosyl vanillyl alcohol and 7-Rhamnoglucoside (Hesperidin)	(Premi and Sharma 2017)
Guangxi, China	Leaf	Quercetin-diR, quercetin-G, kaempferol-G, quercetin-G-Ac, kaemferol-G-Ac, Quercetin-Xyl/Api-S and Kaempferol-Xyl/Api-S.	(Wang et al. 2017)
India	Seed	Gallic acid, catechin, p-coumaric acid, ferulic acid, vanillin, caffeic acid, protocatechuic acid, Cinnamic acid, epicatechin and quercetin	(Govardhan, Negi, and Radha 2013)
Africa	Leaf	Quercetin-G-Rha, Quercetin-G, Kaempferol-G-Rha, Quercetin-Xyl-Api-Ac, Quercetin-G-M, Kaempferol-G, Quercetin-G-M, Kaempferol-Xyl-Api-Ac, Quercetin-G-S, Kaempferol-G-M, Kaempferol-G-M and Kaempferol-G-S	(Coppin et al. 2013)
Malaysia	Leaf	Multiflrin-B, apigenin-8-C-glucoside, apigenin-8-C-glucoside, quercetin-3-O-β-D-glucoside, quercetin-3-O-acetyl glucoside, kaempferol-3-O-glucoside and kaempferol-3-O-acetyl glucoside	(Karthivashan et al. 2013)
India, Nicaragua, Niger	Leaf	Catechin, epicatechin, ferulic acid, ellagic acid, myricetin, quercetin, butein, apigenin, kaempferol, isorhamentin, and rhamnetin	(Siddhuraju and Becker 2003)
	Seed	4-(α-L-rhamnopyranosyloxy)-benzylglucosinolate	(Bennett et al. 2003)
Nicaragua	Old and young leaves	4-(α-L-rhamnopyranosyloxy)-benzyl-glucosinolate, 4-(α-L-rhamnopyranosyloxy)-benzylglucosinolate monoacetyl-Isomer I, 4-(α -L-rhamnopyranosyloxy)-benzylglucosinolate monoacetyl-isomer II and 4-(α-L-rhamnopyranosyloxy)-benzylglucosinolate monoacetyl-isomer III	(Bennett et al. 2003)

*diR: dirhamnosyl, G: Glucosyl/Galactosyl moiety, Ac: Acetyl, Xyl: Xylosyl, Api: Apiosyl, S: Succinoyl.

*G: Glucosyl/Galactosyl moiety; Rha: Rhamnosyl; Xyl: Xylosyl; Api: Apiosyl; Ac: Acetyl; M: Malonyl; S: Succinoyl.

Tannins

Tannins are water-soluble phenolic compounds that are known for their capacity to complexes with alkaloids, proteins, and other molecules, for which they have also been considered as antinutrient compounds. Its antioxidant properties have been extensively reported. *M. oleifera* leaves contain low amounts of tannins. They were said to contain 0.05 mg/g of tannins. Nevertheless, this content can be increased up to 20.6 mg/g when dried. (Ademiluyi et al. 2018).

Tannins have been related to anti-cancer, anti-inflammatory, anti-HIV replication, antibacterial, anti-atherosclerosis, and anti-hepatotoxic activities (Vergara-Jimenez, Almatrafi, and Fernandez 2017). It has been found that freeze-dried leaves have 12 mg/g of tannins. Tannin concentration in dry and freeze-dried leaves are similar to those found in other plants such as berries. Nevertheless, they are considered lower compared to other medicinal plants (Leone et al. 2015). Tannins have also been found in *M. oleifera* flower and pod methanol, ethanol chloroform, acetone, and aqueous extracts. Nevertheless, concentrations have not yet been reported (Gull et al. 2016).

As for *M. oleifera* seed, raw seeds have tannins in levels of up to 2.42 mg/g, which are reduced to 1.8 and 1.42 when the seed is either germinated or fermented, respectively (Ijarotimi, Adeoti, and Ariyo 2013). It is well reported that germination and fermentation techniques significantly reduce phytochemical components of plant seeds due to high enzymatic activity. Compared to other seeds and grains such as groundnut, sorghum, and pigeon pea, tannin content is low.

Carotenoids

Carotenoids are pigments distributed in nature. They are responsible for the characteristic color of some fruits and leaves. Also, carotenoids have high antioxidant capacity, which has been related to potential preventive effect against some diseases. In this regard, some authors have reported that *M. oleifera* has important amounts of carotenoids (Table 9).

M. oleifera fresh leaves have a high content of trans-zeaxanthin, trans-β-carotene, and trans-lutein (6, 18, and 37 mg/100 g, respectively) (Saini, Shetty, et al. 2014). These phytochemicals content is directly influenced by climate factors such as precipitation, solar radiation, temperature, tree age, and other factors such as soil composition. As for this, *M. oleifera* leaf carotenoids are mainly increased by UV solar radiation exposure (Vázquez-León et al. 2017).

Table 9. Carotenoids found in *Moringa oleifera*

Plant part	Compound	Reference
Leaves	Trans-zeaxanthin, Trans-β-carotene, Trans-lutein,	(Saini, Shetty, et al. 2014, Moyo et al. 2011)
	β-carotene	
	Neoxanthin, violaxanthin, β-eryptoxinthin, β-caroteneepoxide, β-Carotene	(Teixeira et al. 2014)
	Lycopene, β-carotene	(Tang et al. 2017)
Flowers	All-E-zeaxanthin, All-E-luteoxanthin, All-E-β-carotene, 13-Z-lutein, 15-Z-β-carotene, All E-Lutein	(Saini, Shetty, and Giridhar 2014)
Fruits	All-E-zeaxanthin, All-E-luteoxanthin, All-E-β-carotene, 13-Z-lutein, 15-Z-β-carotene, All E-Lutein	(Saini, Shetty, and Giridhar 2014)

Carotenoids composition not only differs from one anatomical part to another, but it also depends on the tree cultivar. Carotenoids from leaves, flowers, and fruits of eight *M. oleifera* cultivars have been quantified and identified (Saini, Sivanesan, and Keum 2016). It has been reported that the higher carotenoid content corresponds to leaves. E-Lutein and all-E-β-carotene are the main carotenoids prevalent in *M. oleifera* fruits and leaves, being the first one the one with the higher concentration. Also, neoxanthin, violaxanthin, β-eryptoxinthin, β-caroteneepoxide, β-Carotene, and lutein have been identified in *M. oleifera* leaves (Teixeira et al. 2014).

Comparing the content of 13-Z-lutein, all-E-luteoxanthin, 15-Z-β-carotene, and all-E-zeaxanthin in different cultivars, these compounds are found in higher concentrations in the Bhagya (KDM-1) (Moyo et al. 2011). On the other hand, *M. oleifera* leaves from South Africa possess the highest β-carotene content.

Similarly, Tang et al. (2017) reported a high content of lycopene and β-carotene in the ethanolic extract of *M. oleifera* leaves. Ethanolic leaf extract has a more top carotenoid composition when compared to other *M. oleifera* parts. For example, the seed. Recently, it has been found that phytoconstituents are influenced by an abiotic or biotic factor such as climatic conditions, chemical and physical changes, and elicitors. Thus, the effect of different elicitors on *M. oleifera* carotenoids has been studied. In this regard, Saini, Harish Prashanth, et al. (2014) reported the effectiveness of methyl jasmonate in enhancing *M. oleifera* leaves carotenoids content. Referring to the above, the importance of

M. oleifera in terms of carotenoid content, is due to their high concentrations reported in different parts of the plant, compared to other vegetable sources (Saini, Shetty, and Giridhar 2014). Although carotenoids presence in flowers, fruits, and leaves have been reported, they have not been found in other parts of *M. oleifera*, like stem bark (Kumbhare, Guleha, and Sivakumar 2012). Carotenoids with high antioxidant activity have been linked to diseases prevention, making *M. oleifera* leaves a good source for their obtaining (Atawodi et al. 2010, Tang et al. 2017, Teixeira et al. 2014).

Glucosinolates and Isothiocyanates

Glucosinolates are natural compounds coming from secondary plant metabolism and responsible for the pungency of plants such as mustard and cabbage and the bitter flavor of many cruciferous vegetables. Glucosinolates are precursors to isothiocyanates through myrosinase enzymatic activity. This reaction takes place in *Brassicaceae* order, to which *M. oleifera* belongs. Therefore, glucosinolates and isothiocyanates have been found in different parts of the *M. oleifera* tree (Table 10) (Jaja-Chimedza et al. 2017, Liu et al. 2018, Waterman et al. 2014).

The main glucosinolate found in *M. oleifera* seed is 4-(R-L-rhamnopyranosyloxy)-benzyl glucosinolate, a very atypical compound, being It corresponding isothyocinaiate, glucomoringin (4(α-L-rhamnosyloxy)-benzyl isothiocyanate) isothiocyanate (Amaglo et al. 2010, Jaja-Chimedza et al. 2017, Brunelli et al. 2010).

In both old and young *M. oleifera* leaves several glucosinolates have been identified 4-(R-L-rhamnopyranosyloxy)-benzyl glucosinolate monoacetyl-isomer I, 4-(R-L-rhamnopyranosyloxy)-benzyl glucosinolate monoacetyl-isomer II, 4-(R-L-rhamnopyranosyloxy)-benzyl glucosinolate monoacetyl-isomer III, while in roots the main glucosinolates identified are benzyl-glucosinolate and 4-(R-L-rhamnopyranosyloxy)-benzylglucosinolate (Fahey 2005, Jaja-Chimedza et al. 2017).

In *M. oleifera* leaves ethanolic extracts other compounds have been identified: pterygospermin, niazimicin, niaziminin, and 4-(L-rhamnosyloxy) benzyl isothiocyanate (Anwar et al. 2007, Gupta et al. 2018).

Amaglo et al. (2010) have reported a predominant presence of 4-O-(α-L-rhamnopyranosyloxy)-benzylglucosinolate in all *M. oleifera* parts, except in the roots where benzylglucosinolate was identified in a higher proportion.

Table 10. Glucosinolates and isothiocyanates compound found in *M. oleifera*

Plant part	Compounds	Reference
Bark	4-(α-L- rhamnopyranosyloxy) benzylglucosinolate	(Paikra, Dhongade, and Gidwani 2017)
Fruit	S-methyl-N-(Cheenpracha et al.) -thiocarbamate	(Cheenpracha et al. 2010)
	4-[(2´-O-acetyl-α-L-rhamnosyloxy) benzyl] isothiocyanate	
	4-[(3´-Oacetyl-α-L-rhamnosyloxy) benzyl] isothiocyanate	
Flowers	isolated 4-(4′-O-acetyl-α-L-rhamnosyloxy) benzyl isothiocyanate	(Amaglo et al. 2010, dos Santos et al. 2018)
	4-(4′-O-acetyl-2′,3′-dimethoxy-α-l-rhamnosyloxy) benzyl isothiocyanate 4-hydroxybenzylglucosinolate 4-O-(α-L-acetylrhamnopyranosyloxy)- benzyl isomer I 4-O-(α-L-acetylrhamnopyranosyloxy)- benzyl isomer II 4-O-(α-L-acetylrhamnopyranosyloxy)- benzyl isomer III	
Leaves	4-(R-L-rhamnopyranosyloxy)-benzyl glucosinolate monoacetyl-Isomer I 4-(R-L-rhamnopyranosyloxy)-benzyl glucosinolate monoacetyl-isomer II 4-(R-L-rhamnopyranosyloxy)-benzyl glucosinolate monoacetyl-isomer III	(Bennett et al. 2003)
	4-[(α-L-rhamnosyloxy) benzyl] isothiocyanate 4-[(4´-O-acetyl-α-L-rhamnosyloxy) benzyl] isothiocyanate	(Waterman et al. 2014)
	4-hydroxybenzylglucosinolate	(Amaglo et al. 2010)
	4-(L-rhamnosyloxy) benzyl isothiocyanate Niaziminin Niazimicin	(Anwar et al. 2007, Gupta et al. 2018, Mbikay 2012)
Petioles	4-hydroxybenzylglucosinolate 4-O-(α-L-acetylrhamnopyranosyloxy)- benzyl isomer I 4-O-(α-L-acetylrhamnopyranosyloxy)- benzyl isomer II 4-O-(α-L-acetylrhamnopyranosyloxy)- benzyl isomer III	(Amaglo et al. 2010)
Pods	4-O-(α-L-rhamnopyranosyloxy)-benzylglucosinolate	(Amaglo et al. 2010)
Roots	Benzyl-glucosinolate	(Amaglo et al. 2010, Bennett et al. 2003)
	4-(R-L-rhamnopyranosyloxy)-benzylglucosinolate	
Seeds	4(α-L-rhamnosyloxy)-benzyl isothiocyanate	(Brunelli et al. 2010, Bennett et al. 2003)
	4-(R-L-rhamnopyranosyloxy)-benzyl glucosinolate	
	4-O-(α-L-rhamnopyranosyloxy)-benzylglucosinolate	(Amaglo et al. 2010)
Stems	4-O-(α-L-rhamnopyranosyloxy)-benzyl 4-O-(α-L-acetylrhamnopyranosyloxy)- benzyl isomer III	(Amaglo et al. 2010)

Similarly, they reported the presence of 4-O-(α-L-acetylrhamnopyranosyloxy)- benzyl isomer III in the *M. oleifera* stems, as well as four compounds in petioles, leaves, and flowers (4-hydroxy-benzylglucosinolate, 1-3 (4-O-(α-L-acetylrhamnopyranosyloxy)- benzyl isomer) and 4-O-(α-L-rhamnopyranosyloxy)-benzylglucosinolate in pods and seed.

Recently, new compounds have been identified in *M. oleifera* fruits, where three new phenolic glucosides have been found: (S-methyl-N-thiocarbamate, 4-[(2´-O-acetyl-α-L-rhamnosyloxy) benzyl] isothiocyanate and 4-[(3´-Oacetyl-α-L-rhamnosyloxy)benzyl]isothiocyanate) (Cheenpracha et al. 2010).

As for *M. oleifera*, isothiocyanates that have been both identified and isolated are 4-(4′-O-acetyl-α-L-rhamnosyloxy)benzyl isothiocyanate and 4-(4′-O-acetyl-2′,3′-dimethoxy-α-l-rhamnosyloxy)benzyl isothiocyanate (dos Santos et al. 2018).

M. oleifera bark, such as the previously mentioned tree parts, also have important concentration of these compounds, for instance, 4-(α-L-rhamnopyranosyloxy) benzylglucosinolate (Paikra, Dhongade, and Gidwani 2017).

Saponins

Saponins are a class of chemical compounds containing a sugar unit linked to an aglycone or a triterpene, which gives them various properties such as foaming and emulsification. Harmful effects due to saponin high amounts ingest have been identified over both human beings and animals' regular growth. However, in small quantities, they can confer beneficial effects; for example, the reduction of cholesterol absorption and, therefore, plasma levels (Devisetti, Sreerama, and Bhattacharya 2016). Likewise, it has been found that saponins possess important characteristics such as anticancer activity. Therefore, they are compounds widely studied. The presence of saponins among *M. oleifera* leaves phytochemical profile has been reported (Vergara-Jimenez, Almatrafi, and Fernandez 2017). *M. oleifera* possesses negligible amounts of antinutritional factors such as tannins. Nevertheless, high levels of crude saponins (5 to 18%) have been detected. Freeze-dried *M. oleifera* leaves contain between 64 to 81 g/kg of saponins (Vergara-Jimenez, Almatrafi, and Fernandez 2017). This high saponin concentration has been associated with the antimicrobial properties of these leaves (Oluduro 2012).

According to Divi, Bellamkonda, and Dasireddy (2012) the aqueous extracts of *M. oleifera* leaves possess some phytochemicals compounds like saponins and catechol-derived compounds. Also, saponins have been found in leaves flour, suggesting that these chemical compounds are resistant to industrial processes (Devisetti, Sreerama, and Bhattacharya 2016).

The effectiveness of different solvents (water, methanol, ethanol, ethyl acetate, acetone, chloroform, and n-hexane) in terms of *M. oleifera* leaf saponins extraction, has been evaluated. Saponins extraction is potentialized by the use of n-hexane, chloroform, ethanol, and methanol solvents, and extraction with n-hexane showed the highest yield and specificity (Maqsood et al. 2017).

In addition to *M. oleifera* leaves, the root and steam also have important amounts of saponins, suggesting that *M. oleifera* could have a potential beneficial effect on different diseases (Ugwoke et al. 2017). *M. oleifera* seed flour contains saponins in the order of 9.83 mg/100 g, and this amount is decreased when the seed is either germinated or fermented, where the concentration drops to 8.29 and 7.50 mg/100 g, respectively (Ijarotimi, Adeoti, and Ariyo 2013). The content of saponin in *M. oleifera* is significantly lower compared to other medicinal plants such as *Madhuca utilis*. It has been determined that different processing such as roasting and boiling, increases saponin content by up to 2-fold (Mbah, Eme, and Paul 2012). It is well known that these compounds are not heat-labile and that their concentrations may remain the same, or even increase (by concentration) after heat processing times of around 20 h (Van Le et al. 2015).

Saponins have also been found in *M. oleifera* pods, where 13 saponin components have been identified. Saponin content is also linked to both abiotic and biotic factors, as well as to the extraction conditions, such as time, method, and solvent (Vázquez-León et al. 2017, Vongsak et al. 2013).

Alkaloids

Alkaloids are secondary plant metabolites containing carbon, hydrogen, nitrogen, and usual oxygen as part of their structure (Hussain et al. 2018). Alkaloids biosynthesis is mainly induced in response to herbivores attack on the plant, and their presence is more frequent in leaves, flowers, seeds, and roots (Kutchan 1995). These molecules have been considered as anti-nutrients for their action over the nervous system, where they disrupt or increase electrochemical transmission promoting cardiac pulse acceleration, paralysis, and even death (Sinha and Khare 2017). Despite the adverse effects supported by alkaloids, beneficial health effects have been attributed to them. For example, antitumorigenic, antiviral, anticholinergic, analgesic, diuretic, antiulcer, antihypertensive, and anti-inflammatory activities (Alves de Almeida et al. 2017). Each plant contains a unique mixture of these compounds, promoting different health effects (Krstin, Peixoto, and Wink 2015). As for *M. oleifera,* alkaloids have been found in leaves, flowers, seeds, and roots (Table 11).

Table 11. Alkaloid compounds found in *Moringa oleifera* tree parts

Plant part	Compounds	Reference
Leaves	*N*,α-l-rhamnopyranosyl vincosamide, pyrrolemarumine 4″-*O*-α-l-rhamnopyranoside and moringinine	(Panda et al. 2013)
Flowers	Pterigospermin	(Moura et al. 2011)
Seeds	Moringine	(Gopalakrishnan et al. 2016)
Roots	Moringine, moringinine, and spirochin	(Abd El-Hack et al. 2018, Nellis 1997)

M. oleifera leaves alkaloids average content is 0.68 mg/g. This amount is affected by the tree height, since the lower the tree, the more susceptible the leaves are to suffer from physical damage and by herbivore attacks reaching concentrations of alkaloids around 0.8 mg/g (Nweze and Nwafor 2014, Cabrera-Carrion et al. 2017). The two alkaloids identified in *M. oleifera* leaves are *N*,α-l-rhamnopyranosyl vincosamide, and pyrrolemarumine 4″-*O*-α-l-rhamnopyranoside. As for the first one, a dose of 40 mg/kg during a week in rats was able to reduce cardiac lipid peroxidation and to increase the cellular antioxidant levels, suggesting this compound as a cardio-protective phytochemical (Panda et al. 2013). The mechanism of action of this alkaloid is by increasing glutathione peroxidase and superoxide dismutase activities as well as reducing malondialdehyde in cardiac tissue. *N*,α-l-rhamnopyranosyl vincosamide is then suggested to replace or to lower the dosage level of cardioprotective established drugs (Cheraghi et al. 2017).

As for *M. oleifera* flowers, their antibacterial and antifungal activity has been attributed to pterigospermin (Moura et al. 2011). Pterigospermin has also found to possess pharmacological epinephrine-like effect, stimulating the heart and dilating bronchi vessels, so it would be useful to prove their efficacy over cardiac failure and asthma.

M. oleifera seeds and roots are both the fractions with the higher alkaloid content and the less consumed ones for the bitter taste attributed to these compounds. *M. oleifera* seeds contain an average amount of alkaloids of 0.1733 mg/g (Ijarotimi, Adeoti, and Ariyo 2013) where the alkaloid moringine has been identified (Leone et al. 2016). Moringine is also found in the tree root bark, the fraction with the highest alkaloid content, which represents up to 0.2% of its weight (Gopalakrishnan et al. 2016).

The root bark also contains another alkaloid known as moringinine. Both moringinine and moringine have high hypotensive effects (Abd El-Hack et al. 2018). Consuming more than 46 mg/kg body weight of root bark extract is known to affect liver and kidney function, and also cause violent uterine contractions that in some cases are fatal (Mazumder et al. 1999). These two alkaloids also relax muscles and stimulate the central nervous system in the same way as LSD (Nellis 1997). Moringinine alone has also been found in *M. oleifera* leaves and suspected to mediate their hypoglycemic effect. Also, it was found to normalize elevated serum levels of glucose, triacylglycerol, and cholesterol (Mbikay 2012). Moringinine was later identified as benzylamine.

For the above mentioned adverse effects, the bark was usually removed from the root. However, it has been found that root flesh contains an alkaloid called spirochin. Spirochin causes nerve paralysis and tachycardia at doses higher than 35 mg/kg. On the other hand, this alkaloid is a prophylactic and antiseptic agent against wound infections caused by gram-positive bacteria, especially for *staphylococcus* and *streptococcus* (Nellis 1997). As for pods and stems, they contain irrelevant amounts of alkaloids.

Phytates

Phytic acid is the primary storage form of phosphorus in seeds. For a long time, phytic acid was considered as an anti-nutrient since it can bind minerals and proteins, making them not available for absorption in the gut, which promotes indigestion and flatulence (Omoruyi et al. 2013, Igwilo et al. 2010). On the other hand, phytic acid secondary effects have been considered as beneficial in terms of health. For example, it reduces free radical production in the gastrointestinal tract, an effect associated with a lower colon cancer incidence (Udeh et al. 2018). Phytic acid is mainly found in leaves and seeds. *M. oleifera* leaves have an average phytate content of 1.53 mg/g when fresh (Richter, Siddhuraju, and Becker 2003). Although, the exact amount depends to a large extent on its cultivation conditions, as well as in the leaf processing. Drying and grinding, for example, increase the amount of all components, including that of phytic acid, which reaches a concentration of 23 to 63.97 mg/g (Richter, Siddhuraju, and Becker 2003, Gallaher et al. 2017).

On the other hand, boiling, simmering and blanching the leaves before consumption reduces phytic acid content by 85.44, 57.3, and 39.8%, respectively, improving nutrient absorption. The above because high temperatures denaturalize phytic acid, while those that include water leach it (Sallau et al. 2012). Increasing or decreasing phytic acid concentration will depend on the consumer´s needs. For example, it is known to binds α-amylase leading to incomplete starch digestion, benefiting diabetic patients.

M. oleifera seeds reach up to 1.75 mg/g. Similar phytic acid concentration to that in millet, peas, peanuts, cashew, and nuts. But the seed with the highest phytic acid concentration is that of soybean, 2.220 mg/g (Gupta, Gangoliya, and Singh 2015). Phytates in *M. oleifera* seeds have been associated with increased cooking times (Nwokolo, Bragg, and Kitts 1976). An option to reduce the phytic acid content in *M. oleifera* seeds is defatting them, a process that decreases this compound by up to 35% (Olagbemide and Philip 2014). Germination and fermentation of *M. oleifera* seeds also reduce phytic acid content by up to 49 and 67%, respectively (Ijarotimi, Adeoti, and Ariyo 2013).

As for roots, it occurs at shallow levels of 0.07 mg/g. Negligible levels have also been reported in stems and flowers (Igwilo et al. 2014). Amongst the antinutritional factors found in *M. oleifera*, glycosylates, and phytate are the ones present in the most significant amounts (Makkar and Becker 1997).

Oxalates

Oxalic acid (oxalate) is a secondary metabolite found in small amounts in different plant constituents. Oxalic acid forms water-soluble salts with Na^+, K^+, and NH^+ ions and binds to minerals such as Ca^{2+}, Fe^{2+}, and Mg^{2+}, making them unavailable for absorption. For the above, it has been considered as an antinutritional compound (Israr, Frazier, and Gordon 2013). *M. oleifera* leaves are regarded as a rich source of oxalates compared to other greens since the dry leaves have an average content of 11.2 mg/g (Nambiar and Seshadri 2001, Radek and Savage 2008). In vivo assays using rats have shown that after 7 d of consuming *M. oleifera* leaves, calcium absorption and retention is decreased by around 25 and 40%, respectively, an effect associated with oxalate content (Pankaja and Prakash 1994). It has been determined that 38% of the total calcium in *M. oleifera* leaves is already associated with oxalate, being part of this non-absorbed calcium fraction (Olson et al. 2016). Heat processing is useful to decrease oxalate content in *M. oleifera* leaves. For example, boiling, simmering, and blanching may reduce its content by 85.32, 80.95, and 61.90%, respectively. The reduction is mainly due to soluble oxalate leaving the food matrix (Nikmaram et al. 2017). Oxalic acid is also present *M. oleifera* seeds in high amounts of 10.5 mg/g (Saini, Sivanesan, and Keum 2016). On the other hand, meager amounts have been measured in roots and pods, with values of 391.1 ug/kg and 0.1 mg/g, respectively (Sonbarse, Sharma, and Parvatam 2017, Posmontier 2011).

Phytosterols

Phytosterols are plant-derived bioactive compounds with a chemical structure very similar to cholesterol (Table 12). This term refers to both sterols and their saturated derivatives called stanols (Mo et al. 2013). Although about 250 phytosterols have been identified, the sterols and stanols most commonly found in plants are β-sitosterol, campesterol, and stigmasterol and β-sitostanol, and campestanol, respectively (Cabral and Klein 2017). Because of their similarity to cholesterol, they all diminish cholesterol absorption in the small bowel, reducing its presence in blood serum (Yi et al. 2016).

Table 12. Phytosterol compounds found in *Moringa oleifera* tree parts

Plant part	Compounds	Reference
Leaves	Stigmasterol, β-sitosterol, 5-α-cholestane and campesterol	(Cabral and Klein 2017)
Seed	β-sitosterol, stigmasterol, campesterol, and Δ5-avenasterol	(Tsaknis et al. 1999, Nadeem and Imran, 2016, Leone et al. 2016)
Stem bark	Not identified	(Arora and Onsare 2014, Kumbhare, Guleha, and Sivakumar 2012)

M. oleifera leaves phytosterol profile is characterized by the presence of stigmasterol, β-sitosterol, 5-α-cholestane, and campesterol, making up around 49.55, 27.48, 15.31 and 7.66% of the total phytosterol profile respectively (Tshingani et al. 2017). Among the most important sterols is β-sitosterol, due to its similarity to cholesterol, it has been proven effective against inflammation reactions, viral damage, and ulcer, as well as a potent anti-cancer and boost immune system molecule (Paniagua-Pérez et al. 2017). Due to the β-sitosterol high content in *M. oleifera* leaves (90 mg/g), the powder obtained from them has been incorporated into cocoa, substituting 20% of the formulation to produce chocolate snacks with health benefits (Rajanandh and Kavitha 2010, Gopalakrishnan et al. 2016)

M. oleifera seed oil is also a source rich in phytosterols. The total sterols of *M. oleifera* oil are composed in 92% by β-sitosterol, stigmasterol, campesterol, and Δ5-avenasterol with average amounts of 0.46, 0.23, 0.16 and 0.85 mg/g respectively (Nadeem and Imran 2016, Leone et al. 2015b). *M. oleifera* seed oil phytosterol profile differs from that of olive and other popular vegetable conventional oils as it has more campesterol, Δ5-avenasterol, and stigmasterol than canola and sunflower oil (Nadeem and Imran 2016). Phytosterols have also been found in *M. oleifera* stem bark petroleum extracts, while its presence has not been detected in pod husks (Arora and Onsare 2014, Kumbhare, Guleha, and Sivakumar 2012).

EFFECTS OF *MORINGA OLEIFERA* TREE PARTS OVER VARIOUS DISEASES

The use of different plants to treat and prevent diseases has been registered since the beginning of civilizations. Regarding the *M. oleifera* tree, the consumption of their different parts, as a whole or as extracts, has been associated with the improvement or healing of various medical conditions (Figure 2).

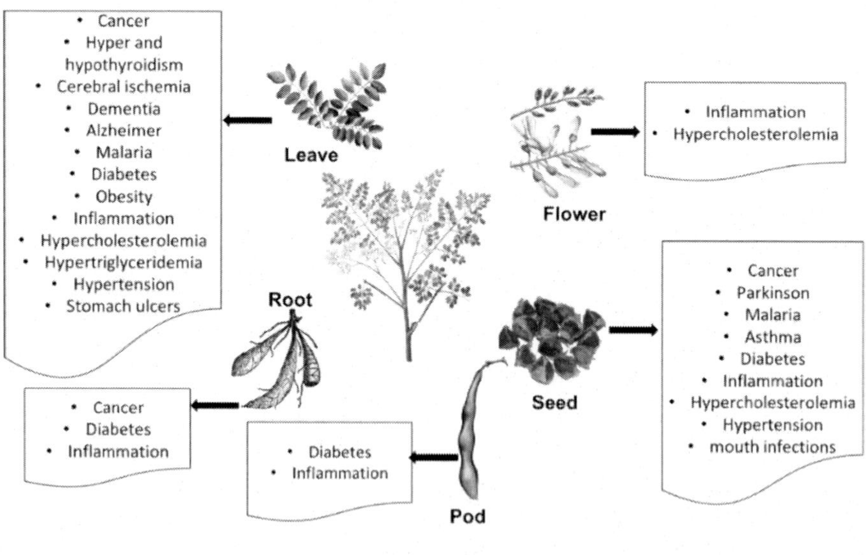

Figure 2. Beneficial effects of the different parts of the *Moringa oleifera* on various diseases.

Nowadays, the therapeutic use of the *M. oleifera* tree has been extended to various parts of the world. It has been of scientific interest to find and to identify the molecules responsible for the healing properties attributed to each part of the tree, to understand the mechanisms that lie in their high efficiency and provide a scientific basis for their use. For the above, different analyses using both *in vivo* and *in vitro* models have been carried out. In this section, the role played by each part of the *M. oleifera* tree on different types of diseases is discussed.

Diabetes

Diabetes mellitus, known as the epidemic of the century, is a disease consequence of metabolism abnormalities. As for type 1 diabetes, it is due to autoimmune system attack and destruction of β-pancreatic cells located on islets of Langerhans , while the main risk factors for type II diabetes are obesity, overweight, impaired glucose tolerance, high blood pressure, among others (Muhammad, Asmawi, and Khan 2016, Yassa and Tohamy 2014). Diabetes is of great concern due to the multiple problems that arise during its progression.

As for β-pancreatic cells, they could be vulnerable due to some enzymes, such as superoxide dismutase and catalase, being weakly expressed, which promotes diabetes to appear (Jaiswal et al. 2013). Therefore, the activity of hypoglycemic agents has been studied over *in vivo* and *in vitro* diabetes I models. Among them, the study of diabetic rats induced by streptozotocin, where Yassa and Tohamy (2014) reported the beneficial effect of *M. oleifera* leaves on hyperglycemia. In a dose of 200 mg/kg the leaves reduced fasting plasma glucose levels and avoided histopathological damage of islet cells in adult diabetic rats, also it increased the stained area of positive purple Gomori modified for β-cells and reduced the percentage area of collagen fiber in comparison to control (Yassa and Tohamy 2014, Van Dyke et al. 2010).

Similarly, *M. oleifera* leaves aqueous extract that has shown a positive effect when it comes to insulin resistance over a murine type I diabetic model induced with streptozotocin. The above have been associated with antihyperlipidemic and antihyperglycemic activity, mainly by an increase in glucose intake (Divi, Bellamkonda, and Dasireddy 2012).

The intake of *M. oleifera* leaves have an effect over postprandial glucose levels and fasting blood glucose, reducing them to average rates in diabetic rats, showing a high antidiabetic and hypoglycemic potential (Jaiswal et al. 2013). This effect is also extended to insulin and low-density lipoprotein cholesterol and triglycerides levels, which are increased and decreased, respectively (Tang et al. 2017).

Jaiswal et al. (2013) reported that *M. oleifera* leaves aqueous extract influenced some enzymes linked to the hepatic damage caused by diabetes, such as superoxide dismutase, catalase, lipoxygenase, and glutathione-transferase. The activity of these enzymes increased by the addition of leaf extract in different organs (spleen, pancreas, brain, liver, and kidney) of diabetic rats induced by streptozotocin. The above suggests *M. oleifera* leaves extract as a possible adjuvant therapy to protect the liver from oxidative stress caused by diabetes.

As for *M. oleifera* stem root and bark, their ethanolic extract have shown an increase of glucose intake when given in a single diary dose of 250 mg/kg to diabetic rats for two weeks, demonstrating also antidiabetic potential and increasing the importance of studying the different parts of *M. oleifera* tree and its effects over this disorder (Kar, Choudhary, and Bandyopadhyay 2003).

Just as type I diabetes, type 2 is a disease of high prevalence and importance. Therefore, alternatives such as the use of natural extracts have been taken into consideration. Different anatomical parts of medicinal plants have been evaluated in terms of inhibiting the activity of α-amylase and α-glucosidase, enzymes participating in glucose intestinal absorption (Duckworth 2001, Jimoh 2018).

M. oleifera leaves inhibit α-amylase and α-glucosidase activity in a concentration of 14.29 μg/ml with an IC50 of 6.49 and 4.73 μg/ml for each enzyme, respectively. The inhibitory effect over both enzymes is attributed to the high phenolic content of the extract, which is mainly constituted by gallic acid, ellagic acid, chlorogenic acid, quercetin, isoquercetin, rutin and kaempferol (Giridhari, Malathi, and Geetha 2011, Jimoh 2018, Kumari 2010).

Metwally et al. (2017) reported the effect of ethanolic leaves-extract of *M. oleifera* over the insulin resistance value and the serum glucose level in obese female rats, concluding that the extract decreased the amount of insulin resistance and decreased the level of glucose in the blood compared to untreated obese group. *M. oleifera* ethanolic leaves extract administered at 600 mg/kg body weight, reduced total weight of obese rats after 12 weeks.

Other parts of the *M. oleifera* tree have also shown antidiabetic effects. In this regard, *M. oleifera* seed powder fed to streptozotocin-induced rat model maintained normal fasting blood glucose levels, as well as the histological health of the pancreas and kidney (Al-Malki and El Rabey 2015).

According to Hafizur et al. (2018), a potential insulin secretory activity is attributed to all *M. oleifera* anatomical parts, which makes it an alternative source for diabetes treatment. The above is mainly attributed to PKA-mediated insulin secretion from pancreatic β cells, which causes a decrease in blood glucose levels. Specifically, *M. oleifera* leaf extracts suppress the expression of enzymes such as glucose-6-phosphatase and pyruvate carboxylase which are related to gluconeogenesis, being able to reduce liver damage (Abd El Latif et al. 2014, Udechukwu et al. 2018)

As far as it is known, no adverse effect has been reported over the use of *M. oleifera extracts* neither in human nor animal models (Hafizur et al. 2018, Stohs and Hartman 2015). In Table 13, the main effects of *M. oleifera* plant over diabetic models are summarized.

Table 13. Hypoglycemic effects of *M. oleifera* plant in animal studies

Part of the plant	Phytochemical	Animal model	Mechanism of action	References
Leaves	Gallic acid, ellagic acid, chlorogenic acid, quercetin, isoquercetin, rutin and kaempferol	Adult rats and humans	↓Fasting plasma glucose levels ↓Damaged islet cells ↓Glucose-6-phosphatase and pyruvate carboxylase Inhibiting α-amylase and α-glucosidase	(Yassa and Tohamy 2014)
Leaves aqueous extract	-	Rats	↑Glucose intake ↑ Superoxide dismutase, catalase, lipoxygenase and glutathione-transferase	(Jaiswal et al. 2013)
Stem root and bark ethanolic extracts	-	Rats	↑Glucose intake	(Kar, Choudhary, and Bandyopad hyay 2003)
Ethanolic leaves extract	-	Rats	↓Insulin resistance ↓Glucose blood concentration	(Metwally et al. 2017)
Seed	-	Male rats	↓Glucose blood concentration	(Al-Malki and El Rabey 2015)

Obesity

Obesity is a medical condition in which prevalence is increasing around the world, especially in developed countries. This disease is widely related to excessive fat intake, which leads to increased blood cholesterol, causing multiple health complications, such as cardiovascular diseases and metabolic syndrome. Various plant extracts have been studied for its ability to positively influence obesity complications.

One of them is *M. oleifera*. It has been found that different parts of the tree show a lipid modulatory effect (Udechukwu et al. 2018). Also, methanolic leaves extract have had significant effects over obese rats, decreasing pro-inflammatory adipokines levels, proteins associated to appetite regulation, energy expenditure, insulin sensitivity, lipid uptake and oxidative capacity (Grundy 2016, Metwally et al. 2017, Bais, Singh, and Sharma 2014)

Metwally et al. (2017) reported that by feeding female obese rats with *M. oleifera* leaves ethanolic extract, the atherogenic index and the cardiac risk index was reduced, at the time that the bodyweight was decreased. Also, the extract was reported to decrease the leptin levels as well as the resistin mRNA levels. On the contrary, a higher concentration of adiponectin mRNA was detected.

As for human assays, *M. oleifera* leaves ethanolic extract has been found to reduce body weight in obese people significantly. It has been reported the effect of *M. oleifera* leaves isothiocyanates over obese mice when fed 66 mg/ kg of body weight for 12 weeks. It was found that these phytochemicals prevented mice from developing fatty liver disease. Also, they inhibited gluconeogenesis. The latter effect is attributed to the upregulation of genes such as G69 (glucose-6-phosphatase). Nevertheless, although lipolysis was not significantly affected, genes promoting these processes such as PRDM16, ADRB3, PGC-1α were upregulated, suggesting a future lipolysis phenomenon (Waterman et al. 2015).

Hepatic lipid accumulation and liver weight are decreased in mice by both consuming fermented and non-fermented *M. oleifera* leaves for ten weeks by the upregulation of genes involved in liver lipid metabolism. Fermented extracts also reduce proinflammatory cytokine expression. Comparing both extracts, the fermented ones showed a higher beneficial effect (Joung et al. 2017). The main effects of *M. oleifera* plant over obese in vivo models are summarized in Table 14.

Table 14. Anti-obesity effects of *M. oleifera* plant in animal studies

Part of the plant	Phytochemical	Animal model	Mechanism of action	References
Methanolic leaves extract	-	Obese Rats	↓Pro-inflammatory adipokines	(Bais, Singh, and Sharma 2014)
Ethanolic leaf extract	-	Female obese rats	↓Body weight ↓Leptin ↓Resistin ↑Adiponectin	(Metwally et al. 2017)
Leaves	4-(R-L-rhamnopyranosyloxy)-benzyl glucosinolate monoacetyl-Isomer I, 4-(R-L-rhamnopyranosyloxy)-benzyl glucosinolate monoacetyl-isomer II and 4-(R-L-rhamnopyranosyloxy)-benzyl glucosinolate monoacetyl-isomer III	Obese mice	↓Fatty liver disease ↓Gluconeogenesis ↑lipolysis genes expression	(Waterman et al. 2014)
Fermented leaves	-	Obese mice	↓Hepatic lipid accumulation ↓Liver weight	(Joung et al. 2017)

Inflammation

Inflammation is an immune response triggered by microbial agents, physical trauma, or noxious chemical substances (Alhakmani, Kumar, and Khan 2013). Also, it could be linked to free radical prevalence, which could affect many organs. In this regard, it has been studied the effect of some plant's bioactive compounds over the different mechanisms that free radicals exert over inflammation processes (Cheenpracha et al. 2010, dos Santos et al. 2018). *M. oleifera* has a variety of bioactive compounds such as carotenoids, glucosinolates, and isothiocyanates, which have been linked to potential health effects. For example, antitumor and anti-inflammatory substances (Cheenpracha et al. 2010, Fahey 2005, Guevara et al. 1999).

Cheenpracha et al. (2010) reported the effect of 4-[(2´-O-acetyl-α-L-rhamnosyloxy) benzyl]isothiocyanate, 4-[(3´-Oacetyl-α-L-rhamnosyloxy) benzyl]isothiocyanate and other acetylated isothiocyanate derivates isolated from *M. oleifera* fruit (pod) over a lipopolysaccharide-induced murine model. These compounds reduced nitric oxide content, and in consequence, inflammation was highly decreased. Due to the phytochemical composition of

M. oleifera flowers, it has been reported that their ethanolic extract can exert an anti-inflammatory effect over in vitro models, even similar to that of the commercial drug sodium diclofenac (Alhakmani, Kumar, and Khan 2013). A benzyl isothiocyanate (4-(4′-*O*-acetyl-α- l- rhamnosyloxy) benzylisothiocyanate) from *M. oleifera* flowers decreased vascular extravasation in a formalin-induced murine model with temporomandibular joint inflammation (dos Santos et al. 2018).

Regarding *M. oleifera* leaves, their extracts also have been found to possess anti-inflammatory effects. They have a modulatory effect over cell signaling proteins like interleukin-6, interleukin-8, and TNF-α, in which production levels were induced in human macrophages (Kooltheat et al. 2014). Isothiocyanates isolated from *M. oleifera* leaves promoted the inhibition of inflammatory markers and genes related to inflammation when applied in murine macrophages (Waterman et al. 2014).

The antioxidant capacity of *M. oleifera* leaves might be one of the main responsible mechanisms for its anti-inflammatory properties as chronic inflammation is characterized by the oxidative stress-induced activation of NF-kB. *M. oleifera* leaves have shown to inhibit LPS-induced NO production. Furthermore, they reduce PGE_2 production and hinder the COX-2 protein expression. Additionally, *M. oleifera* leaves reduce the LPS-induced pro-inflammatory cytokines production (TNF-a, IL-1 b, and IL-6) in a dose-dependent manner and have the ability to raise the IL-10 production. The anti-inflammatory effect could be attributed to the phytochemical content of *M. oleifera*, such as polyphenols, as these molecules have been widely known for their anti-inflammatory properties (Fard et al. 2015).

According to Cáceres et al. (1992), seeds and roots infusions of *M. oleifera* attenuated the increase of hind paw edema by carrageenan-induced murine model, suggesting that these infusions possess similar anti-inflammatory effects that those of commercial drugs (Brilhante et al. 2017). Also, *M. oleifera* ethanolic and butanolic seeds extract have been proved over inflammation-induced Wistar rats and Guinea pigs, showing anti-inflammatory effects (Mahajan et al. 2009, Mahajan, Mali, and Mehta 2007).

Isothiocyanates isolated from *M. oleifera* leaves had higher anti-inflammatory *in vivo* and *in vitro* effect than potent anti-inflammatory compounds such as turmeric-derived curcumin (Udechukwu et al. 2018). Nevertheless, it has been reported that *M. oleifera* leaves isothiocyanates have a minor anti-inflammatory effect when compared to whole leaves extracts. The anti-inflammatory effect could be due to the presence of other phytochemicals such as polyphenols, saponins, carotenoids, which are related to a high antioxidant potential.

M. oleifera extracts from seeds, bark, flowers, leaves, and roots have shown anti-inflammatory effects over a carrageenan-induced murine model (Paikra, Dhongade, and Gidwani 2017). This anti-inflammatory activity could be due to compounds present in *M. oleifera* extracts interfering in the inflammation signaling (Gupta et al. 2018). The main effects of *M. oleifera* plant over inflammation models are summarized in Table 15.

Table 15. The anti-inflammatory effects of *M. oleifera* plant in animal studies

Part of the plant	Phytochemical	Model/assay	Mechanism of action	References
Pods	4-[(2´-O-acetyl-α-L-rhamnosyloxy) benzyl]isothiocyanate and 4-[(3´-Oacetyl-α-L-rhamnosyloxy)benzyl]isothiocyanate	Lipopolysaccharide-induced murine model	↓Nitric oxide content	(Cheenpracha et al. 2010)
Flowers	-	Enzymatic	↓Cycloxygenase-1 and cycloxgenase-2	(Alhakmani, Kumar, and Khan 2013)
Leaves	-	Human macrophages and murine macrophages	↓Interleukin-6, interleukin-8 and TNF-α ↓LPS-induced NO production ↓ PGE_2 production ↓ COX-2 protein expression	(Kooltheat et al. 2014, Waterman et al. 2014, Karthivashan et al. 2013)
Seeds and roots	-	Wistar rats and Guinea pigs	↓Attenuated the increase of hind paw edema	(Brilhante et al. 2017)

Hypercholesterolemia

Hypercholesterolemia is a physiological state characterized by having high plasma cholesterol levels. This health condition is considered as a risk factor for the development of coronary artery disease, heart attack, stroke, among other disorders (Martinez-Hervas and Ascaso 2019). Hypercholesterolemia can be classified as primary (where there is a mutation in the gene that specifies the function of low-density lipoprotein cholesterol (LDL) receptors) and secondary (which is caused by the reduction of LDL receptor as a result of a high-calorie diet intake) (MacPherson et al. 2016).

M. oleifera leaves, seeds, and fruits, have been studied for its hypocholesterolemic effect (Ghasi, Nwobodo, and Ofili 2000, Pandu, Cherupanalli, and Muthukumar 2018, Mehta et al. 2003). *In vivo* experiments have shown that *M. oleifera* has hypocholesterolemic activity even at low doses. For example, 1 mg/g *M. oleifera* leaves extract can reduce serum, liver, and kidney cholesterol concentrations in rats (Ghasi, Nwobodo, and Ofili 2000). Also, a concentration of 200 mg/kg per day *M. oleifera* fruits (pods) mixed with banana pulp reduces the cholesterol levels in rabbit's liver, heart, and aorta (Mehta et al. 2003).

The cholesterol-lowering effects of *M. oleifera* have been partly attributed to its content of β-sitosterol. Plant sterols can lower cholesterol absorption through many mechanisms. One of them is sterol in competition with cholesterol for intestinal absorption since sterols are structurally similar to cholesterol molecules and have an affinity for mixed micelles (Mannarino, Ministrini, and Pirro 2014). Furthermore, cholesterol has been detected in faces, showing the inhibition of its absorption (Mehta et al. 2003).

Besides sterols content, *M. oleifera* is characterized for its high content of phenolic acids and flavonoids (Adedayo et al. 2018, Oyeleye et al. 2019). These molecules have demonstrated to improve liver cells function. Also, they have shown to decrease liver and plasma cholesterol levels as reported by Pandu, Cherupanalli, and Muthukumar (2018). Moreover, these authors stated that the plasma cholesterol-lowering effect might be ascribed to inhibition of cholesterol reabsorption via activation of AMPK enzyme. Furthermore, phenolic compounds of *M. oleifera* can reduce LDL oxidation, thus, preventing cellular uptake of oxidized LDL; this was demonstrated by serum reduction levels of malondialdehyde (Helmy et al. 2017, Pandu, Cherupanalli, and Muthukumar 2018). In this regard, oxidation of LDL is caused by the oxidative stress induced by a high-fat diet.

Furthermore, the rise in oxidative stress and dyslipidemia, correlate positively with the atherogenic index, the one reduced by *M. oleifera* different parts (Pandu, Cherupanalli, and Muthukumar 2018). Moreover, flavonoids can reduce triglyceride levels through its participation in the inhibition of hepatic apolipoprotein B secretion. Also, flavonoids have been reported as signaling molecules involved in the regulation of the signal transduction pathways of the sterol regulatory element and binding proteins, which could, in turn, activate the LDL receptor gene, raising its levels (Oyeleye et al. 2019). Thus, besides the cholesterol-lowering effects, *M. oleifera* can reduce the triglycerides, and low-density lipoprotein cholesterol (LDL-C) levels caused by a high-fat diet or high fat and cholesterol diet in rats (Helmy et al. 2017, Pandu, Cherupanalli, and Muthukumar 2018). Furthermore, *M. oleifera* showed to maintain or raise the levels of high-density lipoprotein cholesterol (HDL-C) and reduced the atherogenic index (El Rabey et al. 2017) significantly.

Additionally, *M. oleifera* seed has shown to improve liver and heart enzyme activity (El Rabey et al. 2017), restore liver cells functions, and mediate the atherosclerosis regression (Pandu, Cherupanalli, and Muthukumar 2018). Finally, *M. oleifera* biological properties can be enhanced through fermentation. As for this, *M. oleifera* seeds fermented by *Rhizopus stolonifera* have shown a higher lowering effect in HDL and LDL cholesterol levels than unfermented *M. oleifera* seeds (Adedayo et al. 2018). The main effects of hypercholesterolemia of *M. oleifera* plant are summarized in Table 16.

Table 16. Hypocholesterolemic effect of *M. oleifera* plant in animal studies

Part of the plant	Phytochemical	Animal Model	Hypercholesterolemic effect	Reference
Leaf ethanolic extract	Phenolic compounds	Albino rats		(Helmy et al. 2017)
Seed	Bound phenolic and catechin	C57BL6 mice	↓Atherogenic index ↑Antioxidant enzymes and molecules in liver and serum ↓Plasma and liver cholesterol ↓Plasma and liver triglycerides	(Pandu, Cherupanalli, and Muthukumar 2018)
M. oleifera fermented seeds		Wistar rats		(Adedayo et al. 2018)
Fruits		Rabbits	↓Body weight ↓Lipids in liver, heart, and aorta ↓Atherogenic index ↑Lipids in feces Hypolipidemic effect and anti-atherosclerotic	(Mehta et al. 2003)
Leaves	Not mentioned	Wistar rats	↓Cholesterol in serum, liver, and kidney.	(Ghasi, Nwobodo, and Ofili 2000)
Seeds	Not mentioned, probably β-sitosterol	Albino rats	↓Serum cholesterol, triglycerides, LDL and VLDL ↑HDL	(El Rabey et al. 2017)
Seeds and leaves	Phenolic compounds (phenolic acids and flavonoids)	Wistar rats	↓Total cholesterol, triglycerides, LDL ↑HDL ↓Atherogenic index	(Oyeleye et al. 2019)

VLDL: Very low-density lipoproteins; HDL: High-density lipoproteins; LDL: Low-density lipoproteins.

Hypertriglyceridemia

Hypertriglyceridemia is a multifactorial disease caused by others, such as familiar hyperlipidemia, dysbetalipoproteinemia, obesity, HIV, renal disease, and diabetes. And also, by health habits like excessive alcohol intake and a high caloric diet. It is characterized by serum high triglyceride concentrations above 150 mg/dL (Karanchi and Wyne, 2017).

M. oleifera leaves (300 or 600 mg/kg body weight) reduce triglycerides levels over in *vivo* models. As the concentration of phenolic compounds and flavonoids is high in this plant material, it can be speculated that these molecules are responsible for the effect on lipid concentrations and metabolisms (Olayaki et al. 2015). However, more studies regarding the effect of isolated and mixture compounds present in *M. oleifera,* as well as the structure-activity relationship, needs to be performed.

M. oleifera leaves can help in hepatic steatosis treatment. *M. oleifera* leaves (15 g/100 g or 10g/100 g) added to a guinea pig high cholesterol diet, alter the expression of genes associated with hepatic lipids synthesis. This effect promotes the concentrations of cholesterol and triglycerides in the serum. Furthermore, *M. oleifera* reduces the concentration of inflammatory cytokines in the liver (Almatrafi et al. 2017).

M. oleifera leaves (400 mg/kg) reduced the hepatic lipid accumulation *in vivo* and restored the plasma triglyceride levels compared to the negative control (rats without any treatment). The authors implied that β-sitosterol might be implicated in this effect. The mechanisms by which *M. oleifera* decreases lipid accumulation in the liver remain unclear and need to be further investigated (Muhammad et al. 2019). *M. oleifera* could help in the treatment of non-alcoholic fatty liver disease and hepatic steatosis due to its effect on lipid accumulation in the liver. The major effects of *M. oleifera* in triglycerides are summarized in Table 17.

Table 17. Hypo-triglyceride effect of *M. oleifera* leaves in animal studies

Animal model	Major effects	Reference
Wistar rats	↓Serum triglycerides, LDL and total cholesterol ↑HDL	(Olayaki et al. 2015)
Hartley guinea pigs	↓Cholesterol and triglycerides	(Almatrafi et al. 2017)
Sprague-Dawley rats	↓Hepatic lipid accumulation	(Muhammad et al. 2019)

Cancer

After cardiovascular disease, cancer is the second leading cause of death worldwide (Bray et al. 2018). This disorder is characterized by the deregulation of thousands of genes, promoting for cells to become unable to undergo apoptosis. This way, cancerous cells form tumors that may later be metastatic (Heymach et al. 2018). Cancer traditional treatments promote toxic effects to healthy cell and loss of effectiveness to cancerous cells, so a lot of new drugs have been tested. For example, the ones coming from natural plants, which offer an alternative with minimal adverse effects to cancer patients.

M. oleifera is one of the medicinal plants from which different chemical compounds have been extracted and tested over cancer models. These phytochemicals have been obtained from their roots, seeds, barks, and mainly leaves and proved both over *in vivo* and *in vitro* models. *M. oleifera* leaves ethanolic extract inhibits liver (HepG2), breast (MCF7) and colorectal (HCT 116) cancer cell growth by up to 67.96, 74.35, 76.37% respectively with minimal effect over normal cells. The inhibitory effects may be associated with high amounts of eugenol, and D-allose presents in high amounts in ethanolic *M. oleifera* leaves extract (Abd-Rabou et al. 2017). It is known that eugenol inhibits cancer-related oncogenes, such as NF-kβ and cyclin D1, while D-allose inhibits the expression of GLUT1, cutting off cell energy sources (Al-Sharif, Remmal, and Aboussekhra 2013, Noguchi et al. 2016)

The effectiveness of *M. oleifera* leaves ethanolic extract is even higher when they are nano encapsulated in PLGA-CS-PEG, improving cell growth inhibition by up to 18%. The improved effect may be due to nanocapsules enhancing water solubility, bioavailability, and stability of bioactive compounds (Rao and Naidu 2016). Besides ethanolic extracts, also water has been tested as a solvent for *M. oleifera* leaves phytochemicals extraction. Water extracts somehow resembles closer the phytochemical profile obtained when homemade infusions of *M. oleifera* leaves are elaborated. The most abundant compounds in an aqueous extract of *M. oleifera* leaves are quercetin and kaempferol.

The application of 200 μg/ml/48 h of *M. oleifera* aqueous extract achieved a cell growth inhibition of 85% in KB human tumor cell lines by apoptosis induction via p53 overexpression, ROS excessive generation and a reduction in Nrf2 protein expression (Sreelatha et al. 2011). This mechanism was also observed in cancerous lung cells (HepG2 and A549), where *M. oleifera* aqueous extracts achieved 52 and 67% of growth inhibition (Jung, Lee, and Kang 2015, Tiloke et al. 2016). Quercetin and kaempferol high toxic effects over cancerous cells are not transposable to normal cells, where they exert no harm. It has also been documented that quercetin induces the expression of p53, Bax, and Puma at the time that cleaves caspase-3 and -9 and Parp (Rauf et al. 2018). On the other hand, kaempferol activates Bcl-2 proteins, increasing mitochondrial membrane permeability, and cytosolic levels of cytochrome C (Lee et al. 2014).

Aqueous *M. oleifera* extracts have also been tested in combination with conventional chemotherapy medications, such as cisplatin, to which pancreatic cells have presented resistance. Cisplatin plus aqueous extract achieves a cell growth inhibition of more than 90% in the PANC-1 cell line by inducing G1 cell cycle arrest and reducing the expression of key NF-κB family protein, p65, p-IkBα and IkBα proteins promoting apoptosis. The inhibition of both combined substances is much higher compared to the 10% that nowadays offers cisplatin by itself (Berkovich et al. 2013). Combining phytochemicals with chemotherapy drugs helps to reduce the needed amount of the latter, and therefore, the side effects of the whole treatment.

The aqueous extracts of *M. oleifera* leaf have been considered as a safe option of the anticancer drug since acute toxicity assays over male Wistar albino mice, estimated an LD50 of 1585 mg/kg for single oral administration. *M. oleifera* seed extracts have also been tested against different types of cancer. Hexane *M. oleifera* seed extract inhibits mammalian cancer cell line proliferation (MCF7) with an IC50 of 130 μg/ml, and no toxic effect over normal mammalian cells was detected. This effect is mainly due to phenolic compounds and hexadecenoic acid (palmitic acid) (Adebayo et al. 2017). Palmitic acid, the most saturated fatty acid and linked to adverse health effects, has been proven to interfere with DNA topoisomerase I (Ravi and Krishnan 2017).

Also, aqueous *M. oleifera* seed extracts rich in lectins have been studied over cancer *in vitro* models inhibiting the growth of lung (NCI-H292) and colon (HT-29) cancer by 42.7 and 51.3% respectively. Nevertheless, the rich lectin extract showed itself cytotoxicity to immune cells (Araújo et al. 2013). Lectins promote the detection of immunoglobulin G and immunoglobulin A antibodies, so it has been proposed the elimination of these proteins from the diet (Vojdani 2015). In addition to alcoholic and aqueous extracts, the oil fraction of the seed has been tested over different types of cancer, including HepG2, MCF7, HCT 116, and Caco-2 cell lines. This extract rich in oleic (>70%), gadoleic, and palmitoleic acids induced mitochondrial apoptosis over the cancer cell lines, while it minimally affected BHK-21 normal cells (Abd-Rabou et al. 2016). *M. oleifera* seeds, an abundant and cheap source, contain up to 41% of oil. It has a very similar fatty acid profile to olive oil so that it could be a good substitute for it (Leone et al. 2016).

M. oleifera root has also been tested against cancer, especially the fraction corresponding to the bark that contains the two alkaloids moringine (identical to benzylamine) and moringinine. They were found to act as sex hormones by interacting with hormone receptor-related and neoplastic growth-related cytokine pathways as well as interacting with the G protein-linked signal transduction system. This mechanism puts *M. oleifera* root bark alkaloids as suitable phytochemicals for epithelial ovarian cancer treatment (Bose 2016). Other compounds of *M. oleifera* root bark with anticancer activities are eugenol, isopropyl isothiocyanate, D-allose, and hexadecanoic acid ethyl ester found in its ethanolic extracts. These compounds have anticancer activity over MDA-MB-231 and HCT-8 cancer cell lines via arresting the cell cycle in G2/M, inducing apoptosis, and decreasing cell motility and colony formation (Al-Asmari et al. 2015). The main effects of hypercholesterolemia of *M. oleifera* plant are summarized in table 18.

Table 18. Anti-cancer effect of *M. oleifera* plant in animal studies

Part of the plant	Phytochemical	Model	Mechanism of action	References
Leaves ethanolic extract	Eugenol and D-allose	HepG2, MCF7 and HCT 116	↓NF-kB, cyclin D1 expression ↓GLUT1	(Al-Sharif, Remmal, and Aboussekhra 2013, Noguchi et al. 2016)
Aqueous leaves extract	Quercetin and kaempferol	KB human tumor cell lines, HepG2 and A549	↑p53, Bax and Puma overexpression overexpression ↓Caspase-3, -9 and Parp ↓Nrf2 expression	(Sreelatha et al. 2011)
Leaves aqueous extract + cisplatin		PANC-1 cell line and Wistar albino mice	↓NF-κB family protein, p65, p-IkBα and IkBα expression	(Berkovich et al. 2013)
Hexane seed extract	Hexadecenoic acid (palmitic acid)	MCF7	Interference with DNA topoisomerase I	(Adebayo et al. 2017)
Seed oil	Oleic, gadoleic and palmitoleic acids acid	HepG2, MCF7, HCT 116, and Caco-2	Mitochondrial apoptosis	(Abd-Rabou et al. 2016)
Root bark	Eugenol, isopropyl isothiocyanate, D-allose, and hexadecanoic acid ethyl ester	MDA-MB-231 and HCT-8	Arresting cell cycle in G2/M Decreasing cell motility and colony formation	(Al-Asmari et al. 2015)

Hyper and Hypothyroidism

Hyperthyroidism and hypothyroidism are disorders where the synthesis and secretion of thyroid hormones by the thyroid gland are either excessive or insufficient. The most common causes for hyperthyroidism and hypothyroidism are Grave immune disease, thyroiditis, and toxic multinodular goiter (Kravets 2016) and iodine deficiency/excess and thyroidectomy, respectively (Brandt et al. 2018).

A molecular marker widely used to measure the capacity of a phytochemical in regulating the functioning of the thyroid gland is triiodothyronine (T3). T3 is the major thyroid hormone and responsible for the majority of metabolic effects on the organisms. For example, calorigenesis referred to as the increase in oxygen consumption and maintenance of the basal metabolic rate (Orman et al. 2018).

T3 levels have been measured on *in vivo* models (rats) after *M. oleifera* leaves aqueous extract exposure, finding contradictory results. On the one hand, the aqueous extract was suggested as a possible regulator over hyperthyroidism disease by decreasing serum T3 concentration as 30% of its synthesis was inhibited (Tahiliani and Kar 2000). On the other hand, it was found that aqueous extracts increase thyroid activity by increasing both T3 and thyroxine (T4) levels, suggesting, on the contrary, that *M. oleifera* leaf extracts may be used for treating hypothyroidism condition (Tabassum, Kullu, and Sinha 2013). Contrasting results may be given by distinct phytochemical concentrations and profiles in the extracts due to different extraction methods. While the one reported reducing T3 levels was extracted for 24 h at 25ºC, the other was extracted by a Soxhlet apparatus, where higher temperatures are applied. It is known that these higher temperatures in Soxhlet extraction increase the risk for some compounds to be thermal degraded; for example, polyphenols and alkaloids (Zhang, Lin, and Ye 2018). Therefore, it would be beneficial to determine the profile of compounds in each of the extracts and to elucidate their mechanism of action on T3 secretion. The effects mentioned above have not yet been attributed to any particular phytochemical of *M. oleifera* leaves. However, regarding T3 decrease, it is known that quercetin, found in aqueous extracts of *M. oleifera* leaves, decreases its plasma levels (Pistollato et al. 2018).

M. oleifera leaves ethanolic extract normalizes thyroid-stimulating hormone (TSH) level in rats induced with hypothyroidism by increasing its concentration (Mohamed et al. 2019). It is possible that this effect is mainly due to rutin, the glycoside combining of the flavonol quercetin and disaccharide rutinose, known to increase TSH in plasma levels and found in m. oleifera leaves alcoholic extracts (Pistollato et al. 2018). The main effects of hyper-cholesterolemia of *M. oleifera* plant are summarized in table 19.

Table 19. Hyper and hypothyroid effect of *M. oleifera* plant in animal studies

Part of the plant	Phytochemical	Model	Mechanism of action	References
Leaves aqueous extract	Quercetin	Rats induced either with Hyper or hypothyroidism	Normalization of triiodothyronine and thyroxine blood levels	(Tahiliani and Kar 2000, Tabassum, Kullu, and Sinha 2013)
Leaves ethanolic extract	Rutin	rats induced with hypothyroidism	↑Thyroid-stimulating hormone (TSH) levels	(Pistollato et al. 2018)

Hypertension

Hypertension is a multifactorial disease characterized by a blood pressure above 140 mmHg or a diastolic pressure above 90 mmHg (Bolívar 2013). It is known that hypertension leads to cardiac complications — for example, myocardial infarction, cognitive impairment, and stroke. *M. oleifera* seed powder reduces nocturnal heart rate and cardiac triglyceride level, at the time that improves diastolic cardiac function and plasmatic prostacyclin and significantly reduced fibrosis in hypertensive rats. Also, after the treatment, the anterior left ventricular wall interseptal and diastole thickness was reduced. These effects are attributed to an increased expression of peroxisome proliferator-activated receptor (PPAR)-α. (Randriamboavonjy et al. 2016). *M. oleifera* leaves aqueous extracts decreases high blood pressure and tachycardia over hypertensive male Wistar rats. Also, at concentrations of 60 mg/kg/day, it relaxed precontracted arterial beds, reduced the impairment of acetylcholine-induced relaxation and decreases the hyperreactivity of adrenergic-mediated contraction, as well as it increased antioxidant activity by CAT and SOD upregulation. Methanolic extract of *M. oleifera* leaves reduced heart/body weight ratio, which is inversely related to nitric oxide production (Adedapo, Falayi, and Oyagbemi 2015).

Phenolic constituents such as ellagic acid, chlorogenic acid, gallic acid, kaempferol, isoquercetin, rutin, and quercetin found in both seeds and leaves have been related to the modulation of the activity of enzymes linked to hypertension, such as an angiotensin-I converting enzyme (Oyeleye et al. 2019).

Cerebroprotective Effect of *Moringa oleifera*

Cerebral Ischemia

Cerebral ischemia is caused by acute occlusion of cerebral arteries that last more than 5 minutes, causing neuron death within the perfusion territory of the affected vessels (Sun et al. 2018). Stroke is the most common cause of disability, the second most frequent cause of dementia, and the fourth most prevalent cause of death in the developed world (Garcia-Ptacek et al. 2018). Cerebral ischemia may be caused by heart disease, blood clots, heart attack, low blood pressure, ventricular tachycardia, etc.

After right middle cerebral artery occlusion, rats that were consuming the hydroalcoholic extracts of *M. oleifera* leaves for two weeks experimented a protective effect against brain damage. This extract protected rat striatum and hippocampus and also, the infarction volume in both cortex and subcortex area (Kirisattayakul et al. 2013). These effects are both associated with the reduction of the oxidative stress promoted by cerebral blood flow reduction. The antioxidant effect is associated with polyphenols found in the extracts. The most abundant polyphenols identified in *M. oleifera* hydroalcoholic extracts are quercetin, kaempferol, and apigenin (Coppin et al. 2013, Karthivashan et al. 2013). *M. oleifera* leaves Hydroalcoholic extracts have also shown a protective effect over dementia *in vivo* models.

Dementia

Dementia causes cortical-subcortical degeneration of ascending cholinergic neurons and large pyramidal cells in the cerebral cortex that results in disturbing emotions, mood, perception, thought, motor activity and alters personality making people more dependent and vulnerable (Cunningham et al. 2018, Sutin et al. 2018). Dementia has both components, genetic and environmental. As for this disease, the hydroalcoholic extract of *M. oleifera* leaves also exerts a brain-protective effect; for instance, consuming them for two weeks decreases free radical content in rat brain injected with a neurotoxin. These polyphenols increase superoxide dismutase and catalase activity, which results in decreased oxidative stress and enhanced chlorogenic function. Also, it improves spatial memory and reduces neurodegeneration by decreasing acetylcholinesterase and malondialdehyde levels. (Sutalangka et al. 2013). The most common type of dementia is Alzheimer´s disease (AD) (Ferencz and Gerritsen 2015).

Alzheimer

Alzheimer's disease is characterized by progressive dementia, starting with memory loss that progresses until it undermines the patient. It all begins with neuronal cell death on the entorhinal cortex, located in the hippocampus, being involved both genetic and environmental components in this disease onset, mainly the age (Kumar and Tsao 2018). Since Alzheimer's is a disease with multiple symptoms and a not very clear etiopathology, the development of drugs with various targets has been promoted, as is the case of phytochemicals (Mahaman, Huang, Kessete Afewerky, et al. 2018). *M. oleifera* is a plant with multiple health benefits associated with its different physiological parts. As for Alzheimer disease, leaves methanolic, ethanolic and aqueous extracts healing capacity have been tested over *in vivo* rat models.

One of the targets in these studies has been oxidative stress, a process that is known to initiate and enhance this disease start. In this regard, *M. oleifera* methanolic leaf extracts both works as a preventive and as a treatment substance in homocysteine-induced Alzheimer disease by decreasing oxidative stress both by neutralizing free radicals and by enhancing the endogenous enzymatic defense system (Huang, Zhang, and Chen 2016). Homocysteine is accumulated and plays a critical role in the development of Alzheimer's disease by oxidative stress induction, DNA damage, NMDA receptor activation, and by modifying both Aβ and tau pathways (Mahaman, Huang, Kessete Afewerky, et al. 2018). As for this, *M. oleifera* leaf methanolic extracts components, decrease the Hyc-induced tau hyperphosphorylation at the same time that reduces Aβ production (Mahaman, Huang, Wu, et al. 2018). Finally, the activity of PSD93, PSD95, Synapsin 1, and Synaptophysin are recovered. All of the above results in the reduction of neurodegeneration. Although the above effects were not attributed to any particular compound in the methanolic extract, it is known that it contains antioxidant compounds such as gallic, chlorogenic, ellagic, and ferulic acids. Moreover, it is known that gallic acid, for example, inhibits Aβ production (Hajipour et al. 2016).

On the other hand, alcoholic extracts restore to near or normal levels monoamines concentration (norepinephrine, dopamine, and serotonin), which are decreased in the cerebral cortex, hippocampus, and caudate nucleus during this disease (Ganguly and Guha 2008). As mentioned above, environmental components are determining factors in this disease start and progression, for example, the exposure to nicotine, mainly by active smokers. It has been found that anthraquinone, terpenoids, tannins, luteolin, and phenols found in *M. oleifera* leaf aqueous extracts can prevent the chromatolysis, distortion of the cerebellar cortical cells and neurobehavioral deficit. Also, after nicotine treatment, which decreased SOD activity, *M. oleifera* aqueous leaves extract was able to restore SOD activity (Omotoso et al. 2018). The main effects of Alzheimer's disease of *M. oleifera* plant are summarized in Table 20.

Table 20. Alzheimer's disease curative effect of *M. oleifera* plant in animal studies

Part of the plant	Phytochemical	Model	Mechanism of action	References
Methanolic leaf extract	Gallic, chlorogenic, ellagic and ferulic acids	Rat	↓Oxidative stress ↑Endogenous enzymatic oxidants defense system ↓Hyc-induced tau hyperphosphorylation ↓Aβ production Recovery of PSD93, PSD95, Synapsin 1 and Synaptophysin production	(Mahaman, Huang, Wu, et al. 2018, Mahaman, Huang, Kessete Afewerky, et al. 2018, Hajipour et al. 2016)
Alcoholic leaf extract	-	Rat	Restore normal levels of norepinephrine, dopamine and serotonin	(Ganguly and Guha 2008)

Parkinson

Parkinson's disease is a progressive neurodegenerative disorder characterized by both motor and nonmotor symptoms, including muscular rigidity, resting tremor, slowing of movements, loss of smell, mood disorders, sleep dysfunction, constipation, etc. (DeMaagd and Philip 2015). It is characterized by the loss or degeneration of around 70% of dopamine-secreting neurons in the substantia nigra, mainly caused by oxidative stress and the formation of protein aggregates (Lewy bodies) in neurons. The most common treatment for Parkinson's disease is the replacement of dopamine with L-Dopa (precursor to dopamine, norepinephrine, and epinephrine). Nevertheless, its effectiveness diminishes after prolonged intake, and also it causes dyskinesia. So safer strategies with fewer side effects have been sought, for example, the use of phytochemicals from *M. oleifera*. The glucosinolate glucomoringin ([4-(α-L-rhamnopyranosyloxy)benzyl]) and its respectively isothiocyanate moringin ([4-(α-L-rhamnopyranosyloxy)benzyl C), are among *M. oleifera* phytochemicals studied for Parkinson disease treatment. Both compounds have been isolated from *M. oleifera* seeds. Both, and specially moringin, have high efficacy countering the inflammatory pathway of this disorder by reducing the expression of TNF-α, IL-1β, and toll-like receptor 4 (TLR4), all implicated as main effectors in neurodegeneration caused by neuroinflammation during Parkinson disease (Leal et al. 2013). Moringin also reduces apoptosis of midbrain dopaminergic neurons by reducing free radical production, which lowers cleaved caspase-9 levels. Also, it attenuates p53 and STAT-1 expression (Giacoppo et al. 2017, Shahpiri et al. 2016). And even when treated with the free radical H2O2, neurons pretreated with moringin resisted to apoptosis. This isothiocyanate protects both cytoskeleton and cytoplasmic inclusion, conserving surface morphological features, and the overall integrity of neurons (Jaafaru et al. 2018). Based on the positive effects of moringin, it is suggested as a candidate for both preventing and treating this disease. There are other phytochemicals such as polyphenols and terpenes with well-established antiparkinsonian effects, so it would be useful to isolate them from the different parts of *M. oleifera* tree and to test them against Parkinson disease (Shahpiri et al. 2016).

Infectious Diseases

Infection is a condition characterized by a pathogen, such as a virus or a microorganism, invading and growing within a host, which may result in impaired biological functions when the pathogen agent colonizes one or more tissues. Infection usually occurs through anatomical orifices such as genital openings, mouth, eyes, and wounds (Ashida et al. 2011). *M. oleifera* stem bark is a potential medicine for infections such as urinary tract, where its consumption (40 ml daily during seven days) cured up to 70% of infected patients versus only 40% that were cured without any drugs. The improvement was due to the herb noticeable effect over microorganisms such as *Escherichia coli*, *Klebsiella pneumoniae,* and *Proteus mirabilis* (Maurya and Singh 2014). Different parts of *M. oleifera* tree extract has also shown a curative effect over mouth infections. It has been found that leaves ethanolic extract to inhibit *Staphylococcus aureus* and *Streptococcus mutans* growth as well as fungi such as *Candida albicans* (Elgamily et al. 2016). *M. oleifera* leaves ethanolic extracts affects an antibiotic against multidrug-resistant gram-negative bacteria at minimum concentrations ranging from 128 to 1024 μg/ml. These low amounts achieved up to 75% growth inhibition of 19 tested bacteria, including

Escherichia coli, *Enterobacter aerogenes*, *Klebsiella pneumoniae*, *and Pseudomonas aeruginosa* resistant strains. The aforementioned might be attributed mainly to their phytochemical content being constituted primarily to polyphenols, triterpenes, and steroids (Dzotam, Touani, and Kuete 2015). It is thought that the compounds exerting the effect are mainly isothiocyanates, with known activities against human pathogens. They inhibit bacterial quorum sensing, affect the pyocyanin production, and exert anti-biofilm activity. They also affect cellular membrane integrity and potential (Romeo et al. 2018). The effect of the different parts and extracts of *M. oleifera* tree over beneficial microorganisms living in the gastrointestinal tract has not been reported yet. The main results of *M. oleifera* tree in infectious diseases are summarized in Table 21.

Table 21. Infection curative effect of *M. oleifera* plant in animal studies

Part of the plant	Phytochemical	Infection type	Model	Mechanism of action	References
Stem bark		Urinary tract	Patients	↓*Escherichia coli*, *Klebsiella pneumoniae* and *Proteus mirabilis*	(Maurya and Singh 2014)
Leaves ethanolic extract	-	Mouth	*In vitro* pathogens	↓*Staphylococcus aureus*, *Streptococcus mutans and Candida albicans*	(Elgamily et al. 2016)
	Polyphenols, triterpenes and steroids	-	multidrug-resistant gram-negative bacteria	↓*Escherichia coli*, *Enterobacter aerogenes*, *Klebsiella pneumoniae and Pseudomonas aeruginosa*	(Dzotam, Touani, and Kuete 2015)

An infectious disease of high incidence worldwide is malaria, known as the infection of red blood cells. Human Malaria is caused by the bite of a female Anopheles mosquito infected by four different *Plasmodium* species: *P. malariae*, *P. falciparum*, *P. ovale,* and *P. vivax*. Although it is endemic in Canada and the United States, nowadays 90% of the cases occur in Africa, where there was registered an estimated 435 000 deaths in 2017 (Angelo et al. 2017). Fever is the most characteristic symptom of malaria, although other ones arise, for example, chills, headache, vomiting, nausea, and diarrhea (O'Connell 2017). The pathology is caused by merozoites invading and multiplying in the circulating erythrocytes (Chan et al. 2017).

The malaria parasite has shown increasing resistance to conventional drugs, so new approaches have been studied, including the use of phytochemicals, for example, those coming from both *M. oleifera* leaves and seeds. For instance, artesunate, a commercial drug, has been proved in combination with aqueous *M. oleifera* leaf extracts over *Plasmodium*-infected mice for four days achieving a malaria suppression of up to 91%, while *M. oleifera* leaf extracts had an effectiveness of 50% when given alone. The high efficacy is associated with terpenoids, flavonoids, alkaloids, quinines, quercetin and kaempferol, all known to have antimalarial activity, mainly quinine. As for flavonoids, they exert inhibitory activity over hemozoin formation, letting heme, very toxic to the malaria parasite, free. Finally, quercetin, kaempferol, and gypenoside inhibit the nuclear transcription factor-kappa B (NF-κB), important in malaria growth and development (Somsak et al. 2016). The extraction of the aforementioned compounds was improved by a microwave-associated water extraction method, increasing the effectiveness of the aqueous leaf extract alone by 70%, achieving 85% of inhibition to *Plasmodium*. By this, the use of drugs such as artesunate may be reduced (Somsak et al. 2016).

Regarding *M. oleifera* seeds, their methanolic extract rich in quercetin and kaempferol causes mortality in more than 90% of pupas and larvae of the malaria vector *Anopheles stephensi* (*A. stephensi*). The above is attributed to the antioxidant action of phenolic hydroxyl groups of quercetin and kaempferol (Prabhu et al. 2011). The advantage of this extract as a possible agent to treat mosquitoes polluted water is that it is not toxic to human begins or animals, making possible its use both household and as water treatment compound for risk communities. The main effects of malaria disease of *M. oleifera* plant are summarized in table 22.

Table 22. Malaria disease curative effect of *M. oleifera* plant in animal studies

Part of the plant	Phytochemical	Model	Mechanism of action	References
Aqueous leaf extracts + artesunate	Terpenoids, flavonoids, alkaloids, quinines, quercetin, and kaempferol	*Plasmodium*-infected mice	↓Hemozoin formation ↓Nuclear transcription factor-kappa B (NF-κB)	(Somsak et al. 2016)
Ethanolic seed extract	Quercetin and kaempferol -	*Anopheles stephensi* pupas and larvae	↓Of 90% in Anopheles stephensi viability	(Prabhu et al. 2011)

Diarrhea

Diarrhea is a condition characterized by continuous watery stools, which promotes excessive loose of water, triggering dehydration. It could be acute or chronic, as well as infectious or non-infectious, depending on the symptoms and duration (Chiejina and Samant 2017). Hexane, chloroform, acetate, and methanol extracts of *M. oleifera* leaf exhibited a high antibacterial effect against pathogen bacteria, causing diarrhea. Mainly over *Escherichia coli*, *Shigella dysenteriae, Salmonella* sp., *Enterobacter* sp., *Klebsiella pneumoniae,* and *Serratia marcescens*. The zones of inhibition of samples isolated from diarrheic patients were found to decrease from 8.0 to 23.2 mm. This result reinforces *M. oleifera* different parts as a natural antimicrobial with various potential applications in pharmaceutical (Rahman et al. 2010). *In vivo* studies have also been carried out, and it was found that *M. oleifera* leaves at concentrations of 300 mg/kg body weight decreases purging frequency and amount. The compounds responsible for this effect have not yet been identified (Misra, Srivastava, and Srivastava 2014). The main effects of the *M. oleifera* plant over diarrhea disease are summarized in table 23.

Table 23. The anti-diarrheic therapeutic effect of *M. oleifera* plant in animal studies

Part of the plant	Model	Mechanism of action	References
Hexane, chloroform, acetate, and methanol leaf extracts	Samples isolated from diarrheic patients	↓*Escherichia coli*, *Shigella dysenteriae, Salmonella* sp., *Enterobacter* sp., *Klebsiella pneumoniae,* and *Serratia marcescens*	(Rahman et al. 2010)
Leaves flour	Diarrheic patients	↓Purging frequency and amount.	(Misra, Srivastava, and Srivastava 2014)

Stomach Ulcers

Ulcers are caused by two factors: anti-inflammatory painkillers or a *Helicobacter pylori* infection. Here, mucous, the membranes lining both the stomach and the duodenum, is inflamed. After the inflammation process, gastric acid is produced excessively, damaging the natural protective membrane barrier (Fashner and Gitu 2015). *M. oleifera* leaf aqueous extract protects ulcer formation by modulating 5-HT secretion through the enterochromaffin cell (located in the lumen) via 5-HT receptors in the gastrointestinal tract when given in a dose of 300 mg/kg to albino rats induced to ulceration using aspirin. 5-HT is a neurotransmitter located in the digestive system and helps in the mucus-secreting process (Debnath et al. 2011). Also, this extract protects health mucosa from lesions and erosion by increasing mucus globules production. No active agents have yet been reported (Ijioma et al. 2018). *M. oleifera* leaf ethanolic extracts have also shown ulcer protective effect when given in doses of 500 mg/kg to albino rats. It decreases ulcer and acid-pepsin secretion. It was also detected a reduction in CAT, LPO, and SOD activity due mainly to the extract antioxidant properties (Verma et al. 2012). *M. oleifera* root bark ethanolic extract reduces ulcer index by up to 86% when supplied at doses of 350 to 500 mg/kg for 15 d to rats. It also reduces the free acidity, total acidity, and ulcer index at the time that increases the pH of gastric content (Choudhary, Bodakhe, and Gupta 2013). *M. oleifera* seeds possess an antiulcer effect similar to omeprazole over ulcerous rats when administered at 200 mg/kg. It reduces the gastric index and increased gastric pH juice (Kansara and Singhal 2013). The seed extracts also have healing effects over ulcerative colitis symptoms in mice. The healing effects are mainly due to isothiocyanates acting through the Nrf2-signaling pathway. It has been reported that these extracts reduce colonic inflammation and histopathological scores in acute ulcerative colitis. Also, the secretion of pro-inflammatory cytokines, nitric oxide, and myeloperoxidase was reduced. These by enhancing iNOS expression and downregulating pro-inflammatory gene expression (Kim et al. 2017).

Asthma

Asthma is a multifactorial and heterogeneous disease where the respiratory pathway is obstructed due to chronic airway inflammation. It usually comes in episodes characterized by difficulty to breathe, cough, rhonchus, wheezing, and chest tightness (Horak et al. 2016). Asthma is a widespread chronic disease worldwide that starts from childhood promoted by sensitization and inhaled allergens, such as pollen, animal dander, and those coming from cockroaches, fungi, and house dust mites (Baldacci et al. 2015). Around 235 million people have asthma worldwide, mainly children. It has been found that *M. oleifera* seeds are efficient against asthma symptoms and complications.

M. oleifera seed flour produces significant improvement in patients with mild-to-moderate asthma by enhancing the total amount of air exhaled from the lungs and its rate by 33 and 32% respectively. Additionally, the flour produces no adverse effects. First, the effects were not attributed to any specific compound, but due to *M. oleifera* seed easy availability and low cost, different extracts were obtained to find the responsible phytochemical (Mehta and Agrawal 2008). Ethanol and n-butanol extracts from *M. oleifera* seeds showed effective against this disease when proved over guinea pigs induced to suffer asthma attacks (bronchospasms). Ethanolic seed extracts were found to prolong the onset of pre-convulsive dyspnea and to reduce the elevated white blood cells eosinophil and monocyte counts in the Broncho-Alveolar Lavage fluid of guinea pigs (Goyal, Goyal, and Mehta 2009). As for n-butanol extract, it was able to decrease the tidal volume, increase respiratory rate as well as to inhibit airway inflammation (Mahajan et al. 2009). The compound responsible for *M. oleifera* seed n-butanolic extract anti-asthmatic effects is β-sitosterol. It suppresses the increase in cytokine levels (TNFα, IL-4, and IL-5) both in serum and in bronchoalveolar lavage fluid. The anti-asthmatic actions exerted by β-sitosterol might be mediated by inhibiting the cellular responses and subsequent release/synthesis of Th2 cytokines (Mahajan and Mehta 2011). The main effects of *M. oleifera* plants in asthma disease are summarized in Table 24.

Table 24. Asthma disease curative effect of *M. oleifera* plant in animal studies

Part of the plant	Phytochemical	Model	Mechanism of action	References
Seed flour	-	Asthmatic human patients	↑The total amount of air exhaled from the lungs	(Mehta, Agrawal, and Medicine 2008)
Ethanol seed extracts	-	Guinea pigs induced to bronchospasms	Prolong the onset of pre-convulsive dyspnea ↓White blood cells eosinophil and monocyte counts	(Goyal, Goyal, and Mehta 2009)
Butanol seed extracts	β-sitosterol	Guinea pigs induced to bronchospasms	↓Tidal volume ↑Respiratory rate ↓Airway inflammation ↓TNFα, IL-4, and IL-5 ↓Th2 cytokines	(Mahajan and Mehta 2011)

CONCLUSION

Moringa family is composed of 13 species. Among them, *Moringa oleifera,* known as the tree of life or the miracle tree, has been by far the most studied one. The health benefits of the different anatomical parts of the *M. oleifera* tree have been known and exploited by ancient civilizations and have transcended to the present time. Consequently, although it was originally distributed only in the sub-Himalayan tracts of Northern India, nowadays, it is found in many countries with tropical and subtropical climates.

For its multiple benefits, *M. oleifera* has been incorporated from different traditional dishes such as infusions and soups to new food formulations such as weaning food, bread, and yogurts and even as an ingredient of complementary food. So far, these new formulations have been intended for infants and scholar dishes for children in developing countries aiming to dissipate malnutrition. However, it is expected that these dishes will soon reach new markets around the world. *M. oleifera* extracts have also been incorporated into supplements to increase macro and micronutrient intake and particularly for their potential to cure and prevent common diseases such as cancer, diabetes, obesity, and hypercholesterolemia, as well as other more specific to some regions such as malaria.

Up to now, there have been studied and identified the diseases to which each part of the tree exerts beneficial effects, by using both in vivo and in vitro models. Although the most studied parts are leaves and seeds, all three fractions have been found to possess specific nutrients promoting healing activities. All *M. oleifera* parts are high sources of protein and fiber, and in micronutrients such as vitamins A, C, and E. *M. oleifera* leaves and pods contain more vitamin A and C compared to carrots and citric respectively. Also, polyphenols are abundant, but the profile will depend on the extraction solvent, being the most utilized ethanol and methanol and even the origin, maturity stage, and climatic conditions. Other particular compounds of the tree have also been found, for example, the alkaloids moringine and moringinine, both with hypoglycemic and hypotensive effects.

Despite the many studies evidencing *M. oleifera* capacity both preventing and curing a wide variety of diseases, supporting the traditional claims, the majority of them have not been adequately validated by placebo-controlled or randomized clinical trials, as well as they have not been published in highly recognized journals. So further scientific research and more rigorous standards are needed. Also, if moringa bioactive compounds are to be used as biopharmaceutical agents, it is important to evaluate the toxicity, pharmacokinetics, and effective doses of these extracts/molecules.

REFERENCES

Abd-Rabou, Ahmed A, Aboelfetoh M Abdalla, NA Ali, and KM Zoheir. 2017. "*Moringa oleifera* root induces cancer apoptosis more effectively than leave nanocomposites and its free counterpart." *Asian Pacific Journal of Cancer Prevention* 18 (8):2141. Doi;10.22034/APJCP.2017.18.8.2141

Abd-Rabou, Ahmed A, Khairy MA Zoheir, Mohamed S Kishta, Aziza B Shalby, and Mohamed Ezzo I. 2016. "Nano-micelle of *Moringa oleifera* seed oil triggers mitochondrial cancer cell apoptosis." *Asian Pacific Journal of Cancer Prevention* 17 (11):4929. doi:10.22034/APJCP.2016.17.11. 4929.

Abd El-Hack, Mohamed, Mahmoud Alagawany, Ahmed Elrys, El-Sayed Desoky, Hala Tolba, Ahmed Elnahal, Shaaban Elnesr, and Ayman Swelum. 2018. "Effect of Forage *Moringa oleifera L.*(moringa) on Animal Health and Nutrition and Its Beneficial Applications in Soil, Plants and Water Purification." *Agriculture* 8 (9):145. doi:10.3390/agriculture8090145.

Abd El Latif, Amira, Badr El Said El Bialy, Hamada Dahi Mahboub, and Mabrouk Attia Abd Eldaim. 2014. "*Moringa oleifera* leaf extract ameliorates alloxan-induced diabetes in rats by regeneration of β cells and reduction of pyruvate carboxylase expression." *Biochemistry and Cell Biology* 92 (5):413-419. doi:10.1139/bcb-2014-0081.

Abdulkadir, Abdulaziz Rabiu, Dhiya Dalila Zawawi, and Md Sarwar Jahan. 2016. "Proximate and phytochemical screening of different parts of *Moringa oleifera*." *Russian Agricultural Sciences* 42 (1):34-36. doi:10.3103/S106836741601002X.

Abdulkarim, SM, Long K, Lai OM, Muhammad SKS, and Ghazali HM. 2005. "Some physico-chemical properties of *Moringa oleifera* seed oil extracted using solvent and aqueous enzymatic methods." *Food Chemistry* 93 (2):253-263. doi:10.1016/j.foodchem.2004.09.023.

Adebayo, Ismail Abiola, Hasni Arsad, Mohd Razip Samian. 2017. "Antiproliferative effect on breast cancer (MCF7) of *Moringa oleifera* seed extracts." *African Journal of Traditional, Complementary, and Alternative Medicines* 14 (2):282-287. doi:10.21010/ajtcam.v14i2.30.

Adedapo, Adeolu Alex, Olufunke Olubunmi Falayi, and Ademola Adetokunbo Oyagbemi. 2015. "Evaluation of the analgesic, anti-inflammatory, anti-oxidant, phytochemical and toxicological properties of the methanolic leaf extract of commercially processed *Moringa oleifera* in some laboratory animals." *Journal of Basic and Clinical Physiology and Pharmacology* 26 (5):491-499. doi:10.1515/jbcpp-2014-0105.

Adedayo, Majekodunmi R., Jacob K. Akintunde, Alhassan Sani, and Aline A. Boligon. 2018. "Effect of dietary supplement from mono-culture fermentation of *Moringa oleifera* seeds by Rhizopus stolonifer on hematology and markers linked to hypercholesterolemia in rat model." *Food Science & Nutrition* 6 (7):1826-1838. doi:10.1002/fsn3.729.

Ademiluyi, Adedayo O., Olubukola H. Aladeselu, Ganiyu Oboh, and Aline A. Boligon. 2018. "Drying alters the phenolic constituents, antioxidant properties, α-amylase, and α-glucosidase inhibitory properties of Moringa (*Moringa oleifera*) leaf." *Food Science & Nutrition* 6 (8):2123-2133. doi:10.1002/fsn3.770.

Al-Asmari, Abdulrahman Khazim, Sulaiman Mansour Albalawi, Md Tanwir Athar, Abdul Quaiyoom Khan, Hamoud Al-Shahrani, and Mozaffarul Islam. 2015. "*Moringa oleifera* as an anti-cancer agent against breast and colorectal cancer cell lines." *PLoS One* 10 (8):e0135814. doi:10.1371/journal.pone.0135814.

Al-Malki, Abdulrahman L., and Haddad A. El Rabey. 2015. "The Antidiabetic effect of low doses of *Moringa oleifera Lam.* seeds on streptozotocin induced diabetes and diabetic nephropathy in male rats" *BioMed Research International* 2015:13. doi:10.1155/2015/381040.

Al-Sharif, Ibtehaj, Adnane Remmal, and Abdelilah Aboussekhra. 2013. "Eugenol triggers apoptosis in breast cancer cells through E2F1/survivin down-regulation." *Cancer* 13 (1):600. doi:10.1186/1471-2407-13-600.

Alhakmani, Fatma, Sokindra Kumar, and Shah Alam Khan. 2013. "Estimation of total phenolic content, in–vitro antioxidant and anti–inflammatory activity of flowers of *Moringa oleifera*." *Asian Pacific Journal of Tropical Biomedicine* 3 (8):623-627. doi:10.1016/S2221-1691(13)60126-4.

Almatrafi, M. Manal, Marcela Vergara-Jimenez, G. Ana Murillo, H. Gregory Norris, N. Christopher Blesso, and L. Maria Fernandez. 2017. "Moringa leaves prevent hepatic lipid accumulation and inflammation in Guinea Pigs by Reducing the Expression of Genes Involved in Lipid Metabolism." *International Journal of Molecular Sciences* 18 (7). doi:10.3390/ijms18071330.

Alves de Almeida, Ana Cristina, Felipe Meira de-Faria, Ricardo José Dunder, Luis Paulo Bognoni Manzo, Alba Regina Monteiro Souza-Brito, Anderson Luis-Ferreira. 2017. "Recent trends in pharmacological activity of alkaloids in animal colitis: potential use for inflammatory bowel disease." *Evidence-Based Complementary and Alternative Medicine* 2017:0-24. doi:10.1155/2017/8528210.

Amabye, Teklit Gebregiorgis. 2015. "Chemical compositions and nutritional value of *Moringa oleifera* available in the market of Mekelle." *Journal of Food and Nutrition Sciences* 3 (5):187-190 doi:10.11648/j.jfns.20150305.14.

Amaglo, Newton K., Richard N. Bennett, Rosario B. Lo Curto, Eduardo A. S. Rosa, Vincenzo Lo Turco, Angela Giuffrida, Alberto Lo Curto, Francesco Crea, and Gladys M. Timpo. 2010. "Profiling selected phytochemicals and nutrients in different tissues of the multipurpose tree *Moringa oleifera L.*, grown in Ghana." *Food Chemistry* 122 (4):1047-1054. doi:10.1016/j.foodchem.2010.03.073.

Anand, Krishnan, Charlette Tiloke, Alisa Phulukdaree, B Ranjan, A Chuturgoon, S Singh, Robert Moonsamy Gengan. 2016. "Biosynthesis of palladium nanoparticles by using *Moringa oleifera* flower extract and their catalytic and biological properties." *Journal of Photochemistry and Photobiology B* 165:87-95. doi:10.1016/j.jphotobiol.2016.09.039.

Angelo, Kristina M, Michael Libman, Eric Caumes, Davidson H Hamer, Kevin C Kain, Karin Leder, Martin P Grobusch, Stefan H Hagmann, Phyllis Kozarsky, and David G Lalloo. 2017. "Malaria after international travel: a GeoSentinel analysis, 2003–2016." *Malaria Journal* 16 (1):293. doi:10.1186/s12936-017-1936-3.

Anwar, Farooq, Sajid Latif, Muhammad Ashraf, and Anwarul Hassan Gilani. 2007. "*Moringa oleifera*: a food plant with multiple medicinal uses." *Phytotherapy Research: An International Journal Devoted to Pharmacological and Toxicological Evaluation of Natural Product Derivatives* 21 (1):17-25. doi:10.1002/ptr.2023.

Araújo, Larissa Cardoso Corrêa, Jaciana Santos Aguiar, Thiago Henrique Napoleão, Fernanda Virgínia Barreto Mota, André Luiz Souza Barros, Maiara Celine Moura, Marília Cavalcanti Coriolano, Luana Cassandra Breitenbach Barroso Coelho, Teresinha Gonçalves Silva, and Patrícia Maria Guedes Paiva. 2013. "Evaluation of cytotoxic and anti-inflammatory activities of extracts and lectins from *Moringa oleifera* seeds." *PLoS One* 8(12):1-15 doi:10.1371/journal.pone.0081973.

Arise, AK, RO Arise, MO Sanusi, OT Esan, SA Oyeyinka . 2014. "Effect of *Moringa oleifera* flower fortification on the nutritional quality and sensory properties of weaning food." *Croatian Journal of Food Science and Technology* 6 (2):65-71. doi:10.17508/CJFST.2014.6.2.01.

Arora, Daljit Singh and Jemimah Gesare. 2014. "*In vitro* antimicrobial evaluation and phytoconstituents of *Moringa oleifera* pod husks."

Industrial Crops and Products 52:125-135. https://doi.org/10.1016/j.indcrop.2013.09.016. doi:10.1016/j.indcrop.2013.09.016.

Asghari, Gholamreza, Abbasali Palizban, and Behnosh Bakhshaei. 2015. "Quantitative analysis of the nutritional components in leaves and seeds of the Persian *Moringa peregrina* (Forssk.) Fiori." *Pharmacognosy Research* 7 (3):242. doi:10.4103/0974-8490.157968.

Ashida, Hiroshi, Hitomi Mimuro, Michinaga Ogawa, Taira Kobayashi, Takahito Sanada, Minsoo Kim, and Chihiro Sasakawa. 2011. "Cell death and infection: a double-edged sword for host and pathogen survival." *Journal of Cellular Biology* 195 (6):931-942. doi:10.1083/jcb.201108081.

Atawodi, Sunday E., Joy C. Atawodi, Gabriel A. Idakwo, Beate Pfundstein, Roswitha Haubner, Gerd Wurtele, Helmut Bartsch, and Robert W. Owen. 2010. "Evaluation of the Polyphenol Content and Antioxidant Properties of Methanol Extracts of the Leaves, Stem, and Root Barks of *Moringa oleifera Lam.*" *Journal of Medicinal Food* 13 (3):710-716. doi:10.1089/jmf.2009.0057.

Avilés-Gaxiola, Sara, Cristina Chuck-Hernández, and Sergio O Serna Saldivar. 2018. "Inactivation methods of trypsin inhibitor in legumes: a review." *Journal of Food Science* 83 (1):17-29. doi:10.1111/1750-3841.13985.

Bais, Souravh, Guru Sewak Singh, and Ramica Sharma. 2014. "Antiobesity and Hypolipidemic Activity of *Moringa oleifera* Leaves against High Fat Diet-Induced Obesity in Rats." *Advances in Biology* 2014:9. doi:10.1155/2014/162914.

Baldacci, S, S Maio, S Cerrai, G Sarno, N Baïz, M Simoni, I Annesi-Maesano, G Viegi, and G Viegi . 2015. "Allergy and asthma: Effects of the exposure to particulate matter and biological allergens." *Respiratory Medicine* 109 (9):1089-1104. doi:10.1016/j.rmed.2015.05.017.

Barakat, Hassan, Galal A Ghazal. 2016. "Physicochemical properties of *Moringa oleifera* seeds and their edible oil cultivated at different regions in Egypt." *Food and Nutrition Sciences* 7 (06):472. doi:10.4236/fns.2016.76049.

Barichella, M., G. Pezzoli, S. A. Faierman, B. Raspini, M. Rimoldi, E. Cassani, S. Bertoli, A. Battezzati, A. Leone, L. Iorio, V. Ferri, G. Pinelli, C. Pusani, C. Bolliri, R. Cilia, S. Caronni, P. De Marco, and E. Cereda. 2018. "Nutritional characterisation of Zambian *Moringa oleifera*: acceptability and safety of short-term daily supplementation in a group of malnourished girls." *International Journal of Food Science and Nutrition*:1-9. doi:10.1080/09637486.2018.1475550.

Bennett, Richard N, Fred A Mellon, Nikolaus Foidl, John H Pratt, M Susan Dupont, Lionel Perkins, and Paul A Kroon. 2003. "Profiling glucosinolates and phenolics in vegetative and reproductive tissues of the multi-purpose trees *Moringa oleifera L.*(Horseradish tree) and *Moringa stenopetala* L." *Journal of Agricultural and Food Chemistry* 51 (12):3546-3553. doi:10.1021/jf0211480.

Berkovich, Liron, Gideon Earon, Ilan Ron, Adam Rimmon, Akiva Vexler, and Shahar Lev-Ari. 2013. "*Moringa oleifera* aqueous leaf extract down-regulates nuclear factor-kappaB and increases cytotoxic effect of chemotherapy in pancreatic cancer cells." *BMC Complementary and Alternative Medicine* 13 (1):212. doi:10.1186/1472-6882-13-21.

Bolívar, Juan J. 2013. "Essential hypertension: an approach to its etiology and neurogenic pathophysiology." *International Journal of Hypertension* 2013:1-11. https://doi.org/10.1155/2013/547809.

Bose, CK. 2016. "Anti cancer effect of Moringa (*Moringa oleifera Lam.*) root extract in OAW 42 (ovarian cancer) cell line." *European Journal of Cancer* 2016:27. doi:10.1093/annonc/mdw585.02.

Boukandoul, Silia, Susana Casal, and Farid Zaidi. 2018. "The potential of some moringa species for seed oil production." *Agriculture* 8 (10):150. doi:10.3390/agriculture8100150.

Brandt, Agnieszka, Michal Ajzensztejn, Sophia Sakka, Moira Cheung, and Tony Hulse. 2018. "Impact of iodine deficiency on thyroid function in vegan siblings." *British Society for Paediatric Endocrinology and Diabetes* 58. doi:10.1530/endoabs.58.P042:

Bray, Freddie, Jacques Ferlay, Isabelle Soerjomataram, Rebecca L Siegel, Lindsey A Torre, and Ahmedin Jemal. 2018. "Global cancer statistics 2018: GLOBOCAN estimates of incidence and mortality worldwide for 36 cancers in 185 countries." 68 (6):394-424. CA: *A Cancer Journal For Clinicians*. doi:10.3322/caac.21492.

Brilhante, Raimunda Sâmia Nogueira, Jamille Alencar Sales, Vandbergue Santos Pereira, Débora de Souza Collares Maia Castelo-Branco, Rossana de Aguiar Cordeiro, Célia Maria de Souza Sampaio, Manoel de Araújo Neto Paiva, João Bosco Feitosa dos Santos, José Júlio Costa Sidrim, and Marcos Fábio Gadelha Rocha. 2017. "Research advances on the multiple uses of *Moringa oleifera*: A sustainable alternative for socially neglected population." *Asian Pacific Journal of Tropical Medicine* 10 (7):621-630. doi:10.1016/j.apjtm.2017.07.002.

Brunelli, Dario, Michele Tavecchio, Cristiano Falcioni, Roberta Frapolli, Eugenio Erba, Renato Iori, Patrick Rollin, Jessica Barillari, Carla Manzotti,

Paolo Morazzoni, and Maurizio D'Incalci. 2010. "The isothiocyanate produced from glucomoringin inhibits NF-kB and reduces myeloma growth in nude mice in vivo." *Biochemical Pharmacology* 79 (8):1141-1148. doi:10.1016/j.bcp.2009.12.008.

Cabral, Carlos Eduardo, and Márcia Regina Simas Torres Klein. 2017. "Phytosterols in the treatment of hypercholesterolemia and prevention of cardiovascular diseases." *Arquivos Brasileiros de Cardiologia* 109 (5):475-482. doi:10.5935/abc.20170158.

Cabrera-Carrion, Jose L, Carmita Jaramillo-Jaramillo, Fausto Dután-Torres, Jorge Cun-Carrion, Pedro A Garcia, and Astudillo Rojas. 2017. "Variation of alkaloid, phenol, flavonoid, and tanin content in *Moringa oleifera Lam.* as a function of plant age and height." *Biogro* 29 (1):53-60.

Cáceres, Armando, Amarillis Saravia, Sofia Rizzo, Lorena Zabala, Edy De Leon, and Federico Nave. 1992. "Pharmacologie properties of *Moringa oleifera*. 2: Screening for antispasmodic, antiinflammatory and diuretic activity." *Journal of Ethnopharmacology* 36 (3):233-237. doi:10.1016/0378-8741(92)90049-W.

Castillo-Lopez, Ramón Ignacio, Josefina Leon-Felix, MA Angulo-Escalante, Roberto Gutierrez-Dorado, María Dolores Muy-Rangel, and José Basilio Heredia. 2017. "Nutritional and phenolic characterization of *Moringa oleifera* leaves grown in Sinaloa, Mexico." *Pakistan Journal of Botany* 49 (1):161-168.

Coppin, Julia P., Yanping Xu, Hong Chen, Min-Hsiung Pan, Chi-Tang Ho, Rodolfo Juliani, James E. Simon, and Qingli Wu. 2013. "Determination of flavonoids by LC/MS and anti-inflammatory activity in *Moringa oleifera*." *Journal of Functional Foods* 5 (4):1892-1899. doi:10.1016/j.jff.2013.09.010.

Cunningham, Nicola A, Tom R Cunningham, Jane M Roberston, and Patricia C Heyn. 2018. "Understanding and measuring the wellbeing of carers of People with dementia." *The Gerontologist* 2018:1-13. doi:10.1093/geront/gny018.

Chan, Jo-Anne, Danielle I Stanisic, Michael F Duffy, Leanne J Robinson, Enmoore Lin, James W Kazura, Christopher L King, Peter M Siba, Freya JI Fowkes, and Ivo Mueller. 2017. "Patterns of protective associations differ for antibodies to P. falciparum-infected erythrocytes and merozoites in immunity against malaria in children." *European Journal of Immunology* 47 (12):2124-2136. doi:10.1002/eji.201747032.

Cheenpracha, Sarot, Eun-Jung Park, Wesley Y. Yoshida, Chaz Barit, Marisa Wall, John M. Pezzuto, and Leng Chee Chang. 2010. "Potential anti-inflammatory phenolic glycosides from the medicinal plant *Moringa oleifera* fruits." *Bioorganic & Medicinal Chemistry* 18 (17):6598-6602. doi:10.1016/j.bmc.2010.03.057.

Cheraghi, Mostafa, Mehrdad Namdari, Hadis Daraee, and Babak %J Journal of microencapsulation Negahdari. 2017. "Cardioprotective effect of magnetic hydrogel nanocomposite loaded N, α-L-rhamnopyranosyl vincosamide isolated from *Moringa oleifera* leaves against doxorubicin-induced cardiac toxicity in rats: In vitro and in vivo studies." *Journal of Microencapsulation* 34 (4):335-341. doi:10.1080/02652048.2017.1311955.

Chiejina, Maria, and Hrishikesh Samant. 2017. "Diarrhea, Viral." In *StatPearls https://www.ncbi.nlm.nih.gov/books/NBK470525/.*

Chin, Chai-Yee, Juriyati Jalil, Pei Yuen Ng, and Shiow-Fern Ng. 2018. "Development and formulation of *Moringa oleifera* standardised leaf extract film dressing for wound healing application." *Journal of Ethnopharmacology* 212:188-199. doi:10.1016/j.jep.2017.10.016.

Choudhary, Manoj Kumar, Surendra H Bodakhe, and Sanjay Kumar Gupta. 2013. "Assessment of the antiulcer potential of *Moringa oleifera* root-bark extract in rats." *Journal of Acupuncture and Meridian Studies* 6 (4):214-220. doi:10.1016/j.jams.2013.07.003.

Debnath, Siddhartha, Debasis Biswas, Koushik Ray, and Debjani Guha. 2011. "*Moringa oleifera* induced potentiation of serotonin release by 5-HT3 receptors in experimental ulcer model." *Phytomedicine* 18 (2-3):91-95. doi:10.1016/j.phymed.2010.06.003

DeMaagd, George and Ashok Philip. 2015. "Parkinson's disease and its management: part 1: disease entity, risk factors, pathophysiology, clinical presentation, and diagnosis." *Pharmacy and Therapeutics* 40 (8):504.

Devisetti, Rajesh, Yadahally N. Sreerama, and Sila Bhattacharya. 2016. "Processing effects on bioactive components and functional properties of moringa leaves: development of a snack and quality evaluation." *Journal of Food Science and Technology* 53 (1):649-657. doi:10.1007/s13197-015-1962-5.

Dewey, Kathryn G, Zhenyu Yang, and Erick Boy. 2009. "Systematic review and meta-analysis of home fortification of complementary foods." *Maternal & Child Nutrition* 5 (4):283-321. doi:10.1111/j.1740-8709.2009.00190.x.

Dhakar, Ram Chand, Sheo Datta Maurya, Brijendra K Pooniya, Narendra Bairwa, and Manisha Gupta. 2011. "Moringa: The herbal gold to combat malnutrition." *Chronicles of Young Scientists* 2 (3):119. doi:10.4103/2229-5186.90887.

Divi, SM, Ramesh Bellamkonda, and Sarala Kumari Dasireddy. 2012. "Evaluation of antidiabetic and antihyperlipidemic potential of aqueous extract of *Moringa oleifera* in fructose-fed insulin resistant and STZ induced diabetic Wistar rats: A comparative study." *Asian Journal of Pharmaceutical and Clinical Research* 5 (1):67-72. Source: ResearchGate.

dos Santos, Alain Oliveira, Danielle Rocha do Val, Felipe Dantas da Silveira, Francisco Isaac Fernandes Gomes, Hermany Capistrano Freitas, Ellen Lima de Assis, Diana Kelly Castro de Almeida, Igor Iuco Castro da Silva, Francisco Geraldo Barbosa, Jair Mafezoli, Marcos Reinaldo da Silva, Gerly Anne de Castro Brito, Juliana Trindade Clemente-Napimoga, Vicente de Paulo Teixeira de Paulo Teixera Pinto, Gerardo Cristino Filho, Mirna Marques Bezerra, and Hellíada Vasconcelos Chaves. 2018. "Antinociceptive, anti-inflammatory and toxicological evaluation of semi-synthetic molecules obtained from a benzyl-isothiocyanate isolated from *Moringa oleifera Lam.* in a temporomandibular joint inflammatory hypernociception model in rats." *Biomedicine & Pharmacotherapy* 98:609-618. doi:10.1016/j.biopha.2017.12.102.

Duckworth, William C. 2001. "Hyperglycemia and cardiovascular disease." *Current Atherosclerosis Reports* 3 (5):383-391. doi:10.1007/s11883-001-0076-x.

Dzotam, Joachim K, Francesco K Touani, and Victor Kuete. 2015. "Antibacterial and antibiotic-modifying activities of three food plants (*Xanthosoma mafaffa Lam.*, *Moringa oleifera* (*L.*) Schott and *Passiflora edulis* Sims) against multidrug-resistant (MDR) Gram-negative bacteria." *BMC Complementary and Alternative Medicine* 16 (1):9. doi:10.1186/s12906-016-0990-7.

Eilert, U, Wolters B, and A Nahrstedt. 1981. "The antibiotic principle of seeds of *Moringa oleifera* and *Moringa stenopetala*." *Planta Medica* 42 (05):55-61. Source:PubMed.

El Rabey, Haddad A, Jalaluddin A Khan, Fahad M Almutairi, and Mohamed A Elbakry. 2017. "The low dose of drumsticks (*Moringa oleifera L.*) seed powder ameliorates blood cholesterol in hypercholesterolemic male rat." *Indian Journal of Biochemistry and Biophysics* 54(6):306-313. Source: ResearchGate.

Elgamily, Hanaa, Amani Moussa, Asmaa Elboraey, Hoda EL-Sayed, Marwa Al-Moghazy, and Aboelfetoh Abdalla. 2016. "Microbiological assessment of *Moringa oleifera* extracts and its incorporation in novel dental remedies against some oral pathogens." *Open Access Macedonian Journal of Medical Sciences* 4 (4):585. doi:10.3889/oamjms.2016.132.

Fahey, Jed W 2005. "*Moringa oleifera*: a review of the medical evidence for its nutritional, therapeutic, and prophylactic properties. Part 1." *Trees For Life Journal* 1 (5):1-15. doi:10.1201/9781420039078.ch12.

Faizi, Shaheen, Bina Shaheen Siddiqui, Rubeena Saleem, Salimuzzaman Siddiqui, KHALID Aftab, and A-ul-H Gilani. 1992. "Isolation and structure elucidation of novel hypotensive agents, niazinin A, niazinin B, niazimicin and niaziminin A+ B from *Moringa oleifera*: the first naturally occurring thiocarbamates." *Journal of the Chemical Society Perkin Transactions 1*:3237-3237. Source: PubMed.

Fakankun, OA, JO Babayemi, and JJ Utiaruk. 2013. "Variations in the mineral composition and heavy metals content of *Moringa oleifera*." *African Journal of Environmental Science and Technology* 7 (6):371-379. doi:10.5897/AJEST12.228.

Falowo, Andrew B, Felicitas E Mukumbo, Emrobowansan M Idamokoro, José M Lorenzo, Anthony J Afolayan, and Voster Muchenje. 2018. "Multi-functional application of *Moringa oleífera Lam.* in nutrition and animal food products: a review." *Food Research International* 106:317-334. doi:10.1016/j.foodres.2017.12.079.

Fard, Masoumeh, Palanisamy Arulselvan, Govindarajan Karthivashan, Siti Adam, and Sharida Fakurazi. 2015. "Bioactive extract from *moringa oleifera* inhibits the pro-inflammatory mediators in lipopolysaccharide stimulated macrophages." *Pharmacognosy Magazine* 11 (44):556-563. doi:10.4103/0973-1296.172961.

Farzana, Tasnim, Suman Mohajan, Trissa Saha, Md Nur Hossain, and Md Zahurul Haque. 2017. "Formulation and nutritional evaluation of a healthy vegetable soup powder supplemented with soy flour, mushroom, and moringa leaf." *Food Science & Nutrition* 5 (4):911-920. doi:10.1002/fsn3.476.

Fashner, Julia, and Alfred C Gitu. 2015. "Diagnosis and treatment of peptic ulcer disease and *H. pylori* infection." *American Family Physician* 91 (4). doi:10.1016/j.amjmed.2018.12.009.

Ferencz, Beata, and Lotte Gerritsen. 2015. "Genetics and underlying pathology of dementia." *Neuropsychology Review* 25 (1):113-124. doi:10.1007/s11065-014-9276.

Ferreira, Paulo Michel Pinheiro, Davi Felipe Farias, José Tadeu de Abreu Oliveira, and Ana de Fátima Ana de Fátima Urano. 2008. "*Moringa oleifera*: bioactive compounds and nutritional potential." *Revista de Nutrição* 21 (4):431-437. doi:10.1590/S1415-52732008000400007.

Gallaher, Daniel D, Cynthia M Gallaher, Sheilla Natukunda, Tonya C Schoenfuss, Ezekiel Mupere, and Sarah E Cusick. 2017. "Iron Bioavailability from *Moringa oleifera* Leaves Is Very Low." The *FASEB Journal* 786.13-786.13. Source: FASEB.

Ganguly, R, and D Guha. 2008. "Alteration of brain monoamines & EEG wave pattern in rat model of Alzheimer's disease & protection by *Moringa oleifera*." *Indian Journal of Medical Research* 128 (6). Source: PubMed.

Ganguly, Subha. 2013. "Indian ayurvedic and traditional medicinal implications of indigenously available plants, herbs and fruits: a review." *International Journal of Research in Ayurveda & Pharmacy* 4 (4). doi:10.7897/2277-4343.04435.

Garcia-Ptacek, Sara, Beatriz Contreras Escamez, Eva Zupanic, Dorota Religa, Lena von Koch, Kristina Johnell, Mia von Euler, Ingemar Kåreholt, and Maria Eriksdotter. 2018. "Prestroke mobility and dementia as predictors of stroke outcomes in patients over 65 years of age: a cohort study from the Swedish Dementia and Stroke Registries." *Journal of the American Medical Directors Association* 19 (2):154-161. doi:10.1016/j.jamda.2017.08.014.

Ghasi, S., E. Nwobodo, and J. O. Ofili. 2000. "Hypocholesterolemic effects of crude extract of leaf of *Moringa oleifera Lam* in high-fat diet fed wistar rats." *Journal of Ethnopharmacology* 69 (1):21-25. doi:10.1016/S0378-8741(99)00106-3.

Giacoppo, Sabrina, Thangavelu Soundara Rajan, Gina Rosalinda De Nicola, Renato Iori, Patrick Rollin, Placido Bramanti and Emanuela Mazzon. 2017. "The Isothiocyanate Isolated from *Moringa oleifera* Shows Potent Anti-Inflammatory Activity in the Treatment of Murine Subacute Parkinson's Disease." *Rejuvenation Research* 20 (1):50-63. doi:10.1089/rej.2016.1828.

Gidamis, AB, JT Panga, SV Sarwatt, BE Chove, NB %J Ecology of food Shayo, and nutrition. 2003. "Nutrient and antinutrient contents in raw and cooked young leaves and immature pods of *Moringa oleifera, Lam*." *Ecology of Food and Nutrition* 42 (6):399-411. doi:10.1080/03670240390268857.

Giridhari, V. V. A., D. Malathi, and K. Geetha. 2011. "Anti-diabetic properties of drumstick (*Moringa oleifera*) leaf tablets." *International Journal of Health Nutrition* 2 (1):1-5. Source: PubMed.

Glover-Amengor, Mary, Richmond Aryeetey, Edwin Afari, and Alexander Nyarko. 2017. "Micronutrient composition and acceptability of *Moringa oleifera* leaf-fortified dishes by children in Ada-East district, Ghana." *Food science & nutrition* 5 (2):317-323. doi:10.1002/fsn3.395.

Gopalakrishnan, Lakshmipriya, Kruthi Doriya, and Devarai Santhosh Kumar. 2016. "*Moringa oleifera*: A review on nutritive importance and its medicinal application." *Food Science and Human Wellness* 5 (2):49-56. doi:10.1016/j.fshw.2016.04.001.

Govardhan Singh, R. S., Pradeep S. Negi, and C. Radha. 2013. "Phenolic composition, antioxidant and antimicrobial activities of free and bound phenolic extracts of *Moringa oleifera* seed flour." *Journal of Functional Foods* 5 (4):1883-1891. doi:10.1016/j.jff.2013.09.009.

Goyal, Bhoomika R, Ramesh K Goyal, and Anita Mehta Anita. "Investigation into the mechanism of anti-asthmatic action of *Moringa oleifera*." *Journal of Dietary Supplements* 6 (4):313-327. doi:10.3109/19390210903280199.

Grundy, Scott M. 2016. "Overnutrition, ectopic lipid and the metabolic syndrome." *Journal of Investigative Medicine* 64 (6):1082. doi:10.1136/jim-2016-000155.

Guevara, Amelia P., Carolyn Vargas, Hiromu Sakurai, Yasuhiro Fujiwara, Keiji Hashimoto, Takashi Maoka, Mutzuo Kozuka, Yoshohiro Ito, Harukuni Tokuda, and Hoyoku Nishino. 1999. "An antitumor promoter from *Moringa oleifera Lam*." *Mutation Research/Genetic Toxicology and Environmental Mutagenesis* 440 (2):181-188. doi:10.1016/S1383-5718(99)00025-X.

Gull, Iram, Attia Javed, Muhammad Shahbaz Aslam, Roohi Mushtaq, and Muhammad Amin Athar. 2016. "Use of *Moringa oleifera* Flower Pod Extract as Natural Preservative and Development of SCAR Marker for Its DNA Based Identification." *BioMed Research International* 2016. doi:10.1155/2016/7584318.

Gupta, Raj Kishor, Shivraj Singh Gangoliya, and Nand Kumar Singh. 2015. "Reduction of phytic acid and enhancement of bioavailable micronutrients in food grains." *Journal of Food Science and Technology* 52 (2):676-684. doi:10.1007/s13197-013-0978-y.

Gupta, Swati, Rohit Jain, Sumita Kachhwaha, and S. L. Kothari. 2018. "Nutritional and medicinal applications of *Moringa oleifera Lam.*—Review of current status and future possibilities." *Journal of Herbal Medicine* 11:1-11. doi:10.1016/j.hermed.2017.07.003.

Hafizur, Rahman M., Kiran Maryam, Abdul Hameed, Lubna zaheer, Samina Bano, Saima Sumbul, Aisha Sana, Rubeena Saleem, Sehrish Naz, Rizwana S. Waraich, Zaheer Ul-Haq, and Shaheen Faizi. 2018. "Insulin releasing effect of some pure compounds from *Moringa oleifera* on mice islets." *Medicinal Chemistry Research* 27 (5):1408-1418. doi:10.1007/s00044-018-2157-1.

Hajipour, Somayeh, Alireza Sarkaki, Yaghoob Farbood, Akram Eidi, Pejman Mortazavi, and Zohreh Valizadeh. 2016. "Effect of gallic acid on dementia type of Alzheimer disease in rats: electrophysiological and histological studies." *Basic and Clinical Neuroscience* 7 (2):97. doi:10.15412/J.BCN.03070203.

Hani, Norziah M., Amir E. Torkamani, Mohammad H. Azarian, Kamil W. A. Mahmood, and Siti Hawa Ngalim. 2017. "Characterisation of electrospun gelatine nanofibres encapsulated with *Moringa oleifera* bioactive extract." *Journal of the Science of Food and Agriculture* 97 (10):3348-3358. doi:10.1002/jsfa.8185.

Hekmat, Sharareh, Kathryn Morgan, Mohammad Soltani, and Robert Gough. 2015. "Sensory evaluation of locally-grown fruit purees and inulin fibre on probiotic yogurt in mwanza, Tanzania and the microbial analysis of probiotic yogurt fortified with *Moringa oleifera*." *Journal of Health, Population, and Nutrition* 33 (1):60. Source:PubMed.

Helmy, S. A., N. F. S. Morsy, S. M. Elaby, and M. A. A. Ghaly. 2017. "Hypolipidemic Effect of *Moringa oleifera Lam* Leaf Powder and its Extract in Diet-Induced Hypercholesterolemic Rats." *Journal of Medical Food* 20 (8):755-762. doi:10.1089/jmf.2016.0155.

Heymach, John, Lada Krilov, Anthony Alberg, Nancy Baxter, Susan Marina Chang, Ryan B Corcoran, William Dale, Angela DeMichele, Catherine S Magid Diefenbach, and Robert Dreicer. 2018. "Clinical cancer advances 2018: annual report on progress against cancer from the American Society of Clinical Oncology." *Journal of Clinical Oncology* 36 (10):1020-1044. doi:10.1200/JCO.2017.77.0446.

Horak, Fritz, Daniel Doberer, Ernst Eber, Elisabeth Horak, Wolfgang Pohl, Josef Riedler, Zsolt Szépfalusi, Felix Wantke, Angela Zacharasiewicz, and Michael Studnicka. 2016. "Diagnosis and management of asthma–Statement on the 2015 GINA Guidelines." *Wiener* Klinische *Wochenschrift* 128 (15-16):541-554. doi:10.1007/s00508-016-1019-4.

Huang, Wen-Juan, XIA Zhang, and Wei-Wei Chen. 2016. "Role of oxidative stress in Alzheimer's disease." *Biomedical Reports* 4 (5):519-522. doi:10.3892/br.2016.630.

Hussain, Ghulam, Azhar Rasul, Haseeb Anwar, Nimra Aziz, Aroona Razzaq, Wei Wei, Muhammad Ali, Jiang Li, and Xiaomeng Li. 2018. "Role of Plant Derived Alkaloids and Their Mechanism in Neurodegenerative Disorders." *International Journal of Biological Sciences* 14 (3):341. doi:10.7150/ijbs.23247.

Igwilo, IO, FC Ezeonu, JO Ezekwesili-Ofili, SN Igwilo, CI Nsofor, MS Abdulsalami, and E Obi . 2014. "Anti-nutritional Factors in the Roots of a Local Cultivar of *Moringa oleifera* (*Lam*)." *Pakistan Journal of Biological Sciences* 17 (1):114. doi:10.3923/pjbs.2014.114.11.

Igwilo, IO, FC Ezeonu, SC Udedi, CJ Okonkwo, and NA Ozumba . 2010. "Nutrient Composition, protein quality and anti-nutritional factors in the seeds of *Moringa oleifera* grown in Awka, Anambra State, Nigeria." *Natural Products an Indian Journal* 6:167-171. Source: ResearchGate.

Ijarotimi, Oluwole S, Oluwole A Adeoti, and Oluwaseun Ariyo. 2013. "Comparative study on nutrient composition, phytochemical, and functional characteristics of raw, germinated, and fermented *Moringa oleifera* seed flour." *Food Science & Nutrition* 1 (6):452-463. doi:10.1002/fsn3.70.

Ij Ijioma, SN, EN Nwaogazi, AA Nwankwo, H Oshilonya, CM Ekeleme, and LU Oshilonya. 2018. "Histological exhibition of the gastroprotective effect of *Moringa oleifera* leaf extract." *Comparative Clinical Pathology* 27 (2):327-332. doi:10.1007/s00580-017-2594-0.

Inbathamizh, L, Padmini E. 2012. "Gas chromatography-mass spectrometric analyses of methanol extract of *Moringa oleifera* flowers." *International Journal of Chemical and Analytical Science.* 2 (5). Source: ResearchGate.

Israr, Beenish, Richard A Frazier, and Michael H Gordon. 2013. "Effects of phytate and minerals on the bioavailability of oxalate from food." *Food Chemistry* 141 (3):1690-1693. doi:10.1016/j.foodchem.2013.04.13.

Jaafaru MS, Nordin N, Shaari K, Rosli R, Abdull Razis AF (2018) Isothiocyanate from *Moringa oleifera* seeds mitigates hydrogen peroxide-induced cytotoxicity and preserved morphological features of human neuronal cells. *PLoS ONE* 13(5): e0196403. doi:10.1371/journal.pone. 0196403.

Jaiswal, Dolly, Prashant Kumar Rai, Shikha Mehta, Sanjukta Chatterji, Surekha Shukla, Devendra Kumar Rai, Gaurav Sharma, Bechan Sharma, Shahidul khair, and Geeta Watal. 2013. "Role of *Moringa oleifera* in regulation of diabetes-induced oxidative stress." *Asian Pacific Journal of Tropical Medicine* 6 (6):426-432. doi:10.1016/S1995-7645(13)60068-1.

Jaja-Chimedza A, Graf BL, Simmler C, Kim Y, Kuhn P, Pauli GF, et al. (2017) "Biochemical characterization and anti-inflammatory properties of an isothiocyanate-enriched moringa (*Moringa oleifera*) seed extract." *PloS One* 12(8): e0182658. doi:10.1371/journal.pone.0182658.

Jimoh, Tajudeen O. 2018. "Enzymes inhibitory and radical scavenging potentials of two selected tropical vegetable (*Moringa oleifera* and *Telfairia occidentalis*) leaves relevant to type 2 diabetes mellitus " *Revista Brasileira de Farmacognosia*. 28:73-79. doi:10.1016/j.bjp.2017.04.003.

Joung, Hyunchae, Bobae Kim, Hyunjoon Park, Kyuyeon Lee, Hee-Hoon Kim, Ho-Cheol Sim, Hyun-Jin Do, Chang-Kee Hyun, and Myoung-Sool Do.

2017. "Fermented *Moringa oleifera* decreases hepatic adiposity and ameliorates glucose intolerance in high-fat diet-induced obese mice." *Journal of Medicinal Food* 20 (5):439-447. doi:10.1089/jmf.2016.3860.

Jung, Il Lae, Ju Hye Lee, and Se Chan. 2015. "A potential oral anticancer drug candidate, *Moringa oleifera* leaf extract, induces the apoptosis of human hepatocellular carcinoma cells." *Oncology Letters* 10 (3):1597-1604. doi:10.3892/ol.2015.3482.

Kansara, Swati S, and Manmohan Singhal. 2013. "Evaluation of antiulcer activity of *Moringa oleifera* seed extract." *Journal of Pharmaceutical Science and Bioscientific Research*. 3 (1):20-25. Source: SemanticScholar.

Kar, Ajit, B. K. Choudhary, and N. G. Bandyopadhyay. 2003. "Comparative evaluation of hypoglycaemic activity of some Indian medicinal plants in alloxan diabetic rats." *Journal of Ethnopharmacology* 84 (1):105-108. doi:10.1016/S0378-8741(02)00144-7.

Karanchi H, Wyne K. Hypertriglyceridemia. [Updated 2019 Feb 17]. 2019 Jan. In: *StatPearls [Internet]*. Treasure Island (FL): StatPearls Publishing. Available from: https://www.ncbi.nlm.nih.gov/books/NBK459368/.

Karthivashan, Govindarajan, Masoumeh Tangestani Fard, Palanisamy Arulselvan, Faridah Abas, and Sharida Fakurazi. 2013. "Identification of Bioactive Candidate Compounds Responsible for Oxidative Challenge from Hydro-Ethanolic Extract of *Moringa oleifera* Leaves." *Journal of Food Science* 78 (9):C1368-C1375. doi:10.1111/1750-3841.12233.

Kim, Youjin, Alex G Wu, Asha Jaja-Chimedza, Brittany L Graf, Carrie Waterman, Michael P Verzi, and Ilya Raskin. 2017. "Isothiocyanate-enriched moringa seed extract alleviates ulcerative colitis symptoms in mice." *PloS one*. 12 (9):e0184709. doi:10.1371/journal.pone.0184709.

Kirisattayakul, Woranan, Jintanaporn Wattanathorn, Terdthai Tong-Un, Supaporn Muchimapura, Panakaporn Wannanon, Jinatta Jittiwat. 2013. "Cerebroprotective effect of *Moringa oleifera* against focal ischemic stroke induced by middle cerebral artery occlusion." *Oxidative Medicine and Cellular Longevity*. Article ID 951415, 10 pp. doi:10.1155/2013/951415.

Kooltheat, Nateelak, Rungnapa Pankla Sranujit, Pilaipark Chumark, Pachuen Potup, Nongnit Laytragoon-Lewin, and Kanchana Usuwanthim. 2014. "An Ethyl Acetate Fraction of *Moringa oleifera* Lam. Inhibits Human Macrophage Cytokine Production Induced by Cigarette Smoke." *Nutrients* 6 (2):697-710. doi: 10.3390/nu6020697.

Kravets, IGOR. 2016. “Hyperthyroidism: diagnosis and treatment.” *American Academy of Family Physician*. 93(5): 363-70. Source: PubMed.

Krstin, Sonja, Herbenya Silva Peixoto, Michael Wink. 2015. "Combinations of alkaloids affecting different molecular targets with the saponin digitonin can synergistically enhance trypanocidal activity against *Trypanosoma brucei brucei*." *Antimicrobial Agents and Chemoterapy*. 59 (11) 7011-7017. doi:10.1128/AAC.01315-15.

Kumar, Anil, and Jack W Tsao. [Updated 2018 Dec 18]. 2018. "Alzheimer Disease." In *StatPearls [Internet]*. Treasure Island (FL): StatPearls Publishing 2019 Jan. Available from: https://www.ncbi.nlm.nih.gov/books/NBK499922/.

Kumari, D. Jalaja. 2010. "Hypoglycemic effect of *Moringa oleifera* and *Azadirachta indica* in type-2 diabetes." *Bioscan*. 5 (2):211-214. Source: ResearchGate.

Kumbhare, M. R., V. Guleha, and T. Sivakumar. 2012. "Estimation of total phenolic content, cytotoxicity and in–vitro antioxidant activity of stem bark of *Moringa oleifera*." *Asian Pacific Journal of Tropical Disease*. 2 (2):144-150. doi:10.1016/S2222-1808(12)60033-4.

Kumssa, Diriba B, Edward JM Joy, Scott D Young, David W Odee, E Louise Ander, and Martin R Broadley. 2017. "Variation in the mineral element concentration of *Moringa oleifera* Lam. and *M. stenopetala* (Bak. f.) Cuf.: Role in human nutrition." *PloS one*. 12 (4):e0175503. doi:10.1371/journal.pone.0175503.

Kutchan, Toni M. 1995. "Alkaloid Biosynthesis [mdash] The Basis for Metabolic Engineering of Medicinal Plants." *The Plant Cell*. 7(7), 1059–1070. doi:10.1105/tpc.7.7.1059.

Lalas, Stavros, and John J Tsaknis. 2002. "Extraction and identification of natural antioxidant from the seeds of the *Moringa oleifera* tree variety of Malawi." *Journal of the American Oil Chemists' Society*. 79 (7):677-683. doi:10.1007/s11746-002-0542-2.

Leal, María Celeste, Juan Cruz Casabona, Mariana Puntel, and Fernando Pitossi. 2013. "Interleukin-1β and tumor necrosis factor-α: reliable targets for protective therapies in Parkinson's Disease?." *Frontiers in Cellular Neuroscience*. 7:53. doi:10.3389/fncel.2013.00053.

Lee, Hyun Sook, Han Jin Cho, Rina Yu, Ki Won Lee, Hyang Sook Chun, and Jung Han Yoon Park. 2014. "Mechanisms underlying apoptosis-inducing effects of Kaempferol in HT-29 human colon cancer cells." *International Journal of Molecular Sciences*. 15 (2):2722-2737. doi:10.3390/ijms15022722.

Leone, Alessandro, Alberto Spada, Alberto Battezzati, Alberto Schiraldi, Junior Aristil, and Simona Bertoli. 2015. "Cultivation, Genetic, Ethnopharmacology, Phytochemistry and Pharmacology of *Moringa oleifera* Leaves: An Overview." *International Journal of Molecular Sciences* 16 (6): 12791-12835. doi:10.3390/ijms160612791.

Leone, Alessandro, Alberto Spada, Alberto Battezzati, Alberto Schiraldi, Junior Aristil, and Simona Bertoli. 2016. "*Moringa oleifera* seeds and oil: Characteristics and uses for human health." *International Journal of Molecular Sciences.* 17 (12):2141. doi:10.3390/ijms17122141.

Liu, Yang, Xiao-yue Wang, Xue-min Wei, Zi-tong Gao, and Jian-ping Han. 2018. "Values, properties and utility of different parts of *Moringa oleifera*: An overview." *Chinese Herbal Medicines.* 10 (4):371-378. doi:10.1016/j.chmed.2018.09.002.

MacPherson, Matthew, Jeffrey Burgess, Brain McMillan, Todd Daviau, and Srinivas M. Tipparaju. 2016. "Chapter 11 - Artificial Neural Networks in Drug Transport Modeling and Simulation–I." In *Artificial Neural Network for Drug Design, Delivery and Disposition*, edited by Munish Puri, Yashwant Pathak, Vijay Kumar Sutariya, Srinivas Tipparaju and Wilfrido Moreno, 221-241. Boston: Academic Press. doi:10.1016/B978-0-12-801559-9.00011-9.

Mahajan, Shailaja G, Aryamitra Banerjee, Bhupendrasinh F Chauhan, Harish Padh, Manish Nivsarkar, and Anita A. Mehta. 2009. "Inhibitory effect of n-butanol fraction of *Moringa oleifera* Lam. seeds on ovalbumin-induced airway inflammation in a guinea pig model of asthma." *International Journal of Toxicology.* 28 (6):519-527. doi:10.1177/1091581809345165.

Mahajan, Shailaja G, and Anita A. Mehta. 2011. "Suppression of ovalbumin-induced Th2-driven airway inflammation by β-sitosterol in a guinea pig model of asthma." *European Journal of Pharmacology.* 650 (1):458-464. doi:10.1016/j.ejphar.2010.09.075.

Mahajan, Shailaja G., Ravindra G. Mali, and Anita A. Mehta. 2007. "Effect of *Moringa oleifera* Lam. Seed Extract on Toluene Diisocyanate-Induced Immune-Mediated Inflammatory Responses in Rats." *Journal of Immunotoxicology.* 4 (2):85-96. doi:10.1080/15476910701337472.

Mahaman, Yacoubou Abdoul Razak, Fang Huang, Henok Kessete Afewerky, Tanko Mahamane Salissou Maibouge, Bishwajit Ghose, and Xiaochuan Wang. 2018. "Involvement of calpain in the neuropathogenesis of Alzheimer's disease." *Medicinal Research Reviews.* 39(2), 608-630. doi:10.1002/med.21534.

Mahaman, Yacoubou Abdoul Razak, Fang Huang, Mengjuan Wu, Yuman Wang, Zhen Wei, Jian Bao, Maibouge Tanko Mahamane Salissou, Dan Ke, Qun Wang, and Rong Liu. 2018. "*Moringa oleifera* Alleviates

Homocysteine-Induced Alzheimer's Disease-Like Pathology and Cognitive Impairments." *Journal of Alzheimer's Disease*. 63(3), 1141-1159. doi:10.3233/JAD-180091.

Makkar, HPS, and K Becker. 1997. "Nutrients and antiquality factors in different morphological parts of the *Moringa oleifera* tree." *The Journal of Agricultural Science*. 128 (3):311-322. Source: CambridgeCore.

Mannarino, Massimo R., Stefano Ministrini, and Matteo Pirro. 2014. "Nutraceuticals for the treatment of hypercholesterolemia." *European Journal of Internal Medicine*. 25 (7):592-599. doi:10.1016/j.ejim.2014.06.008.

Maqsood, Muhammad, Rahmatullah Qureshi, Muhammad Arshad, Muhammad Sheeraz Ahmed, and Masroor Ikram. 2017. "Preliminary Phytochemical Screening, Antifungal and Cytotoxic Activities of Leaves Extract of *Moringa oleifera* Lam. From Salt Range, Pakistan." *Pakistan Journal of Botany* 49 (1):353-359. URL: http://www.pakbs.org/pjbot/PDFs/49(1)/46.pdf.

Martinez-Hervas, Sergio, and Juan F. Ascaso. 2019. "Hypercholesterolemia." In *Encyclopedia of Endocrine Diseases (Second Edition)*, edited by Ilpo Huhtaniemi and Luciano Martini, 320-326. Oxford: Academic Press.

Matshediso, Phatsimo G, Ewa Cukrowska, and Luke Chimuka. 2015. "Development of pressurised hot water extraction (PHWE) for essential compounds from *Moringa oleifera* leaf extracts." *Food Chemistry*. 172:423-427. doi:10.1016/j.foodchem.2014.09.047.

Maurya, Santosh Kumar, and Anil Kumar Singh. 2014. "Clinical efficacy of *Moringa oleifera* Lam. stems bark in urinary tract infections." *International Scholarly Research Notices*. Article ID 906843, 7 pp. doi:10.1155/2014/906843

Mazumder, Upal Kanti, Malaya Gupta, Sumit Chakrabarti, and Dilipkumar Pal. 1999. "Evaluation of hematological and hepatorenal functions of methanolic extract of *Moringa oleifera* Lam. root treated mice." *Indian Journal of Experimental Biology*. 37(6) 612-614.

Mbah, BO, PE Eme, and AE Paul. 2012. "Effect of drying techniques on the proximate and other nutrient composition of Moringa oleifera leaves from two areas in Eastern Nigeria." *Pakistan Journal of Nutrition* 11 (11):1044. Source: Science Alert.

Mbikay, Majambu. 2012. "Therapeutic Potential of Moringa oleifera Leaves in Chronic Hyperglycemia and Dyslipidemia: A Review." *Frontiers in Pharmacology*. 3 (24). doi:10.3389/fphar.2012.00024.

Mehta, Anita, Babita Agrawal. 2008. "Investigation into the mechanism of action of *Moringa oleifera* for its anti-asthmatic activity." *Oriental Pharmacy and Experimental Medicine.* 8 (1):24-31. doi:10.3742/OPEM.2008.8.1.024.

Mehta, K., R. Balaraman, A. H. Amin, P. A. Bafna, and O. D. Gulati. 2003. "Effect of fruits of *Moringa oleifera* on the lipid profile of normal and hypercholesterolaemic rabbits." *Journal of Ethnopharmacoly.* 86 (2-3):191-5. doi:10.1016/S0378-8741(03)00075-8.

Metwally, Fateheya Mohamed, Hend Mohamed Rashad, Hanaa Hamdy Ahmed, Asmaa Ahmed Mahmoud, Ehab Ragaa Abdol Raouf, and Aboelfetoh Mohamed Abdalla. 2017. "Molecular mechanisms of the anti-obesity potential effect of *Moringa oleifera* in the experimental model." *Asian Pacific Journal of Tropical Biomedicine* 7 (3):214-221. doi:10.1016/j.apjtb.2016.12.007.

Meza-Carranco, Zahidd, Emilio Olivares-Sáenz, Erasmo Gutiérrez-Ornelas, Hugo Bernal-Barragán, Juana Aranda-Ruiz, and Rigoberto E. Vázquez-Alvarado. 2016. "Crecimiento y producción de biomasa de moringa (*Moringa oleifera* Lam.) bajo las condiciones climáticas del Noreste de México. [Growth and production of moringa biomass (Moringa oleifera Lam.) Under the climatic conditions of the Northeast of Mexico]" *Tecnociencia Chihuahua.* 5 (3):143-153. URL: https://vocero.uach.mx/index.php/tecnociencia/article/view/177.

Mgbemena, NM, and GA Obodo. 2016. "Comparative Analysis of Proximate and mineral composition of *Moringa oleifera* root, leave and seed obtained in Okigwe Imo State, Nigeria." *Journal of Molecular Studies and Medicine Research.* 1 (2):57-62. doi:10.18801/jmsmr.010216.07.

Misra, Ankita, Sharad Srivastava, and Manjoosha Srivastava. 2014. "Evaluation of anti diarrheal potential of *Moringa oleifera* (Lam.) leaves." *Journal of Pharmacognosy and Phytochemistry.* 2 (5):43-46. Source: ResearchGate.

Mo, Shunyan, Linlin Dong, W Jeffrey Hurst, and Richard B Van Breemen. 2013. "Quantitative analysis of phytosterols in edible oils using APCI liquid chromatography–tandem mass spectrometry." *Lipids.* 48 (9):949-956. doi:10.1007/s11745-013-3813-3.

Mohamed, Doha A, Sherein S Abdelgayed, Rasha S Mohamed, and Hend A Essa. 2019. "Impact of Safflower Petals and *Moringa* Leaves Extracts in Experimental Hyper and Hypothyroidism in Rats." *International Journal of Pharmacology.* 15:219-228. doi:10.3923/ijp.2019.219.228.

Moura, Maiara C, Emmanuel V Pontual, Francis S Gomes, Thiago H Napoleão, Haroudo S Xavier, Patrícia MG Paiva, and LCBB Coelho. 2011.

"Preparations of *Moringa oleifera* flowers to treat contaminated water." *Advances in Environmental Research*. 21:269-285. ISBN 978-1-61470-007-4. Source: ResearchGate.

Moyo, B., S. Oyedemi, P. J. Masika, and V. Muchenje. 2012. "Polyphenolic content and antioxidant properties of *Moringa oleifera* leaf extracts and enzymatic activity of liver from goats supplemented with *Moringa oleifera* leaves/sunflower seed cake." *Meat Science* 91 (4):441-447. doi:10.1016/j.meatsci.2012.02.029.

Moyo, Busani, Patrick J Masika, Arnold Hugo, and Voster Muchenje. 2011. "Nutritional characterization of Moringa (*Moringa oleifera* Lam.) leaves." *African Journal of Biotechnology*. 10 (60):12925-12933. doi:10.5897/AJB10.1599.

Mozafar, Ahmad. 2018. *Plant vitamins: agronomic, physiological, and nutritional aspects*. CRC Press. 432 pp.

Muhammad, Hafiz Irfan, Mohd Zaini Asmawi, and Nurzalina Abdul Karim Khan. 2016. "A review on promising phytochemical, nutritional and glycemic control studies on *Moringa oleifera* Lam. in tropical and sub-tropical regions." *Asian Pacific Journal of Tropical Biomedicine*. 6 (10):896-902. doi:10.1016/j.apjtb.2016.08.006.

Muhammad, N., K. G. Ibrahim, A. R. Ndhlala, and K. H. Erlwanger. 2019. "*Moringa oleifera* Lam. prevents the development of high fructose diet-induced fatty liver." *South African Journal of Botany*. doi:10.1016/j.sajb.2018.12.003.

Nadeem, Muhammad, Muhammad Imran. 2016. "Promising features of *Moringa oleifera* oil: recent updates and perspectives." *Lipids in Health and Disease*. 15 (1):212. doi:10.1186/s12944-016-0379-0.

Nagarajan, Jayesree, Ramakrishnan Nagasundara Ramanan, Mavinakere Eshwaraiah Raghunandan, Charis M. Galanakis, and Nagendra Prasad Krishnamurthy. 2017. "Chapter 8 - Carotenoids." In *Nutraceutical and Functional Food Components*, edited by Charis M. Galanakis, 268. Academic Press.

Naik, Raghavendra, Sneha D Borkar, Sulochana Bhat, and Rabinarayan Acharya. 2018. "Therapeutic potential of wild edible vegetables- a review." *Journal of Ayurveda and Integrated Medical Sciences*. (ISSN 2456-3110) 2 (6):85-97. doi:10.21760/jaims.v2i06.10930.

Nambiar, Vanisha S, and Subadra Seshadri. 2001. "Bioavailability trials of β-carotene from fresh and dehydrated drumstick leaves (*Moringa oleifera*) in a rat model." *Plant Foods for Human Nutrition*. 56 (1):83-95. doi:10.1023/A:1008132503972.

Nellis, David W. 1997. *Poisonous plants and animals of Florida and the Caribbean*: Pineapple Press Inc.

Nikmaram, Nooshin, Sze Ying Leong, Mohamed Koubaa, Zhenzhou Zhu, Francisco J Barba, Ralf Greiner, Indrawati Oey, and Shahin Roohinejad. 2017. "Effect of extrusion on the anti-nutritional factors of food products: An overview." *Food Control*. 79:62-73. doi:10.1016/j.foodcont.2017.03.027.

Noguchi, Chisato, Kazuyo Kamitori, Akram Hossain, Hiroshi Hoshikawa, Ayako Katagi, Youyi Dong, Li Sui, Masaaki Tokuda, and Fuminori Yamaguchi. 2016. "D-Allose inhibits cancer cell growth by reducing GLUT1 expression." *The Tohoku Journal of Experimental Medicine*. 238 (2):131-141. doi:10.1620/tjem.238.131.

Nweze, Nkechinyere O, and Felix I Nwafor. 2014. "Phytochemical, proximate and mineral composition of leaf extracts of *Moringa oleifera* Lam. from Nsukka, South-Eastern Nigeria." *IOSR Journal of Pharmacy and Biological Sciences* 9(1):99-103. Source: ResearchGate.

Nwokolo, EN, DB Bragg, and WDJ. 1976. "The availability of amino acids from palm kernel, soybean, cottonseed and rapeseed meal for the growing chick." *Poultry Science Kitts*. 55 (6):2300-2304. doi:10.3382/ps.0552300.

O'Connell, Michael. 2017. "Arthropods and Human Disease." In *Stinging Insect Allergy*, 247-268. Springer. doi:10.1007/978-3-319-46192-2_14.

Olagbemide, Peter Taiwo, CNA Philip. 2014. "Proximate analysis and chemical composition of raw and defatted *Moringa oleifera* kernel." *Advances in Life Science and Technology*. 24:92-99. Source: International Knowledge Sharing Platform.

Olayaki, L. A., J. E. Irekpita, M. T. Yakubu, and O. O. Ojo. 2015. "Methanolic extract of *Moringa oleifera* leaves improves glucose tolerance, glycogen synthesis and lipid metabolism in alloxan-induced diabetic rats." *Journal of Basic and Clinical Physiology Pharmacoly*. 26 (6):585-93. doi:10.1515/jbcpp-2014-0129.

Olson, Mark E, and Leonardo O Alvarado-Cárdenas. 2016. "¿Dónde cultivar el árbol milagro, *Moringa oleifera*, en México? Un análisis de su distribución potencial." *Revista Mexicana de Biodiversidad*. 87 (3):1089-1102. doi:10.1016/j.rmb.2016.07.007.

Olson, Mark E, Renuka P Sankaran, Jed W Fahey, Michael A Grusak, David Odee, and Wasif Nouman. 2016. "Leaf protein and mineral concentrations across the "Miracle Tree" genus Moringa." *PloS one*. 11 (7):e0159782. doi:10.1371/journal.pone.0159782.

Olson, Mark E. 2002. "Combining Data from DNA Sequences and Morphology for a Phylogeny of Moringaceae (Brassicales)." *Systematic Botany*. 27 (1):55-73. doi:10.1043/0363-6445-27.1.55.

Oluduro, Anthonia Olufunke. 2012. "Evaluation of antimicrobial properties and nutritional potentials of *Moringa oleifera* Lam. leaf in South-Western Nigeria." *Malaysian Journal of Microbiology* 8 (2):59-67. Source: ResearchGate.

Omoruyi, FO, A Budiaman, Y Eng, FE Olumese, JL Hoesel, A Ejilemele, and AO Okorodudu. 2013. "The potential benefits and adverse effects of phytic acid supplement in streptozotocin-induced diabetic rats." *Advances in Pharmacological Sciences*. vol. 2013, Article ID 172494, 7 pages, 2013. doi:10.1155/2013/172494.

Omotoso, Gabriel Olaiya, Ismail Temitayo Gbadamosi, Olayemi Joseph Olajide, Shakirat Opeyemi Dada-Habeeb, Tolulope Timothy Arogundade, and Emmanuel Olusola Yawson. 2018. "*Moringa oleifera* phytochemicals protect the brain against experimental nicotine-induced neurobehavioral disturbances and cerebellar degeneration." *Pathophysiology*. 25 (1):57-62. doi:10.1016/j.pathophys.2017.12.003.

Orman, Suleyman, Banu Isbilen Basok, Ucler Kisa, Nevin Genc Kahraman, and Ferruh Kemal Isman. 2018. "Effects of thyroid hormone supplementation on oxidative stress after sleeve gastrectomy in rats." *Journal of Turgut Ozal Medical* Center. 25 (4) 743–746. doi:10.5455/annalsmedres.2018.08.170.

Oyeleye, Sunday I., Tosin A. Olasehinde, Ayokunle O. Ademosun, Ayodele J. Akinyemi, and Ganiyu Oboh. 2019. "Horseradish (*Moringa oleifera*) seed and leaf inclusive diets modulates activities of enzymes linked with hypertension, and lipid metabolites in high-fat fed rats." *Pharma Nutrition* 7:100141. doi:10.1016/j.phanu.2018.100141.

Oyeyinka, Adewumi T, and Samson A Oyeyinka. 2018. "*Moringa oleifera* as a food fortificant: Recent trends and prospects." *Journal of the Saudi Society of Agricultural Sciences*. 17 (2):127-136. doi:10.1016/j.jssas.2016.02.002.

Paikra, Birendra Kumar, Hemant Kumar J. Dhongade, and Bina Gidwani. 2017. "Phytochemistry and Pharmacology of Moringa oleifera Lam." *Journal of Pharmacopuncture*. 20 (3):194-200. doi:10.3831/KPI.2017.20.022.

Palada, MC, HG Patricio, AW Ebert, and DL Wu. 2014. "Horticultural characterization of AVRDC moringa germplasm in the Philippines and Taiwan." *XXIX International Horticultural Congress on Horticulture: Sustaining Lives, Livelihoods and Landscapes* (IHC2014):1102. doi:10.17660/ActaHortic.2015.1102.11.

Panda, Sunanda, Anand Kar, Pratibha Sharma, Ashok Sharma. 2013. "Cardioprotective potential of N, α-l-rhamnopyranosyl vincosamide, an indole alkaloid, isolated from the leaves of *Moringa oleifera* in isoproterenol induced cardiotoxic rats: In vivo and in vitro studies." *Bioorganic & Medicinal Chemistry Letters*. 23 (4):959-962. doi:10.1016/j.bmcl.2012.12.060.

Pandey, Kanti Bhooshan, and Syed Ibrahim Rizvi. 2009. "Plant polyphenols as dietary antioxidants in human health and disease." *Oxidative Medicine and Cellular Longevity*. 2 (5):270-278. doi:10.4161/oxim.2.5.9498.

Pandu, Swetha M., Radha Cherupanalli, and Serva P. Muthukumar. 2018. "Effects of bound phenolic from defatted *Moringa oleifera* seed flour on diet-induced hypercholesterolemic mice." *Journal of Food Biochemistry* 42 (5):e12553. doi:10.1111/jfbc.12553.

Paniagua-Pérez, Rogelio, Gabriela Flores-Mondragón, Celia Reyes-Legorreta, Brígida Herrera-López, Isabel Cervantes-Hernández, Osiris Madrigal-Santillán, José Antonio Morales-González, Isela Álvarez-González, Eduardo Madrigal-Bujaidar. 2017. "Evaluation of the anti-inflammatory capacity of beta-sitosterol in rodent assays." *African Journal of Traditional, Complementary, and Alternative Medicines*. 14 (1):123-130. URL: https://www.ajol.info/index.php/ajtcam/article/view/151920.

Pankaja, N, and Jamuna Nahrung Prakash. 1994. "Availability of calcium from kilkeerai (*Amaranthus tricolor*) and drumstick (*Moringa oleifera*) greens in weanling rats." *Food/Nahrung*. 38 (2):199-203. doi:10.1002/food.19940380212.

Paul, C. W., and B. C. Didia. 2012. "The effect of methanolic extract of *Moringa oleifera* Lam. Roots on the histology of kidney and liver of Guinea Pigs." *Asian Journal of Medical Science*. 4:55-60. Source: ResearchGate.

Pistollato, Francesca, Manuel Masias, Pablo Agudo, Francesca Giampieri, and Maurizio J Battino. 2018. "Effects of phytochemicals on thyroid function and their possible role in thyroid disease." *Annals of the New York Academy of Sciences*. doi:10.1111/nyas.13980.

Pontual, Emmanuel Viana, Nataly Diniz de Lima Santos, Maiara Celine de Moura, Luana Cassandra Breitenbach Barroso Coelho, Daniela Maria do Amaral Ferraz Navarro, Thiago Henrique Napoleão, and Patrícia Maria Guedes Paiva. 2014. "Trypsin inhibitor from *Moringa oleifera* flowers interferes with survival and development of Aedes aegypti larvae and kills bacteria inhabitant of larvae midgut." *Parasitology Research*. 113 (2):727-733. doi:10.1007/s00436-013-3702-y.

Posmontier, Bobbie. 2011. "The medicinal qualities of *Moringa oleifera*." *Holistic Nursing Practice*. 25 (2):80-87. doi:10.1097/HNP.0b013e31820dbb27.

Prabakaran, Mayakrishnan, Seung-Hyun Kim, Asokan Sasireka, Murugesan Chandrasekaran, and Ill-Min Chung. 2018. "Polyphenol composition and antimicrobial activity of various solvent extracts from different plant parts of *Moringa oleifera*." *Food Bioscience*. 26:23-29. doi:10.1016/j.fbio.2018.09.003.

Prabhu, K, K Murugan, A Nareshkumar, N Ramasubramanian, and S Bragadeeswaran. 2011. "Larvicidal and repellent potential of *Moringa oleifera* against malarial vector, *Anopheles stephensi* Liston (Insecta: Diptera: Culicidae)." *Asian Pacific Journal of Tropical Biomedicine*. 1 (2):124-129. doi:10.1016/S2221-1691(11)60009-9.

Premi, Monica, and H. K. Sharma. 2017. "Effect of extraction conditions on the bioactive compounds from *Moringa oleifera* (PKM 1) seeds and their identification using LC–MS." *Journal of Food Measurement and Characterization*. 11 (1):213-225. doi:10.1007/s11694-016-9388-y.

Radek, M., and G. P. Savage. 2008. "Oxalates in some Indian Green Leafy Vegetables." *International Journal of Food Sciences and Nutrition* 59 (3):246-260. doi:10.1080/09637480701791176.

Rahman, M. M., M. M. Rahman, S. Akhter, M. A. Jamal, D. R. Pandeya, M. A. Haque, M. F. Alam, and A. Rahman. 2010. "Control of Coliform Bacteria Detected from Diarrhea Associated Patients by Extracts of *Moringa oleifera*." *Nepal Medical College Journal* 12 (1):12-9. Source: PubMed.

Rajanandh, M. G., and J. Kavitha. 2010. "Quantitative Estimation of β-Sitosterol, Total Phenolic and Flavonoid Compounds in the Leaves of *Moringa oleifera*." *International Journal of PharmTech Research* 2 (2):1049-1414. Source: Semantic Scholar.

Randriamboavonjy, Joseph I., Gervaise Loirand, Nathalie Vaillant, Benjamin Lauzier, Sévérine Derbré, Serge Michalet, Pierre Pacaud, and Angela Tesse. 2016. "Cardiac Protective Effects of *Moringa oleifera* Seeds in Spontaneous Hypertensive Rats." *American Journal of Hypertension* 29 (7):873-881. doi:10.1093/ajh/hpw001.

Rani, Nur Zahirah Abd, Khairana Husain, and Endang Kumolosasi. 2018. "Moringa Genus: A Review of Phytochemistry and Pharmacology." *Frontiers in Pharmacology* 9:108-108. doi:10.3389/fphar.2018.00108.

Rao, Pooja J., and Madhav M. Naidu. 2016. "Nanoencapsulation of Bioactive Compounds for Nutraceutical Food." In *Nanoscience in Food and*

Agriculture 2, edited by Shivendu Ranjan, Nandita Dasgupta and Eric Lichtfouse, 129-156. Cham: Springer International Publishing.

Rauf, Abdur, Muhammad Imran, Imtiaz Ali Khan, Mujeeb ur-Rehman, Syed Amir Gilani, Zaffar Mehmood, and Mohammad S. Mubarak. 2018. "Anticancer Potential of Quercetin: A Comprehensive Review." *Phytotherapy Research* 32 (11):2109-2130. doi:10.1002/ptr.6155.

Ravani, Amee, R. V. Prasad, R. R. Gajera, and Dinesh C. Joshi. 2017. "Potentiality of *Moringa oleifera* for Food and Nutritional Security - A Review." *Agricultural Reviews* 38 (3):228-232. doi:10.18805/ag.v38i03.8983.

Ravi, Lokesh, and Krishnan Krishnan. 2017. "Cytotoxic Potential of N-hexadecanoic Acid Extracted from *Kigelia pinnata* Leaves." *Asian Journal of Cell Biology* 12 (1):20-27. doi:10.3923/ajcb.2017.20.27.

Richter, Nahid, Perumal Siddhuraju, and Klaus Becker. 2003. "Evaluation of Nutritional Quality of Moringa (*Moringa oleifera* Lam.) Leaves as an Alternative Protein Source for Nile tilapia (*Oreochromis niloticus L.*)." *Aquaculture* 217 (1):599-611. doi:10.1016/S0044-8486(02)00497-0.

Romeo, Letizia, Renato Lori, Patrick Rollin, Placido Bramanti, and Emanuela Mazzon. 2018. "Isothiocyanates: An Overview of Their Antimicrobial Activity against Human Infections." *Molecules (Basel, Switzerland)* 23 (3):624. doi:10.3390/molecules23030624.

Saha, Goutam, and Mou Sen. 2019. "Moringa Production and Consumption: An Alternative Perspective for Government Policy-Making." In *Transition Strategies for Sustainable Community Systems*, edited by Amar K. J. R. Nayak. India: Springer International Publishing.

Sahay, Surbhi, Upasana Yadav, and Sheetal Srinivasamurthy. 2017. "Potential of *Moringa oleifera* as a Functional Food Ingredient: A Review." *International Journal of Food Science and Nutrition* 2 (5):31-37. Source: ResearchGate.

Saini, R. K., K. V. Harish Prashanth, N. P. Shetty, and P. Giridhar. 2014. "Elicitors, SA and MJ Enhance Carotenoids and Tocopherol Biosynthesis and Expression of Antioxidant Related Genes in *Moringa oleifera* Lam. Leaves." *Acta Physiologiae Plantarum* 36 (10):2695-2704. doi:10.1007/s11738-014-1640-7.

Saini, R. K., N. P. Shetty, M. Prakash, and P. Giridhar. 2014. "Effect of Dehydration Methods on Retention of Carotenoids, Tocopherols, Ascorbic Acid and Antioxidant activity in *Moringa oleifera* Leaves and Preparation of a RTE Product." *Journal of Food Science and Technology* 51 (9):2176-82. doi:10.1007/s13197-014-1264-3.

Saini, Ramesh Kumar, Nandini Prasad Shetty, and Parvatam Giridhar. 2014. "Carotenoid Content in Vegetative and Reproductive Parts of Commercially Grown *Moringa oleifera* Lam. cultivars from India by LC–APCI–MS." *European Food Research and Technology* 238 (6):971-978. doi:10.1007/s00217-014-2174-3.

Saini, Ramesh Kumar, Iyyakkannu Sivanesan, and Young-Soo Keum. 2016. "Phytochemicals of *Moringa oleifera*: A Review of their Nutritional, Therapeutic and Industrial Significance." *3 Biotech* 6 (2):203-203. doi:10.1007/s13205-016-0526-3.

Sallau, A. B., S. B. Mada, S. Ibrahim, and U. Ibrahim. 2012. "Effect of Boiling, Simmering and Blanching on the Antinutritional Content of *Moringa oleifera* Leaves." *International Journal of Food Nutrition and Safety* 2 (1):1-6. Source: ResearchGate.

Sánchez-Machado, Dalia I., José A. Núñez-Gastélum, Cuauhtémoc Reyes-Moreno, Benjamin Ramírez-Wong, and Jaime López-Cervantes. 2010. "Nutritional Quality of Edible Parts of *Moringa oleifera*." *Food Analytical Methods* 3 (3):175-180. doi:10.1007/s12161-009-9106-z.

Santiago, Margaret Thatcher Barros, and Egídio Bezerra Neto. 2017. "Ecophysiology of *Moringa oleifera* Lam in Function of Different Rainfall Conditions." *Revista Geama* 3 (4):236-241. Source: ResearchGate.

Sashidhara, Koneni V., Jammikuntla N. Rosaiah, Ethika Tyagi, Rakesh Shukla, Ram Raghubir, and Siron M. Rajendran. 2009. "Rare Dipeptide and Urea derivatives from Roots of *Moringa oleifera* as Potential Anti-inflammatory and Antinociceptive Agents." *European Journal of Medicinal Chemistry* 44 (1):432-436. doi:10.1016/j.ejmech.2007.12.018.

Shahpiri, Zahra, Roodabeh Bahramsoltani, Hosein Mohammad Farzaei, Fatemeh Farzaei, and Roja Rahimi. 2016. "Phytochemicals as Future drugs for Parkinson's Disease: A Comprehensive Review." *Reviews in the Neuroscience* 27 (6):651-68. doi:10.1515/revneuro-2016-0004.

Shanker, Karuna, Madan M. Gupta, Santosh K. Srivastava, Dnyaneshwar U. Bawankule, Anirban Pal, and Suman P. S. Khanuja. 2007. "Determination of Bioactive Nitrile Glycoside(s) in Drumstick (*Moringa oleifera*) by Reverse Phase HPLC." *Food Chemistry* 105 (1):376-382. doi:10.1016/j.foodchem.2006.12.034.

Siddhuraju, Perumal, and Klaus Becker. 2003. "Antioxidant Properties of Various Solvent Extracts of Total Phenolic Constituents from Three Different Agroclimatic Origins of Drumstick Tree (*Moringa oleifera* Lam.) Leaves." *Journal of Agricultural and Food Chemistry* 51 (8):2144-2155. doi:10.1021/jf020444+.

Sinha, Kavita, and Vikrant Khare. 2017. "Review on: Antinutritional factors in Vegetable Crops." *The Pharma Innovation International Journal* 6 (12):353-358. Source: Index Copernicus.

Somsak, Voravuth, Preeyanuch Borkaew, Chokdee Klubsri, Kittiyaporn Dondee, Panatda Bootprom, and Butsarat Saiphet. 2016. "Antimalarial Properties of Aqueous Crude Extracts of Gynostemma pentaphyllum and *Moringa oleifera* Leaves in Combination with Artesunate in Plasmodium berghei-Infected Mice." *Journal of Tropical Medicine* 2016:6. doi:10.1155/2016/8031392.

Sonbarse, Priyanka Purushottam, Preksha Sharma, and Giridhar Parvatam. 2017. "PGPR's Mix Treatment to Moringa Improved plant growth and Iron Content in Foliage as Substantiated by Biochemical and Molecular Methods." *Journal of Plant Interactions* 12 (1):526-532. doi:10.1080/17429145.2017.1400125.

Sreelatha, S., A. Jeyachitra, and P. R. Padma. 2011. "Antiproliferation and Induction of Apoptosis by *Moringa oleifera* Leaf Extract on Human Cancer Cells." *Food and Chemical Toxicology* 49 (6):1270-1275. doi:10.1016/j.fct.2011.03.006.

Stohs, Sidney J., and Michael J. Hartman. 2015. "Review of the Safety and Efficacy of *Moringa oleifera*." *Phytotherapy Research* 29 (6):796-804. doi:10.1002/ptr.5325.

Sun, Yongjun, Xiaokun Cheng, Jie Hu, and Zibin Gao. 2018. "The Role of GluN2A in Cerebral Ischemia: Promoting Neuron Death and Survival in the Early Stage and Thereafter." *Molecular Neurobiology* 55 (2):1208-1216. doi:10.1007/s12035-017-0395-8.

Sutalangka, Chatchada, Jintanaporn Wattanathorn, Supaporn Muchimapura, and Wipawee Thukham-mee. 2013. "*Moringa oleifera* Mitigates Memory Impairment and Neurodegeneration in Animal Model of Age-Related Dementia." *Oxidative Medicine and Cellular Longevity* 2013:9. doi:10.1155/2013/695936.

Sutin, Angelina, Yannick Stephan, Martina Luchetti, and Antonio Terracciano. 2017. "Self-reported Personality Traits are Prospectively Associated with Proxy-reported Behavioral and Psychological Symptoms of Dementia at the end of Life." *Geriatric Psychiatry* 33(3):489-494. doi:10.1002/gsp.4782.

Tabassum, Wazida, Aruna Roshni Kullu, and M. P. Sinha. 2013. "Effects of Leaf Extracts of *Moringa oleifera* on Regulation of Hypothyroidism and Lipid Profile." *The Bioscan* 8 (2):665-669. Source: SemanticScholar.

Tahiliani, Pankaj, and Anand Kar. 2000. "Role of *Moringa oleifera* Leaf Extract in the Regulation of Thyroid Hormone Status in Adult Male and Female

Rats." *Pharmacological Research* 41 (3):319-323. doi:10.1006/phrs. 1999.0587.

Tan, Woan Sean, Palanisamy Arulselvan, Govindarajan Karthivashan, and Sharida Fakurazi. 2015. "*Moringa oleifera* Flower Extract Suppresses the Activation of Inflammatory Mediators in Lipopolysaccharide-Stimulated RAW 264.7 Macrophages via NF-kB Pathway." *Mediators of Inflammation* 2015:11. doi:10.1155/2015/720171.

Tang, Yujiao, Eun-Ju Choi, Weon Cheol Han, Mirae Oh, Jin Kim, Ji-Young Hwang, Pyo-Jam Park, Sang-Ho Moon, Yon-Suk Kim, and Eun-Kyung Kim. 2017. "*Moringa oleifera* from Cambodia Ameliorates Oxidative Stress, Hyperglycemia, and Kidney Dysfunction in Type 2 Diabetic Mice." *Journal of Medicinal Food* 20 (5):502-510. doi:10.1089/jmf.2016.3792.

Teixeira, Estelamar Maria Borges, Maria Regina Barbieri Carvalho, Valdir Augusto Neves, Maraíza Apareci Silva, and Lucas Arantes-Pereira. 2014. "Chemical Characteristics and Fractionation of Proteins from *Moringa oleifera* Lam. Leaves." *Food Chemistry* 147:51-54. doi:10.1016/ j.foodchem.2013.09.135.

Tiloke, Charlette, Alisa Phulukdaree, Krishnan Anand, Robert M. Gengan, and Anil A. Chuturgoon. 2016. "*Moringa oleifera* Gold Nanoparticles Modulate Oncogenes, Tumor Suppressor Genes, and Caspase-9 Splice Variants in A549 Cells." *Journal of Cellular Biochemistry* 117 (10):2302-2314. doi:10.1002/jcb.25528.

Tsaknis, J., S. Lalas, V. Gergis, V. Dourtoglou, and V. Spiliotis. 1999. "Characterization of *Moringa oleifera* Variety Mbololo Seed Oil of Kenya." *Journal of Agricultural and Food Chemistry* 47 (11):4495-4499. doi:10.1021/jf9904214.

Tshingani, Koy, Philippe Donnen, Henri Mukumbi, Pierre Duez, and Michèle Dramaix-Wilmet. 2017. "Impact of *Moringa oleifera* lam. Leaf Powder Supplementation Versus Nutritional Counseling on the Body Mass Index and Immune Response of HIV Patients on Antiretroviral Therapy: A Single-blind Randomized Control Trial." *BMC Complementary and Alternative Medicine* 17 (1):420-420. doi:10.1186/s12906-017-1920-z.

Udechukwu, Maryann Chinonye, Abbey Lord, Nwodo Uchechukwu and Udenigwe Chibuike Chinedu. 2018. "Potential of *Moringa oleifera* Seeds and Leaves as Functional Food Ingredients for Human Health Promotion." *Journal of Food and Nutrition Research* 57(1):1-13. Source: EBSCO.

Udeh, Henry O., Kwaku G. Duodu, and Afam I. O. Jideani. 2018. "Effect of Malting Period on Physicochemical Properties, Minerals, and Phytic Acid of Finger Millet (*Eleusine coracana*) Flour Varieties." *Food Science & Nutrition* 6 (7):1858-1869. doi:10.1002/fsn3.696.

Ugwoke, C. E. C., K. A. Eze, K. M. Tchimene, and S. P. G. Anze. 2017. "Pharmacognostic Evaluation and Antimicrobial Studies on *Moringa oleifera Lam.* (Moringaceae)." *International Journal of Phramaceutical Sciences and Research* 8 (1):88-94. doi:10.13040/IJPSR.0975-8232.8(1).88-94.

Van Dyke, Knox, Nabil Jabbour, Robert Hoeldtke, Chris Van Dyke, and Mark Van Dyke. 2010. "Oxidative/nitrosative Stresses Trigger Type I Diabetes: Preventable in Streptozotocin Rats and Detectable in Human Disease." *Annals of the New York Academy of Sciences* 1203 (1):138-145. doi:10.1111/j.1749-6632.2010.05563.x.

Van Le, Thi Hong Van, Seo Young Lee, Gwang Jin Lee, Ngoc Khoi Nguyen, Jeong Hill Park, and Minh Duc Nguyen. 2015. "Effects of Steaming on Saponin Compositions and Antiproliferative Activity of Vietnamese Ginseng." *Journal of Ginseng Research* 39 (3):274-278. doi:10.1016/j.jgr.2015.01.006.

Vasanth, K., G. C. Minakshi, K. Ilango, R. Mohan Kumar, Aruna Agrawal, and G. P. Dubey. 2015. "*Moringa oleifera* Attenuates the Release of Pro-inflammatory Cytokines in Lipopolysaccharide Stimulated Human Monocytic Cell Line." *Industrial Crops and Products* 77:44-50. doi:10.1016/j.indcrop.2015.08.013.

Vázquez-León, L. A., D. E. Páramo-Calderón, V. J. Robles-Olvera, O. A. Valdés-Rodríguez, A. Pérez-Vázquez, M. A. García-Alvarado, and G. C. Rodríguez-Jimenes. 2017. "Variation in Bioactive Compounds and Antiradical Activity of *Moringa oleifera* Leaves: Influence of Climatic Factors, Tree Age, and Soil Parameters." *European Food Research and Technology* 243 (9):1593-1608. doi:10.1007/s00217-017-2868-4.

Vergara-Jimenez, Marcela, M. Manal Almatrafi, and L. Maria Fernandez. 2017. "Bioactive Components in *Moringa oleifera* Leaves Protect against Chronic Disease." *Antioxidants* 6 (4). https://doi.org/10.3390/antiox6040091.

Verma, Arti R., M. Vijayakumar, Chandra S. Mathela, and Chandana V. Rao. 2009. "*In vitro* and *In vivo* Antioxidant Properties of Different Fractions of *Moringa oleifera* Leaves." *Food and Chemical Toxicology* 47 (9):2196-2201. doi:10.1016/j.fct.2009.06.005.

Verma, Kumar Vinay, Nripendra Singh, Puja Saxena, and Ritu Singh. 2012. "Anti-ulcer and Antioxidant Activity of *Moringa oleifera* (Lam) Leaves Against Aspirin and Ethanol Induced Gastric ulcer in Rats." *International*

Research Journal of Pharmaceuticals 2 (2):46-57. Source: SemanticsScholar.

Vojdani, A. 2015. "Lectins, Agglutinins, and their Roles in Autoimmune Reactivities." *Alternative Therapies in Health and Medicine* 21 (1):46-51. Source: PubMed.

Vongsak, Boonyadist, Pongtip Sithisarn, and Wandee Gritsanapan. 2013. "Simultaneous HPLC Quantitative Analysis of Active Compounds in Leaves of *Moringa oleifera* Lam." *Journal of Chromatographic Science* 52 (7):641-645. doi:10.1093/chromsci/bmt093.

Vongsak, Boonyadist, Pongtip Sithisarn, Supachoke Mangmool, Suchitra Thongpraditchote, Yuvadee Wongkrajang, and Wandee Gritsanapan. 2013. "Maximizing Total Phenolics, Total Flavonoids Contents and Antioxidant Activity of *Moringa oleifera* Leaf Extract by the Appropriate Extraction Method." *Industrial Crops and Products* 44:566-571. doi:10.1016/j.indcrop.2012.09.021.

Wadhwa, Sheetu, M. S. Panwar, N. Saini, S. S. Rawat, and S. Singhal. 2013. "A Review on Commercial, Traditional Uses Phytoconstituents and Pharmacological Activity of *Moringa oleifera*." *Global Journal of Traditional Medicinal Systems* 2 (1):1-13. Source: ResearchGate.

Wang, Yongqiang, Yujie Gao, Hui Ding, Shejiang Liu, Xu Han, Jianzhou Gui, and Dan Liu. 2017. "Subcritical Ethanol Extraction of Flavonoids from *Moringa oleifera* Leaf and Evaluation of Antioxidant Activity." *Food Chemistry* 218:152-158. doi:10.1016/j.foodchem.2016.09.058.

Waterman, Carrie, Diana M. Cheng, Patricio Rojas-Silva, Alexander Poulev, Julia Dreifus, Mary Ann Lila, and Ilya Raskin. 2014. "Stable, Water Extractable Isothiocyanates from *Moringa oleifera* Leaves Attenuate Inflammation *In vitro*." *Phytochemistry* 103:114-122. doi:10.1016/j.phytochem.2014.03.028.

Waterman, Carrie, Patricio Rojas-Silva, Tugba Boyunegmez Tumer, Peter Kuhn, Allison J. Richard, Shawna Wicks, Jacqueline M. Stephens, Zhong Wang, Randy Mynatt, William Cefalu, and Ilya Raskin. 2015. "Isothiocyanate-rich *Moringa oleifera* Extract Reduces Weight Gain, Insulin Resistance, and Hepatic Gluconeogenesis in Mice." *Molecular Nutrition & Food Research* 59 (6):1013-1024. doi:10.1002/mnfr.201400679.

Yameogo, Charles Windépagnagdé, Marcel Daba Bengaly, Aly Savadogo, Philippe Augustin Nikiema, and Sabadénédyo Alfred Traore. 2011. "Determination of Chemical Composition and Nutritional Values of

Moringa oleifera Leaves." *Pakistan Journal of Nutrition* 10 (3):264-268. Source: SemanticsScholar.

Yassa, Hanan Dawood, and Adel Fathy Tohamy. 2014. "Extract of *Moringa oleifera* leaves ameliorates streptozotocin-induced Diabetes mellitus in adult rats." *Acta Histochemica* 116 (5):844-854. doi:10.1016/j.acthis. 2014.02.002.

Yi, Jinsoo, Tine A. Knudsen, Anne-Louise Nielsen, Lars Duelund, Morten Christensen, Pablo Hervella, David Needham, and Ole G. Mouritsen. 2016. "Inhibition of Cholesterol Transport in an Intestine Cell Model by Pine-Derived Phytosterols." *Chemistry and Physics of Lipids* 200:62-73. doi:10.1016/j.chemphyslip.2016.06.008.

Zeng, B., J. Luo, P. Wang, L. Yang, T. Chen, J. Sun, M. Xie, M. Li, H. Zhang, J. He, Y. Zhang, and Q. Xi. 2019. "The Beneficial Effects of *Moringa oleifera* Leaf on Reproductive Performance in Mice." *Food Science & Nutrition* 7 (2):738-746. doi:10.1002/fsn3.918.

Zhang, Q. W., L. G. Lin, and W. C. Ye. 2018. "Techniques for Extraction and Isolation of Natural Products: A Comprehensive Review." *Chinese Medicine* 13:20. doi:10.1186/s13020-018-0177-x.

In: Medicinal Plants …
Editors: A. Cardador Martínez et al.
ISBN: 978-1-53618-061-9

Chapter 7

RUTACEAE: AN APPROACH TO RUE

Anayantzin Torres-Morales*
Escuela de Ingeniería y Ciencias. Tecnologico de Monterrey.
Querétaro. México

ABSTRACT

Ruta genus is originally from the Mediterranean (North Africa and southern Europe) and minor Asia. It grows spontaneously in stony places, thickets, dry soils, or near cultivated orchards being their cosmopolitan distribution. The plant used in cases of dysmenorrhoea (only in high doses is abortive), as a uterine stimulant, in gargles, in cases of angina, heart palpitations, pleurisy, respiratory complications, and cramps. Phytochemicals present in *Ruta* include furanocoumarins (bergapten, psoralen), flavonoids (rutin, quercetin), and alkaloids (skimmianine, isotaifine, taifine). These compounds have been studied for anticancer, antidiabetic, antioxidant, and anti-inflammatory activities. Moreover, because of the phototoxic activity of *Ruta* furanocoumarins, extracts of *Ruta*, have been used to treat psoriasis. The biological activity of *Ruta* extracts support its use in traditional medicine.

Keywords: *Rutacea*, antidiabetic, anti-inflammatory, anticancer, flavonoids, furanocoumarins

* Corresponding Author's Email: ana_ibt@hotmail.com.

Introduction

Rutaceae is the family name of a plant group that covers, in the majority, *Citrus* (oranges and lemons) and *Ruta* (Rzedowski and Rzedowski 2005). The specific characteristics of this family are either the absence of stipules or the endowed of translucent glands. This family has approximately 150 genera and more than 1500 different species (Rzedowski and Rzedowski 2005). Due to its use in traditional medicine (Eftekhari et al. 2015, Pollio et al. 2008, San Miguel 2003), *Ruta* is an essential genus inside *Rutaceae.*

Ruta is a native of the Mediterranean region; however, it has spread around the world (Eftekhari et al. 2015). This genus shows, mainly, evergreen shrub herbs, and it is widely studied due to its beneficial effects and its use in popular medicine (Dob et al. 2008). The two most diffused species are: *Ruta chalepensis* L. and *Ruta graveolens* L. Both have similar morphology. They have been used in medicine as antispasmodic, vermifuge, diuretic, emmenagogue, and in some cases as abortifacient (Günaydin and Savci 2005, Pollio et al. 2008, Dob et al. 2008, Parray et al. 2012).

According to researchers, the biological activity of *Ruta* relies on the presence of secondary metabolites, including flavonoids, alkaloids, coumarins, and volatile oils (Baumert et al. 1992). These compounds are produced in different parts of the plant, and their biological activities are antioxidant, anti-inflammatory, anti-tumor, antimicrobial, among others (Parray et al. 2012).

Rutaceae

The family *Rutaceae* is one of the largest, with almost 1500 species classified in 150 genera. The plants of this family grow in tropical and sub-tropical parts of the world (Parray et al. 2012). This family is rich in aromatic plants with a wide variety of sizes, such as trees, shrubbery, and herbs. They possess translucent glands and upper ovary with 3 to 5 locules and axillary placentation (Rzedowski and Rzedowski 2005). Inside this family, there are commonly known fruits such as oranges, lemons, and grapes, which belong to the *Citrus* genus. Additionally, there are rue plants, belonging to the *Ruta* genus, which is remarkable for their medicinal properties (Dob et al. 2008, Parray et al. 2012).

Ruta

The *Ruta* genus is native of the Mediterranean region; nonetheless, because of its importance in traditional medicine, this genus has spread around the world. The majority of plants within *Ruta* are evergreen shrub herbs, perennial, with a height of approximately 2 feet (Parray et al. 2012, Eftekhari et al. 2015). There are two main plants that represent the *Ruta* genus, *Ruta chalepensis* L. and *Ruta graveolens* L. Both are frequently known as Rue, and their most significant characteristic is their smell since it is very strong and specific of Rue (Parray et al. 2012, Fredj et al. 2007).

Usually, Rue is used as a vasodilator, analgesic, anti-inflammatory, antispasmodic, diuretic, and to treat pulmonary, gynecologic, and gastrointestinal disorders (Eftekhari et al. 2015). Recent studies have suggested that *Ruta* species can treat dermatologic problems such as vitiligo or psoriasis (Milesi et al. 2001). Furthermore, it is used to treat amenorrhea and dysmenorrhea, thus it can also be employed as an abortifacient (Eftekhari et al. 2015, Parray et al. 2012).

Ruta graveolens L.

Ruta graveolens L. is a perennial plant that can be half-shrubby and can reach a height of approximately 2.5 feet. The fruits of this plant are dry with 4 or 5 lobes that have a grayish brown at the top. The most distinctive characteristic of Rue is its smell, it is strong and unpleasant (Parray et al. 2012). Its flowers are small and present 4 to 5 petals in clusters in greenish yellow color; its leaves are blue-green of approximately 3 to 5 inches long and their shape has spatulate segments (Asgarpanah and Khoshkam 2012)

Rue has many uses; it is mainly used at ornamental, its essential oil (EO) is used as a flavoring agent in food, and as a medicinal plant is considered a key plant for pharmacopeia (Jaradat 2016). The main used parts of Rue are the flowers, leaves, and stems; their applications are several, for instance, to treat rheumatism, arthritis, vitiligo, fertility regulation and psoriasis (Jaradat 2016).

Nowadays, the interest in the extracts is increasing due to the knowledge about the benefits of Rue as a medical plant and the importance of the metabolites that this plant contains and their multiple applications, such as antidote against toxins of snakes and scorpions (Asgarpanah and Khoshkam 2012). Moreover, the EO of *Ruta graveolens* L. is also used with a medical approach because it has spasmolytic, anti-inflammatory and antihistaminic effects (Asgarpanah and Khoshkam 2012).

Ruta chalepensis L.

Ruta chalepensis L., also known as Egyptian Rue, is a malodorous shrublet that presents bi or tripinnatisect leaves with dark green color and leaflets of 6 mm that are narrowly oblong-lanceolate. Its flowers are yellow with 4-5 ciliate petals, 8-10 stames, and a superior ovary. Its fruit is a globose capsule of approximately 7 mm (Boulos 2005). The plant can reach 2 feet in height and sometimes even more. Finally, the aerial parts are the most used with medical approaches (Jaradat 2016).

The medical uses of *Ruta chalepensis* are reported in some parts of Africa, where they employ leaves to treat fever or earache, aerial part as an anti-inflammatory or to treat rheumatism and the roots as abortifacient (Jaradat 2016). The benefits and biological activities of *R. chalepensis* L. are the results of the several metabolites that contain alkaloids, furanocoumarins, flavonoids, amino acids, and saponins. All of these active compounds make *R. chalepensis* L. a highly valuable plant (Günaydin and Savci 2005).

According to the information mentioned above, the interest in extracts and EO from *R. chalepensis* L. has increased, as well as their application in food, perfumery, and drugs. Thus the importance to analyze deeper their composition (Mejri, Abderrabba, and Mejri 2010). A couple of examples of the applications of the metabolites are: the use of EO as antibacterial; the main compound present is 2-undecanone that is proven to be an excellent antibacterial metabolite (Mejri, Abderrabba, and Mejri 2010); and the recent study to employ ethanolic extract of *R. chalepensis* L. as an ecologic alternative to inhibit the corrosion of steel provoked by acids (Khadraoui and Khelifa 2013).

The Use of Rue in Traditional Medicine

There are many applications of *Ruta* species in traditional medicine; some of the observed effects involve the use of the EO and different parts of the herb. In India, the leaves are used to treat rheumatic pains and they are spread in the abdomen to help in dropsy; leaves are also used in an infusion to treat infantile paralysis (Parray et al. 2012).

In Table 1, some beneficial effects of *Ruta* are presented, including the part of the plant and its preparation.

Table 1. Main benefits of genus *Ruta* in traditional medicine, part of the plant used and references

Medical uses	Preparation/Part of plant	References
Inflammation	Leaves pounded in wine	(Pollio et al. 2008, Jaradat 2016, Ratheesh, Sindhu, and Helen 2013, Mancuso et al. 2015)
Nervine disorders	Powdered plant with honey	(Parray et al. 2012)
Skin disorders	Leaves	(Eftekhari et al. 2015, Milesi et al. 2001, Mancuso et al. 2015)
Emmenagogue	Powdered plant with oil and water	(Dob et al. 2008, Wu et al. 2003)
Angina	Leaves of Rue	(Pollio et al. 2008, Wu et al. 2003)
Eyesight	Tincture of leaves	(Parray et al. 2012, Mancuso et al. 2015)
Menstrual problems	Powdered seed	(Parray et al. 2012, Pollio et al. 2008, Jaradat 2016)

Furthermore, the EO of *Ruta* is another important factor in the use of this plant in traditional medicine; some researchers have proven that this EO has cytotoxic and antifungal effects, it also presents anti-inflammatory and antiandrogenic properties (Fredj et al. 2007, Parray et al. 2012). The studies dilucidated that the therapeutic and aromatic properties of *Ruta* are due to the composition of the EO and the active principles inside the plant, which can variate according to the plant species and its geographical origin (San Miguel 2003, Fredj et al. 2007).

BIOLOGICAL ACTIVITIES OF GENUS *RUTA*

The following description of biological activities includes the three most representative plants of *Ruta*: *Ruta chalepensis* L., *Ruta graveolens* L., and *Ruta angustifolia* L.

Anticancer Activity

Ruta genus possesses several phytochemicals with antioxidant capacity, related to anticancer potential (Khlifi et al. 2013, Kinjo et al. 2016, Ouerghemmi et al. 2017).

Pain is a symptom related to breast cancer. Patients with joint pain associated with breast cancer were treated with *R. graveolens* extracts. The individual components of the pain score (frequency, intensity, and the number of sites of pain) decreased significantly in the treated group (Karp et al. 2016). A decrease in pain has also reported in mice and rats- acetic acid-induced writhes model (Loonat and Amabeoku 2014).

Patients with colorectal cancer show an increase in oxidative hemolysis. *Ruta chalepensis* extracts and rutin, the main phytochemical observed in it, were proved by (Acquaviva et al. 2011) to inhibit oxidative hemolysis. Both, *R. chalepensis* extracts and rutin protected erythrocytes from hemolysis. This effect was observed only in the erythrocytes of colorectal patients.

Extracts of *Ruta graveolens* induced cytotoxicity and a decrease in cell proliferation in human colorectal carcinoma even in ultra-diluted molecular preparations, like the ones used in homeopathy (Arora et al. 2013). Moreover, hallmarks of apoptosis were evident including, cell shrinkage, chromatin condensation, and DNA fragmentation in cancer cells treated with homeopathic dilutions (Arora and Tandon 2015).

The methanolic extract of *R. graveolens* was tested on colon, breast, and prostate cancer cells by Fadlalla et al. (2011) decreasing dose-dependently the viability and the clonogenicity of treated cells and induced G_2/M arrest, aberrant mitoses, and caspase-3 activation. It also induced the p53 pathway and focal concentration of the DNA damage response proteins 53BP1 and γ-H2AX. Moreover, the levels of phospho-Akt and cyclin B1 were reduced by the *R. graveolens* extract.

Glioblastoma multiforme is a highly aggressive brain tumor whose prognosis is very poor. Due to early invasion of brain parenchyma, its complete surgical removal is nearly impossible, and even after aggressive combined treatment (association of surgery and chemo- and radiotherapy), five-year survival is only about 10%. Then, natural treatments, including *Ruta* extracts, have been proved. *Ruta* graveolens' effect was mediated by ERK1/2 and AKT activation, and the inhibition of these pathways, via PD98058 and wortmannin, reverted its antiproliferative activity. Rue extract also affects the survival of neural precursor cells (A1) obtained from embryonic mouse CNS. As in the case of glioma cells, rue stimulates the activation of ERK1/2 and AKT in A1 cells, whereas their blockade by pharmacological inhibitors prevents cell death (Gentile et al. 2015).

Anti-cancer drugs generally kill cancer cells by apoptosis but fail to do so when they become resistant and escape apoptosis signals. But these resistant cells can still be killed by autophagy. Therefore, drugs having both apoptotic and autophagic abilities are solicited in effective cancer management. Graveoline isolated from *R. graveolens* extracts induced Beclin-1 associated autophagy in A375 cells and 3-methyladenine, an inhibitor of autophagy did not affect apoptosis. Thus, graveoline-induced both apoptotic and autophagic cell death in skin melanoma cells, a desirable quality effective anti-cancer drug design (Ghosh, Bishayee, and Khuda-Bukhsh 2014, Ghosh et al. 2015).

Human brain cancer and HL-60 leukemia cells, normal B-lymphoid cells were treated by a combination of *R. graveolens* extracts and calcium phosphate. *Ruta graveolens* extract kill glioma brain cancer cells selectively and protect normal lymphocytes by inducing cell division in blood-forming cells (Pathak et al. 2003)

Antidiabetic Activity

Diabetes mellitus is a severe and complicated metabolic disorder widely reported to be accompanied by increased levels of oxidative damage, which are associated with hyperglycemia, hypoinsulinemia, hypercholesterolemia and insulin resistance (Hamdiken, Bouhalit, and Kechrid 2018). Extracts of *R. chalepensis* had presented hypoglycemic effect probably due to the presence of flavonoids and other substances, such as glycosides, alkaloids, saponin, tannins, and triterpenes. *R. chalepensis* also attenuated oxidative stress and oxidative damage. In other words, the findings showed a significant reduction in the formation of thiobarbituric acid reactive substances and an augmentation of GSH concentrations plus an improvement in GSH-Px and GST activities in animals given *R. chalepensis* extracts (Hamdiken, Bouhalit, and Kechrid 2018). Ahmed et al. (2010) reported that *R. graveolens* and rutin to exhibit antihyperglycemic and antihyperlipidemic properties via their insulinogenic effects, decreasing intestinal glucose and cholesterol absorption, improving peripheral insulin action, affecting mediators of insulin resistance, enhancing peripheral glucose uptake and decreasing hepatic glucose output in addition to the ameliorating effect on the antioxidant status in diabetic albino rats. A similar effect was observed in male rats were which were administered orally, increasing doses of methanol extract of *Ruta graveolens* between 0.5 and 2 g/kg.

A significant reduction in blood glucose was observed (519 a 115-112 mg/dL) (Meléndez 2011).

The methanolic extract of *Ruta graveolens* can reduce plasma glucose concentration in hyperglycemic rats experimentally, which supports its potential use as an alternative to traditional medicine.

PHYTOCHEMICALS PRESENT IN *RUTA*

Although the benefits of *Ruta* in health are well known, the analysis of the secondary metabolites and active principles is not well defined, and it is starting, targeting mainly the EO, different extracts of leaves, and aerial parts of the plant. Table 2 describes some active principles, their function, the part of the plant where they are found, and the extract in which each compound is obtained.

Psoralens are furanocoumarins that have been used for many years as photochemotherapy agents for the treatment of psoriasis and vitiligo. Non-polar extracts of *Ruta graveolens* leaf tissue are rich in furanocoumarins; for instance, psoralen concentration is 3.6 μmoles/mg (Ayil-Gutiérrez et al. 2015).

Another furanocoumarin present in *Ruta* is bergapten. It has been claimed that bergapten can help prevent sunlight-related skin cancer since tanned skin is more protective against sunlight damage (Tisserand and Young 2014).

Furanocoumarins such as imperatorin and xanthotoxin have been attributed with anticonvulsant activity (Luszczki et al. 2010).

Alkaloids present in *Ruta* have anti-inflammatory activity (Ulubelen and Öztürk 2006). Besides, quinolone alkaloids from *Ruta graveolens* showed antiparasitic activity (Oliva et al. 2003).

CONCLUSION

Due to the biological activities that present each compound, it is important to know them and especially their mechanism of action to use all the information to improve the actual treatments and try to prevent the development of diseases (Boots, Haenen, and Bast 2008). Moreover, all this information allows the understanding of why the *Ruta* species are used in traditional medicine and why it is important to continue with the investigation about the different species (Parray et al. 2012). Nowadays, these investigations are focus in two main

Table 2. Secondary metabolites from *Ruta* species, their application and the part of the plant used to prepare extracts

Class of organic chemical compounds	Secondary metabolite	Part of the plant	Application	Extract	References
Furanocoumarins	Psoralen	Fruit, leaves	Antimicrobial, fungicide, anti-inflammatory	Ethanol	(Ayil-Gutiérrez et al. 2015, Milesi et al. 2001, Eickhorst, DeLeo, and Csaposs 2007, Günaydin and Savci 2005, Santana et al. 2004)
	Bergapten	Fruit, aerial parts	Fungicide, anti-platelet, anti-inflammatory	Ethanol	(Milesi et al. 2001, Santana et al. 2004, Kostova et al. 1999, Günaydin and Savci 2005)
	Xanthotoxin	Fruit, aerial parts, root	Anti-inflammatory, analgesic	Ethanol	(Milesi et al. 2001, Günaydin and Savci 2005, Haesen, Vörding, and Kho 1971, Kostova et al. 1999)
	Isopimpinellin	Root	Antibacterial, anti-platelet aggregation	Ethanol	(Milesi et al. 2001, Günaydin and Savci 2005, Wolters and Eilert 1981, Wu et al. 2003)
Alkaloids	Isotaifine	Leaves	Antiparasitic, Antiarrhythmic, anthelmintic	Petrol ether	(Jaradat 2016, Günaydin and Savci 2005, Ustalar et al. 2017)
	Skimmianine	Aerial part, root	Anti-inflammatory, anti-platelet, antimicrobial	Methanol	(Steck et al. 1971, Ratheesh, Sindhu, and Helen 2013, Wu et al. 2003, Wolters and Eilert 1981)
Flavonoids	Quercetin	Aerial parts	Antioxidant, anti-inflammatory	Ethanol	(Hamad 2012, Parray et al. 2012, Boots, Haenen, and Bast 2008)
	Rutin	Aerial parts	Antioxidant, antimicrobial, anti-inflammatory, anti-cancer	Ethanol	(Hamad 2012, Parray et al. 2012, Gullón et al. 2017, Yang, Guo, and Yuan 2008)
Volatile oils	2-undecanone	Aerial parts	Antibacterial	Essential oil	(França Orlanda and Nascimento 2015, Yaacob, Abdullah, and Joulain 1989)

species *Ruta graveolens* L. and *Ruta chalepensis* L (Hamad 2012, Parray et al. 2012, Ratheesh, Sindhu, and Helen 2013, Jaradat 2016, Milesi et al. 2001, Günaydin and Savci 2005, El Sayed et al. 2000, Mejri, Abderrabba, and Mejri 2010). Both species contain several secondary metabolites whose biological activity supports the use of *Ruta* in traditional medicine.

References

Acquaviva, R., Iauk, L., Sorrenti, V., Lanteri, R., Santangelo, R., Licata, A., Licata, F., Vanella, A., Malaguarnera, M., Ragusa, S. & Di Giacomo, C. (2011). "Oxidative profile in patients with colon cancer: effects of *Ruta chalepensis* L." *European Review for Medical and Pharmacological Sciences*, no. 15, (2), 181-191.

Ahmed, Osama, Adel Moneim, Ibrahim Yazid & Ayman Mahmoud. (2010). "Antihyperglycemic, antihyperlipidemic and antioxidant effects and the probable mechanisms of action of *Ruta graveolens* infusion and rutin in nicotinamide-streptozotocin-induced diabetic rats." *Diabetologia Croatica*, no. 39-1, *15*.

Arora, S., Aggarwal, A., Singla, P., Jyoti, S. & Tandon, S. (2013). "Anti-proliferative effects of homeopathic medicines on human kidney, colon and breast cancer cells." *Homeopathy*, no. 102, (4), 274-282. doi: 10.1016/j.homp.2013.06.001.

Arora, Shagun & Simran Tandon. (2015). "DNA fragmentation and cell cycle arrest: a hallmark of apoptosis induced by *Ruta graveolens* in human colon cancer cells." *Homeopathy*, no. 104, (1), 36-47. doi: 10.1016/j.homp.2014.10.001.

Asgarpanah, Jinous & Roghaieh Khoshkam. (2012). "Phytochemistry and pharmacological properties of Ruta graveolens L." *Journal of medicinal plants research*, no. 6, (23), 3942-3949.

Ayil-Gutiérrez, Benjamín A., Jesús M Villegas-Mendoza, Zuridai Santes-Hernández, Alma D Paz-González, Maribel Mireles-Martínez, Ninfa M Rosas-García & Gildardo Rivera. (2015). "Ruta graveolens extracts and metabolites against Spodoptera frugiperda." *Natural product communications*, no. 10, (11), 1934578X1501001137.

Baumert, Alfred, Detlef Gröger, Inna N Kuzovkina & Johannes Reisch. (1992). "Secondary metabolites produced by callus cultures of various Ruta species." *Plant cell, tissue and organ culture*, no. 28, (2), 159-162.

Boots, Agnes W., Guido RMM Haenen & Aalt Bast. (2008). "Health effects of quercetin: from antioxidant to nutraceutical." *European journal of pharmacology*, no. 585, (2-3), 325-337.

Boulos, Loutfy. (2005). *A guide to medicinal plants in North Africa*: IUCN. Union internationale pour la conservation de la nature et de ses ressources. [International Union for the Conservation of Nature and Natural Resources].

Dob, Tahar, Dahmane Dahmane, Bénédicte Gauriat-Desrdy & Virgine Daligault. (2008). "Volatile Constituents of the Essential Oil of Ruta chalepensis L. subsp. Angustifolia (Pers.) P. Cout." *Journal of Essential Oil Research*, no. 20, (4), 306-309.

Eftekhari, Z, Zargaran, A., Bahmani, M., Baharvand Ahmadi, B, Baharvand Ahmadi, S, Saki, K. & Mahmoud Rafieian Kopaei. (2015). "*Ruta graveolens* plant: A plant with a range of high therapeutic effect called cardiac plant." *Der Pharmacia Lettre*, no. 7 (11), 172-173.

Eickhorst, Kimberly, Vincent DeLeo & Joan Csaposs. (2007). "Rue the herb: Ruta graveolens-associated phytophototoxicity." *Dermatitis*, no. 18, (1), 52-55.

El Sayed, Khalid, Mansour S. Al-Said, Farouk S. El-Feraly & Samir A. Ross. (2000). "New Quinoline Alkaloids from Ruta chalepensis." *Journal of Natural Products*, no. 63, (7), 995-997. doi: 10.1021/np000012y.

Fadlalla, K., Watson, A., Yehualaeshet, T., Turner, T. & Samuel, T. (2011). "*Ruta graveolens* Extract Induces DNA Damage Pathways and Blocks Akt Activation to Inhibit Cancer Cell Proliferation and Survival." *Anticancer Research*, no. 31, (1), 233-241.

França Orlanda, J. F. & Nascimento, A. R. (2015). "Chemical composition and antibacterial activity of Ruta graveolens L. (Rutaceae) volatile oils, from São Luís, Maranhão, Brazil." *South African Journal of Botany*, no. 99, 103-106. doi: https://doi.org/10.1016/ j.sajb.2015.03.198.

Fredj, Mouna Ben Hadj, Belsem Marzouk, Imed Chraief, Kamel Boukef & Zohra Marzouk. (2007). "Analysis of Tunisian Ruta graveolens L. oils from Jemmel." *Journal of Food Agriculture and Environment*, no. 5, (1), 52.

Gentile, M. T., Ciniglia, C., Reccia, M. G., Volpicelli, F., Gatti, M., Thellung, S., Florio, T., Melone, M. A. B. & Colucci-D'Amato, L. (2015). "*Ruta graveolens* L. induces death of glioblastoma cells and neural progenitors, but not of neurons, via ERK 1/2 and AKT activation." *PLoS ONE*, no. 10, (3). doi: 10.1371/journal.pone.0118864.

Ghosh, S., Bishayee, K. & Khuda-Bukhsh, A. R. (2014). "Graveoline isolated from ethanolic extract of *Ruta graveolens* triggers apoptosis and autophagy in skin melanoma cells: A novel apoptosis-independent autophagic signaling pathway." *Phytotherapy Research*, no. 28, (8), 1153-1162. doi: 10.1002/ptr.5107.

Ghosh, Samrat, Sourav Sikdar, Avinaba Mukherjee & Anisur Rahman Khuda-Bukhsh. (2015). "Evaluation of chemopreventive potentials of ethanolic extract of *Ruta graveolens* against A375 skin melanoma cells *in vitro* and induced skin cancer in mice *in vivo*." *Journal of Integrative Medicine*, no. 13, (1), 34-44. doi: 10.1016/S2095-4964(15)60156-X.

Gullón, Beatriz, Thelmo A. Lú-Chau, María Teresa Moreira, Juan M. Lema & Gemma Eibes. (2017). "Rutin: A review on extraction, identification and purification methods, biological activities and approaches to enhance its bioavailability." *Trends in Food Science & Technology*, no. 67, 220-235. doi: https://doi.org/10.1016/j.tifs.2017.07.008.

Günaydin, Keriman & Sezer Savci. (2005). "Phytochemical studies on *Ruta chalepensis* (LAM.) lamarck." *Natural Product Research*, no. 19, (3), 203-210. doi: 10.1080/ 14786410310001630546.

Haesen, J. P., Zum Vörde Sive Vörding, J. G. M. & Kho, K. F. F. (1971). "Isolation and identification of xanthotoxin from the underground parts of *Ruta graveolens*." *Planta medica*, no. 19, (01), 285-289.

Hamad, Maha Noori. (2012). "Isolation of rutin from Ruta graveolens (Rutaceae) cultivated in Iraq by precipitation and fractional solubilization." *Pharmacie Globale*, no. 3, (4), 1.

Hamdiken, Malika, Samira Bouhalit & Zine Kechrid. (2018). "Effect of *Ruta chalepensis* on Zinc, Lipid Profile and Antioxidant Levels in the Blood and Tissue of Streptozotocin-Induced Diabetes in Rats Fed Zinc-Deficient Diets." *Canadian Journal of Diabetes*, no. 42, (4), 356-364. doi: 10.1016/j.jcjd.2017.08.239.

Jaradat, Nidal. (2016). "*Quantitative Estimations for the Volatile Oil by Using Hydrodistillation and Microwave Accelerated Distillation Methods from Ruta graveolens L. and Ruta chalepensis L. leaves from Jerusalem Area/Palestine.*," no. 4, (1).

Karp, J. C., Sanchez, C., Guilbert, P., Mina, W., Demonceaux, A. & Curé, H. (2016). "Treatment with *Ruta graveolens* 5CH and *Rhus toxicodendron* 9CH may reduce joint pain and stiffness linked to aromatase inhibitors in women with early breast cancer: results of a pilot observational study." *Homeopathy*, no. 105, (4), 299-308. doi: 10.1016/j.homp.2016.05.004.

Khadraoui, A. & Khelifa, A. (2013). "Ethanolic extract of Ruta chalepensis as an eco-friendly inhibitor of acid corrosion of steel." *Research on Chemical Intermediates*, no. 39, (9), 3937-3948.

Khlifi, Daycem, Rabiaa Manel Sghaier, Sameh Amouri, Dhafer Laouini, Mokhtar Hamdi & Jalloul Bouajila. (2013). "Composition and anti-oxidant, anti-cancer and anti-inflammatory activities of *Artemisia herba-alba*, *Ruta chalpensis* L. and *Peganum harmala* L." *Food and Chemical Toxicology*, no. 55, 202-208. doi: 10.1016/j.fct.2013.01.004.

Kinjo, J., Nakano, D., Fujioka, T. & Okabe, H. (2016). "Screening of promising chemotherapeutic candidates from plants extracts." *Journal of Natural Medicines*, no. 70, (3), 335-360. doi: 10.1007/s11418-016-0992-2.

Kostova, Ivanka, Antoaneta Ivanova, Bozhana Mikhova & Iris Klaiber. (1999). "Alkaloids and coumarins from Ruta graveolens." *Monatshefte für Chemie/Chemical Monthly*, no. 130, (5), 703-707.

Loonat, F. & Amabeoku, G. J. (2014). "Antinociceptive, anti-inflammatory and antipyretic activities of the leaf methanol extract of *Ruta graveolens* L. (Rutaceae) in mice and rats." *African journal of traditional, complementary, and alternative medicines: AJTCAM/ African Networks on Ethnomedicines*, no. 11, (3), 173-181. doi: 10.4314/ajtcam.v11i3.25.

Luszczki, J. J., Andres-Mach, M., Glensk, M. & Skalicka-Wozniak, K. (2010). "Anticonvulsant effects of four linear furanocoumarins, bergapten, imperatorin, oxypeucedanin, and xanthotoxin, in the mouse maximal electroshock-induced seizure model: a comparative study." *Pharmacological Reports*, no. 62, (6), 1231-6. doi: 10.1016/s1734-1140(10)70387-x.

Mancuso, Giuseppe, Gigliola Borgonovo, Leonardo Scaglioni & Angela Bassoli. (2015). "Phytochemicals from Ruta graveolens Activate TAS2R Bitter Taste Receptors and TRP Channels Involved in Gustation and Nociception." *Molecules*, no. 20, (10), 18907-18922.

Mejri, Jamel, Manef Abderrabba & Mondher Mejri. (2010). "Chemical composition of the essential oil of Ruta chalepensis L: Influence of drying, hydro-distillation duration and plant parts." *Industrial Crops and Products*, no. 32, (3), 671-673. doi: https://doi.org/ 10.1016/j.indcrop.2010.05.002.

Meléndez, Manuel. (2011). "Efecto antihiperglucemiante del extracto metanólico de ruda (*Ruta graveolens*) en un modelo experimental de ratas hiperglicémicas. [Antihyperglycaemic Effect of the Rue (*Ruta graveolens*) Methanol Extract in an Experimental Model of Hyperglycemic Rats]." *Revista de la Facultad de Ciencias Veterinarias*, no. 52, (2), 119-126.

Milesi, S., Massot, B., Gontier, E., Bourgaud, F. & Guckert, A. (2001). "Ruta graveolens L.: a promising species for the production of furanocoumarins." *Plant Science*, no. 161, (1), 189-199. doi: https://doi.org/10.1016/S0168-9452(01)00413-7.

Oliva, A., Meepagala, K. M., Wedge, D. E., Harries, D., Hale, A. L., Aliotta, G. & Duke, S. O. (2003). "Natural fungicides from *Ruta graveolens* L. leaves, including a new quinolone alkaloid." *Journal of Agricultural and Food Chemistry*, no. 51, (4), 890-6. doi: 10.1021/jf0259361.

Ouerghemmi, Ines, Iness Bettaieb Rebey, Fatma Zohra Rahali, Soumaya Bourgou, Luisa Pistelli, Riadh Ksouri, Brahim Marzouk & Moufida Saidani Tounsi. (2017). "Antioxidant and antimicrobial phenolic compounds from extracts of cultivated and wild-grown Tunisian *Ruta chalepensis*." *Journal of Food and Drug Analysis*, no. 25, (2), 350-359. doi: 10.1016/j.jfda.2016.04.001.

Parray, Shabir Ahmad, Bhat, J. U., Ghufran Ahmad, Najeeb Jahan, Sofi, G. & M IFS. (2012). "*Ruta graveolens*: from traditional system of medicine to modern pharmacology: an overview." *American Journal of Pharm Tech Research*, no. 2, (2), 239-52.

Pathak, S., Multani, A. S., Banerji, P. & Banerji, P. (2003). "Ruta 6 selectively induces cell death in brain cancer cells but proliferation in normal peripheral blood lymphocytes: A novel treatment for human brain cancer." *International Journal of Oncology*, no. 23, (4), 975-982.

Pollio, A., De Natale, A., Appetiti, E., Aliotta, G. & Touwaide, A. (2008). "Continuity and change in the Mediterranean medical tradition: Ruta spp. (rutaceae) in Hippocratic medicine and present practices." *Journal of Ethnopharmacology*, no. 116, (3), 469-482. doi: https://doi.org/10.1016/j.jep.2007.12.013.

Ratheesh, M., Sindhu, G. & Antony Helen. (2013). "Anti-inflammatory effect of quinoline alkaloid skimmianine isolated from Ruta graveolens L." *Inflammation Research*, no. 62, (4), 367-376. doi: 10.1007/s00011-013-0588-1.

Rzedowski, G. C. de. & Rzedowski, J. (2005). *Flora fanerogámica del Valle de México*. [*Fanerochemical flora of the Valley of Mexico*], Instituto de Ecología, AC y Comisión Nacional para el Conocimiento y Usos de la Biodiversidad, Pátzcuaro (Michoacán). [Institute of Ecology, AC and National Commission for the Knowledge and Uses of Biodiversity, Pátzcuaro (Michoacán)].

San Miguel, Elia. (2003). "Rue (Ruta L., Rutaceae) in traditional Spain: frequency and distribution of its medicinal and symbolic applications." *Economic botany*, no. 57, (2), 231-244.

Santana, L., Uriarte, E., Roleira, F., Milhazes, N. & Borges, F. (2004). "Furocoumarins in medicinal chemistry. Synthesis, natural occurrence and biological activity." *Current medicinal chemistry*, no. 11, (24), 3239-3261.

Steck, Warren, Bailey, B. K., Shyluk, J. P. & Gamborg, O. L. (1971). "Coumarins and alkaloids from cell cultures of Ruta graveolens." *Phytochemistry*, no. 10, (1), 191-194.

Tisserand, Robert & Rodney Young. (2014). "5 - The skin." In *Essential Oil Safety (Second Edition)*, edited by Robert Tisserand and Rodney Young, 69-98. St. Louis: Churchill Livingstone.

Ulubelen, Ayhan & Mehmet Öztürk. (2006). "Alkaloids and coumarins from Ruta species." *Natural Product Communications*, no. 1, (10), 1934578X0600101006.

Ustalar, Asli, Mehmet Yilmaz, Agim Osmani & SEMA AŞKIN KEÇELİ. (2017). "Synthesis and antifungal activity of new dihydrofurocoumarins and dihydrofuroquinolines." *Turkish Journal of Chemistry*, no. 41, (1), 80-88.

Wolters, B. & Eilert, U. (1981). "Antimicrobial substances in callus cultures of Ruta graveolens." *Planta medica*, no. 43, (10), 166-174.

Wu, Tian-Shung, Li-Shian Shi, Jhi-Joung Wang, Song-Chou Iou, Hsien-Chang Chang, Yuh-Pan Chen, Yao-Haur Kuo, Ya-Ling Chang & Che-Ming Tenge. (2003). "Cytotoxic and antiplatelet aggregation principles of Ruta graveolens." *Journal of the Chinese Chemical Society*, no. 50, (1), 171-178.

Yaacob, Karim b., Che Mazenah Abdullah & Daniel Joulain. (1989). "Essential Oil of Ruta graveolens L." *Journal of Essential Oil Research*, no. 1, (5), 203-207. doi: 10.1080/10412905.1989.9697787.

Yang, Jianxiong, Juan Guo & Jiangfeng Yuan. (2008). "*In vitro* antioxidant properties of rutin." *LWT-Food Science and Technology*, no. 41, (6), 1060-1066.

In: Medicinal Plants …
Editors: A. Cardador Martínez et al.

ISBN: 978-1-53618-061-9

Chapter 8

GINGER: ANALYSIS OF THE RAW RHIZOME, ESSENTIAL OIL AND ALCOHOL EXTRACT OF TWO VARIETIES GROWN IN ECUADOR

***Migdalia Miranda Martínez*[1,*], *Rafael Viteri Espinoza*[2], *Maribary Monsalve Paredes*[3] *and Gabriela Carrillo Lavid*[3]**

[1]ESPOL Polytechnic University, Escuela Superior Politécnica del Litoral, ESPOL, Facultad de Ciencias Naturales y Matemáticas. Departamento de Ciencias Químicas y Ambientales. Campus Gustavo Galindo. Guayaquil, Ecuador

[2]ESPOL Polytechnic University, Escuela Superior Politécnica del Litoral, ESPOL, Centro de Investigaciones Biotecnológicas del Ecuador, Campus Gustavo Galindo. Guayaquil, Ecuador

[3]Guayaquil University of Ecuador. Faculty of Chemical Sciences

ABSTRACT

Ginger is one of the most used species in traditional and ancestral medicine in different countries. Ginger contains chemical constituents such as gingerol and shogaol, both with scientifically proven pharmacological and nutritive actions. In addition to its essential oil, pharmacological

[*] Corresponding Author's Email: mgmiran@espol.edu.ec.

properties are also reported and employed in the cosmetic and food industries. In Ecuador, two species are known as sweet ginger, and spicy ginger; both are marketed indistinctly, but no studies have been conducted on them. Therefore, the main objective of this work is to establish some physicochemical characteristics of the species commercialized in Ecuador, as well as to extract and characterize their essential oils and alcoholic extracts. The results indicated that the physicochemical parameters of the plant rhizomes presented differences, so it is a variety or another species, which would have to be demonstrated by genetic studies. The essential oils of both species showed a different chemical composition, allowing us to identify 62 compounds for sweet ginger and 92 for spicy ginger. The alcoholic extracts also showed differences in the physicochemical parameters and the qualitative chemical composition.

INTRODUCTION

Zingiberaceae is a family of herbaceous plants that has more than a thousand species distributed in around 50 genera. The most represented are Alpinia (150 species), Amomum (120 species), Zingiber (141 species), Globba (70 species), Turmeric (60 species), Kaempferia (60 species) and Hedychium (50 species). They are perennial, aromatic spicy plants with dispersed secretory cells containing essential oils, various terpenoids, and phenylpropanoid compounds. They are of tropical climate and are present in a good part of the equatorial regions of the world. Zingiber is a genus that contains real gingers, plants with medicinal, and culinary value in many parts of the world. The best known is the *Zingiber officinale*, a plant with branched, tuberose, and aromatic rhizome, which is a traditional spice that is used whole, frosted, or pulverized.

The genus comprises 211 described species, and of these, only 141 accepted. It reproduces asexually, whereby the few varieties of the plant. It is a perennial, creeping, characterized by having a height between 60 and 120 cm, tuberous and coarse rhizome (Ravindran, Babu, and Shiva 2016, Green 2007). Different information about its origin and domestication reveals that the different species of this genus are native to Southeast Asia, and from there, they dispersed throughout the tropical and subtropical regions of the world (Kizhakkayil and Sasikumar 2011). It is indicated that there are two kinds of ginger, the common ginger or scientifically known as *Zingiber officinale*; and the wild ginger or *Zingiber serumber*, being the second one more bitter and dark. This kind of ginger is found in Southeast Asia and India. It is one of the most widely used species in traditional medicine in countries such as India, Japan,

China, Greece, Rome and the Mediterranean (Baliga et al. 2011), due to the presence of compounds such as gingerol and shogaol. Those compounds have antioxidant, anti-inflammatory, anti-emetic and anti-cancer properties, among others (Geiger 2005, Shukla and Singh 2007, Stoilova et al. 2007, Shirin and Prakash 2010, Baliga et al. 2011, Butt and Sultan 2011).

India has 5 types of ginger: the one with long rhizomes known as "Cochin"; the Calicut which is of lesser quality; the most productive being the Hawaiian or cream; the wynad manantody, and the original variety from Brazil that is the most selected for the length of its rhizomes (Benavides Manzano, Cabadiana Guaman, and Cordova Tay Hing 2010).

In Thailand there is a class of ginger scientifically named *Zingiber cassumunar* Robx., also known as *Zingiber purpureum* Rosc., *Zingiber cliffordiae* or *Zingiber montanum*; its main use is in inflammatory treatments because the essential oil contains high levels of terpinen-4- ol. Other studies show that the essential oil obtained from the rhizome of *Zingiber cassumunar* Robx present high activity against yeasts (Tripathi, Dubey, and Shukla 2008).

In addition to the use of the rhizome as food and traditional medicine, the essential oil is widely used in the food and beverage industry, and in the pharmaceutical, cosmetic and perfume industry (Salgado 2011, Sharma, Chirangini, and Kishor 2011, Sasidharan, Venugopal, and Menon 2012).

Emergent interests in exploiting the potential of natural phytochemicals and plant-derived foods with compounds used to restore metabolic balance has been on the rise in the past years. One of the most widely consumed spices is ginger (*Zingiber officinale* Roscoe, Zingiberaceae). It contains numerous phytochemicals and biologically active compounds, like phenolics and flavonoids. Gingerols and Shogaols, identified components found in ginger, have been found to be major bioactive compounds (Wang et al. 2017).

Gingerol, a chemical compound, as well as several gingerols of various chain lengths (n6–n10), are also present in ginger (Figure 1A).

Shogaols, the dehydrated form of gingerols, are mainly contained in semi-dried and thermally treated gingers, a degradation product of the thermally labile gingerols (Figure 1B).

These compounds have shown numerous pharmacological benefits which include improvement of blood glucose tolerance (Lee et al. 2015), enhancement of lipid profile (Saravanan et al. 2014), and modulation of inflammatory factors (Li and Zhou 2015). In regards to obesity control, the use of natural materials has been considered as an effective tool and ginger has shown the most significant effects in both *in-vitro* and *in vivo* studies.

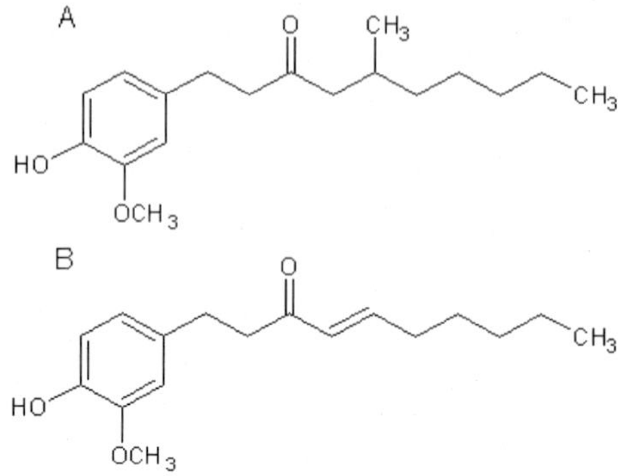

Figure 1. A: Gingerol structure. B: Shogaol structure.

Through the oral administration of the ginger extract to rats fed a high-fat diet (HFD), reduced body weight and serum lipid levels were observed (Misawa et al. 2015). Additionally, that same extract decreased HFD- induced obesity by increasing skeletal muscle fat catabolism and energy expenditure (Nammi, Sreemantula, and Roufogalis 2009). One of the major active compounds of ginger was 6-gingerol which in particular exhibited anti-obesity effects by altering the activities and expressions of some lipid metabolism marker enzymes, such as fatty acid synthase (FAS), acetyl-coA carboxylase, HMG co-A reductase, lecithin choline acyltransferase, and lipoprotein lipase (Brahma Naidu et al. 2016). Furthermore, 6-gingerol suppressed the activity of amylase and pancreatic lipase, leading to a reduction of plasma and tissue lipids (Saravanan et al. 2014).

Anti-obesity effects ginger properties may be related to its anti-inflammatory activity. The studies have shown that ginger extract and 6-gingerol can significantly downregulate mRNA levels of interleukin-6 (IL-6) and tumor necrosis factor (TNF-α) in adipose tissue of male rats fed with ginger extract (Brahma Naidu et al. 2016, Nammi, Sreemantula, and Roufogalis 2009).

Adipogenesis creates a complex process of cell differentiation that leads pre-adipocytes to become adipocytes. 6-gingerol was reported to effectively inhibit the differentiation of pre-adipocytes into adipocytes and prevent triglyceride deposition. Other benefits of 6-gingerol involve the prevention of lipid accumulation, decrease in protein expression during adipogenesis, related transcription factors and the key lipogenic enzymes in 3T3-L1 cells (Tzeng and Liu 2013, Li and Zhou 2015). Another bioactive constituent that had outstanding effects inhibiting adipogenesis of 3T3-L1 pre-adipocytes and decreasing expression of several adipogenic/lipogenic marker proteins was shogaol (Suk et al. 2016). Besides, an analysis of cellular respiration revealed that cultured skeletal muscle myotubes pretreated with ginger extract increased the palmitate-induced oxygen consumption rate, leading to an increase in cellular fatty acid catabolism (Misawa et al. 2015).

In spite of the *in vitro* and animal experiments aforementioned, only a few clinical trials performed on ginger are available for MetSs. This lack of clinical studies may be attributed to numerous factors, including ethical issues, limited commercial support, and the complex chemical composition of ginger (Roufogalis 2014). Additionally, ginger supplementation showed a favorable effect on weight loss and some associated obesity parameters in overweight and obese adults (Ebrahimzadeh Attari et al. 2015, Ebrahimzadeh Attari et al. 2016).

Ecuador enjoys the right climatic conditions and can produce ginger throughout the year, unlike the main world producers that only produce in specific annual periods. The ideal areas for production in Ecuador are the humid tropical and subtropical places of Esmeraldas (San Lorenzo, Quinindé, La Concordia), Santo Domingo de los Tsáchilas (Santo Domingo), Los Ríos (Quevedo), Guayas (El Triunfo), Napo (Tena), Morona Santiago (Macas) and Los Bancos, Pichincha. It is proposed that the common ginger or *Zingiber officinalis* is generally cultivated, although two varieties known as sweet and hot are distinguished, no studies have been conducted to establish their similarities and differences.

The extraction of the essential oils of ginger is done through a process of steam distillation of the dehydrated species (dry rhizomes, unpeeled, and freshly crushed). The essential oil obtained is a product with particular characteristics (liquid: thick, shiny crystalline, color: greenish yellowish, smell: characteristic of the raw material, flavor: slightly spicy), compared with other oils available in the international market. It is also consumed in the food industry as a fragrance and flavoring of food and beverages (Vásquez, Alva, and Marreros 2001).

Some of the components of ginger essential oil have shown a potent inhibitory effect on prostaglandin synthesis *in vitro*; they also inhibit platelet aggregation. Gingerols are antioxidants and inhibitors of lipoxygenase and cycloxygenase, then are potent anti-inflammatory agents. Recent trials have demonstrated the antitumor and anti-proliferative effects of aromatic compounds found in ginger (6- paradol). Its antiemetic activity is observed in nausea caused by the chemotherapy treatment of cancer as it has been proven in dogs and cats (Mao et al. 2019, Srinivasan 2017).

The main objective of this work is to establish some physicochemical characteristics of the species commercialized in Ecuador, as well as to extract and characterize their essential oils and alcoholic extracts, from which you can develop functional products to combat obesity.

MATERIALS AND METHODS

Harvest, Selection, Washing, and Drying

The rhizomes were collected in the province of Esmeraldas, at the Vuelta Larga parish, Coronel Carlos Concha Canton (0° 57'00"N, 79° 40'00"W), in July 2018. The two species are popularly known as sweet ginger and spicy ginger presented macromorphological differences, selecting those rhizomes that had smooth skin and a bright light brown color.

One specimen of each species was sent to the Guay herbarium of the Faculty of Natural Sciences of the University of Guayaquil, for its characterization. Rhizomes were washed thoroughly with distilled water to remove as many impurities as possible, then a portion of them was chopped and dried in an oven at a temperature of 30°C.

Determination of the Physical-Chemical Parameters and Qualitative Chemical Analysis

The physical-chemical parameters of quality (residual moisture, total and insoluble ashes in hydrochloric acid and water and alcohol-soluble substances at 80%) were determined for the dry vegetal material and this the procedures described by WHO, (2011) were used. Phytochemical screening was also performed on the plant rhizomes following the procedure established by Miranda and Cuellar (2000).

Extraction and Analysis of Essential Oils

A part of the rhizome was used fresh for the extraction of essential oils. For this purpose, 200 g of the samples previously cut into 1 cm pieces were weighed. The extraction was performed by hydro-distillation in a Clevenger equipment of 1000 ml capacity, and the extraction was performed for 3 hours. The procedure was repeated until a sufficient amount of essential oil was obtained.

The essentials oils were analyzed by using Agilent Technologies gas chromatography mass-spectrometry equipment (7890A GC system and 5975C inert XL MSD with triple-axis detector). A capillary column DB-5ms UI (30 m x 0.25 mm x 0.25 μ m) and helium as the carrier gas (1.1 ml/min). The injection of 1.0 μ l of sample diluted in hexane was done at a temperature of 250°C with split mode, split ratio 25:1, the detector temperature was 230°C and the oven temperature was maintained at 60°C for 1.0 minutes, then it was increased to 240°C at 2°C/min. The electron ionization to 70 eV and 230°C was used as the ion source, and the data compounds were collected with the full scan mode (40-1000 μ ma). Finally, the compounds were identified by comparison of their mass spectra and mass reference of Wiley 9th with NIST 2011 MS Library.

Obtaining and Analyzing the Alcoholic Extract

The method used to obtain the alcoholic extract was the maceration from the dry and chopped plant material; a ratio of 1:10 m /v was used, and the extraction was performed in an amber glass container. It was left to marinate for 15 days, removing the solvent daily, and the mash was filtered. For the characterization of the extracts, the procedures described by Miranda and Cuellar (2000), the determinations were made in triplicate; the tests carried out were: pH, density, and refractive index.

RESULTS

The botanical identification was made by Dr. Carmen Bonifaz of Elao, of the Guay Herbarium, de la Facultad de Ciencias Naturales, assigning the identifications number 008 and the code GUAY 13,100.

Results of the macro-morphological analysis, as well as the botanical characterization, showed that the species known as sweet ginger, corresponded to the varitey *Zingiber officinale*, which was classified as *Zingiber ssp*., the so-called spicy ginger, was identified as *Zingiber officinale* Roscoe. The physical-chemical parameters determined to plant rhizomes are presented in Table 1.

The results obtained for the qualitative chemical analysis of the species studied are presented in Table 2.

The analytical gaseous chromatogram of the essential oils of the species under study is presented in Figure 2.

The components identified in each essential oil are presented in Tables 3 and 4.

Table 1. Physical and chemical characteristics of the rhizomes understudy

Parameters	Sweet Ginger	Spicy Ginger
Total ashes	1.648	1.467
Soluble Ashes in Water	0.494	1.139
Insoluble Ashes in Hydrochloric Acid	1.976	0.496
Residual Moisture (Azeotropic)	24.966	13.169
Substances Solubles in Water	10.264	3.595
Solubles in Ethanol (90%)	6.461	4.912

Table 2. Results of phytochemical screening

Essay	Metabolites	Sweet Ginger	Spicy Ginger
Baljet	Lactone	(++)	(++)
Liebermann- Buchard	Triterpenes-steroids	(+)	(+)
Sudan	Oils and fats	(+)	(+)
Fehling	Reducing compounds	(+)	(+)
Ferric chloride	Phenols and Tannins	(+)	(+)
Foam	Saponins	(+)	(+)

Table 3. Most abundant compounds identified in the sweet ginger essential oil

No	Compounds	RIlit[a]	RI[b]	%
1	(2R,3R)-2-Methylbutane-1,3-diol	859[*]	808.91	1.78 ± 0.02
2	β-thujene	962	92183	0.36 ± 0.01
3	α-pinene	936	92952	5.66 ± 0.07
4	Camphene	950	944.57	0.51 ± 0.03
5	Sabinene	973	967.77	0.23 ± 0.00
6	β-pinene	978	975.83	13.55 ± 0.18
7	Myrcene	987	986.27	0.63 ± 0.01
8	α-phellandrene	1002	1004.62	0.22 ± 0.00
9	δ 3-carene	1010	1006.43	0.31 ± 0.00
10	o-cymene	976	1022.02	2.54 ± 0.03
11	1,8-Cineol	1024	1030.78	34.4 ± 0.49
12	E-β-ocimene	1041	1041.98	0.03 ± 0.00
13	γ-terpinene	1051	1053.14	0.61 ± 0.01
14	Terpinolene	1082	1080.77	0.12 ± 0.00
15	α-pinene oxide	1096	1094.36	0.04 ± 0.00
16	Linalool	1086	1099.17	0.72 ± 0.01
17	Trans-p-menthane-2-en-1-ol	1123	1120.72	0.06 ± 0.00
18	α-campholenal	1105	1121.99	0.11 ± 0.00
19	L-pinocarveol	1126	1135.05	0.04 ± 0.00

No	Compounds	RIlit[a]	RI[b]	%
20	3-cyclohexene-1-carboxaldehyde, 1,3,4-trimethyl	1171*	1157.67	0.02 ± 0.00
21	Borneol	1150	1166.42	0.41 ± 0.01
22	Trans-pinocanfona	1109*	1168.61	0.04 ± 0.00
23	Terpinen-4-ol	1164	1175.97	1.72 ± 0.02
24	p-Cymen-8-ol	1183*	1184.59	0.02 ± 0.00
25	Myrtanal	1187*	1186.72	0.01 ± 0.00
26	α-Terpineol	1176	1193.10	3.13 ± 0.03
27	Estragol	1175	119496	2.30 ± 0.04
28	Cis-carvotanacetol	1195*	1205.39	0.03 ± 0.00
29	2-hydroxycineol	1227*	1222.17	0.03 ± 0.00
30	Ascaridole	1290	1243.41	0.04 ± 0.00
31	Chavicol	1219	1257.71	0.09 ± 0.00
32	p-menthan-2-en-1,4-diol	1259*	1270.55	0.04 ± 0.00
33	iso-bornyl acetate	1276	1277.42	0.01 ± 0.00
34	p-menthan-1,8-dien-7-ol	1259*	1294.77	0.02 ± 0.00
35	Cis-2,3-pinanediol	1276*	1316.81	0.25 ± 0.00
36	α-terpinenyl acetate	1322*	1340.61	0.40 ± 0.01
37	α-damascona	1343	1344.66	0.02 ± 0.00
38	Eugenol	1331	1346.52	0.09 ± 0.00
39	β-elemene	1389	1381.27	0.02 ± 0.00
40	Methyleugenol	1369	1400.86	18.21 ± 0.33
41	Caryophyllene	1409	1407.57	0.25 ± 0.19
42	α-gurjunene	1413	1438.10	0.05 ± 0.01
43	Humulene	1455	1443.25	0.07 ± 0.00
44	6-methyl-γ-Ionona	1466*	1462.78	0.01 ± 0.00
45	α-selinene	1474*	1471.54	0.08 ± 0.00
46	Junipene	1432*	1476.35	0.03 ± 0.00
47	(-)-α-Selinene	1494	1483.80	0.02 ± 0.00
48	Ionol	1503*	1495.67	0.02 ± 0.00
49	β-bisabolene	1503	1500.54	0.30 ± 0.01
50	(-)-α-panasinsen	1455	1505.40	0.14 ± 0.00
51	δ-cadinene	1520	1508.37	0.02 ± 0.00
52	Elemicine	1522	1543.71	0.03 ± 0.00
53	2(3H)-Furanone, 5-heptyldihydro	1521	1563.70	0.07 ± 0.00
54	Caryophyllene oxide	1578	1567.13	1.23 ± 0.02
55	Epiglobulol	1530*	1576.55	0.02 ± 0.00
56	Humulene-1,2-epoxide	1601*	1594.38	0.25 ± 0.00
57	Aromadendrene oxide-(2)	1678*	1611.51	0.02 ± 0.00
58	α-cadinol	1643	1643.88	0.05 ± 0.00
59	Longifolenaldehyde	1581*	1656.28	0.22 ± 0.00
60	Phenol, 4-(1,1,3,3-tetramethylbuthyl)	1629*	1694.42	0.08 ± 0.01
61	Bencyl benzoate	1730	1753.38	0.44 ± 0.02
62	Docosane	2200	2297.71	0.11 ± 0.01

Area percentage (n= 3) ± standard deviation.

[a] RIlit: retention indices according to tepenoids library Website (1) otherwise stated.

[b] RI= retention indices measured on apolar capillary columns.

* Mass Spectral Library. Wiley 9th Edition/NIST 2011 MS Library. Agilent Technologies (2).

Table 4. Most abundant compounds identified in the spicy ginger essential oil

No	Compounds	RIlit	RI	%
1	Hexanal	832	801.87	0.03 ± 0.00
2	2-heptanol	880	900.56	0.01 ± 0.00
3	α-pinene	936	928.68	0.03 ± 0.00
4	Camphene	950	944.44	0.11 ± 0.00
5	Artemisia ketone	1044	962.85	0.04 ± 0.00
6	β-pinene	978	973.03	0.01 ± 0.00
7	5-Hepten-2-one, 6-methyl	958*	979.94	0.03 ± 0.00
8	Myrcene	987	985.95	0.15 ± 0.00
9	Octanal	981	1002.11	0.02 ± 0.00
10	α-phellandrene	1002	1004.41	0.04 ± 0.00
11	o-Cymene	976	1020.81	0.03 ± 0.00
12	1,8-Cineol	1024	1027.63	1.43 ± 0.00
13	Linalool oxide trans	1058	1065.67	0.02 ± 0.00
14	Terpinolene	1082	1080.70	0.02 ± 0.00
15	trans-3(10)-caren-2-ol	1131*	1096.44	0.15 ± 0.00
16	L-linalool	1086	1100.82	1.55 ± 0.00
17	2-nonanol	1085	1101.88	0.02 ± 0.00
18	Fenchol	1099	1115.77	0.04 ± 0.00
19	trans- p-menth-2-en-1-ol	1123	1120.84	0.05 ± 0.00
20	cis-piperitol	1181	1138.29	0.04 ± 0.01
21	Camphor	1123	1140.07	0.12 ± 0.00
22	Isopulegol	1132	1143.36	0.05 ± 0.00
23	Citronellal	1129	1148.69	0.24 ± 0.00
24	Isoborneol	1142	1157.72	0.09 ± 0.00
25	1-borneol	1160*	1169.12	3.05 ± 0.00
26	4-terpineol	1164	1176.14	0.35 ± 0.00
27	Cryptone	1160	1180.90	0.03 ± 0.00
28	p-cymene-8-ol	1172	1185.36	0.07 ± 0.00
29	Myrtenal	1172	1188.97	0.10 ± 0.00
30	α-terpineol	1176	1193.13	1.29 ± 0.02
31	Decanal	1180	1204.47	0.05 ± 0.02
32	Hydrocinnamic acid, α, β-epoxy-β-methyl	1215*	1217.20	0.03 ± 0.00
33	Nerol	1210	1222.82	0.07 ± 0.01
34	Citronellol	1213	1228.12	0.17 ± 0.01
35	Geranial	1244	1237.80	3.88 ± 0.02
36	trans-2-caren-4-ol	1176*	1244.23	0.04 ± 0.00
37	Geraniol	1235	1250.32	0.14 ± 0.02
38	2-decenal, (Z)	1240	1259.80	0.36 ± 0.01
39	α-citral	1244	1270.10	6.69 ± 0.03
40	2-undecanone	1273	1290.85	0.14 ± 0.00
41	δ-elemene	1340	1328.08	0.02 ± 0.01
42	8-hydroxyneomenthol	1320*	1335.56	0.02 ± 0.00
43	α-copaene	1379	1366.35	0.23 ± 0.00
44	Bornyl acetate	1270	1381.69	0.30 ± 0.00
45	α-bergamotene	1407*	1396.63	0.16 ± 0.01
46	Cariophyllene	1421	1407.32	0.04 ± 0.00
47	β-cubebene	1390	1418.50	0.02 ± 0.00

No	Compounds	RIlit	RI	%
48	γ-elemene	1429	1420.88	0.05 ± 0.00
49	Cedrene	1424	1433.29	0.02 ± 0.00
50	Aromadendrene	1443	1447.10	0.43 ± 0.00
51	(E)-β-farnesene	1446	1449.24	0.21 ± 0.00
52	α-selinene	1494	1463.04	0.11 ± 0.00
53	Germacrene-D	1479	1469.60	0.28 ± 0.00
54	α-curcumene	1473	1479.06	1.46 ± 0.04
55	δ-selinene	1490	1484.60	0.59 ± 0.01
56	γ-muurolene	1474	1489.63	4.35 ± 0.04
57	Zingiberene	1489	1493.16	8.18 ± 0.08
58	(E,E)-α-farnesene	1498	1504.44	7.99 ± 0.03
59	4-epi-cubebol	1490	1508.08	0.47 ± 0.01
60	δ-cadinene	1520	1511.15	0.28 ± 0.01
61	Calamenene	1517	1513.33	0.10 ± 0.01
62	β-sesquiphellandrene	1516	1521.39	8.53 ± 0.04
63	trans-sesquisabinene hydrate	1564	1537.89	0.05 ± 0.01
64	Elemol	1541	1541.26	0.80 ± 0.02
65	Germacrene B	1552	1545.82	0.17 ± 0.02
66	E-nerolidol	1553	1558.86	1.86 ± 0.03
67	7-epi-cis-sesquisabinene hydrate	1523*	1562.94	0.02 ± 0.01
68	Diepicedrene-1-oxide	1551*	1565.47	0.03 ± 0.01
69	cis-sesquisabinene hydrate	1558	1584.59	1.53 ± 0.09
70	Cariophyllene oxide	1578	1592.94	0.13 ± 0.01
71	α-eudesmol	1653	1596.87	0.23 ± 0.01
72	Cubenol	1630	1601.63	0.07 ± 0.01
73	Zingiberenol	1596	1609.81	3.11 ± 0.02
74	(-)-spathulenol	1625	1613.50	0.29 ± 0.01
75	Globulol	1589	1617.47	1.14 ± 0.18
76	γ-eudesmol	1618	1621.33	0.46 ± 0.01
77	α-acorenol	1623	1638.70	0.28 ± 0.00
78	β-eudesmol	1641	1644.10	3.05 ± 0.48
79	α-cadinol	1643	1646.38	0.92 ± 0.00
80	β-bisabolol	1659	1662.38	0.50 ± 0.01
81	Isoaromadendrene epoxide	1623	1678.31	0.53 ± 0.01
82	Cedrenol	1604	1689.74	3.01 ± 0.00
83	trans-nuciferol	1715	1714.72	0.50 ± 0.01
84	trans-farnesal	1735*	1730.31	0.45 ± 0.01
85	α-sinensal	1726	1739.26	0.23 ± 0.01
86	Cuparenol	1763*	1744.52	0.45 ± 0.01
87	Murolan-3,9(11)-diene-10-peroxy	1729*	1770.81	0.04 ± 0.01
88	cis-Z-α-bisabolene epoxide	1704*	1794.52	0.34 ± 0.04
89	Geranyl-p-cymene	2006*	1940.30	0.12 ± 0.00
90	Geranyl-α-terpinene	1962*	1967.05	0.07 ± 0.01
91	Geranillinalool	2008	2015.54	0.09 ± 0.00
92	6-paradol	2232*	2208.93	0.11 ± 0.00

Terpenoids Library Website. http://massfinder.com/wiki/Terpenoids_Library

National Institute of Standards and Technology. Mass Spectral Library. Wiley 9th Edition/NIST 2011 MS Library. Agilent Technologies.

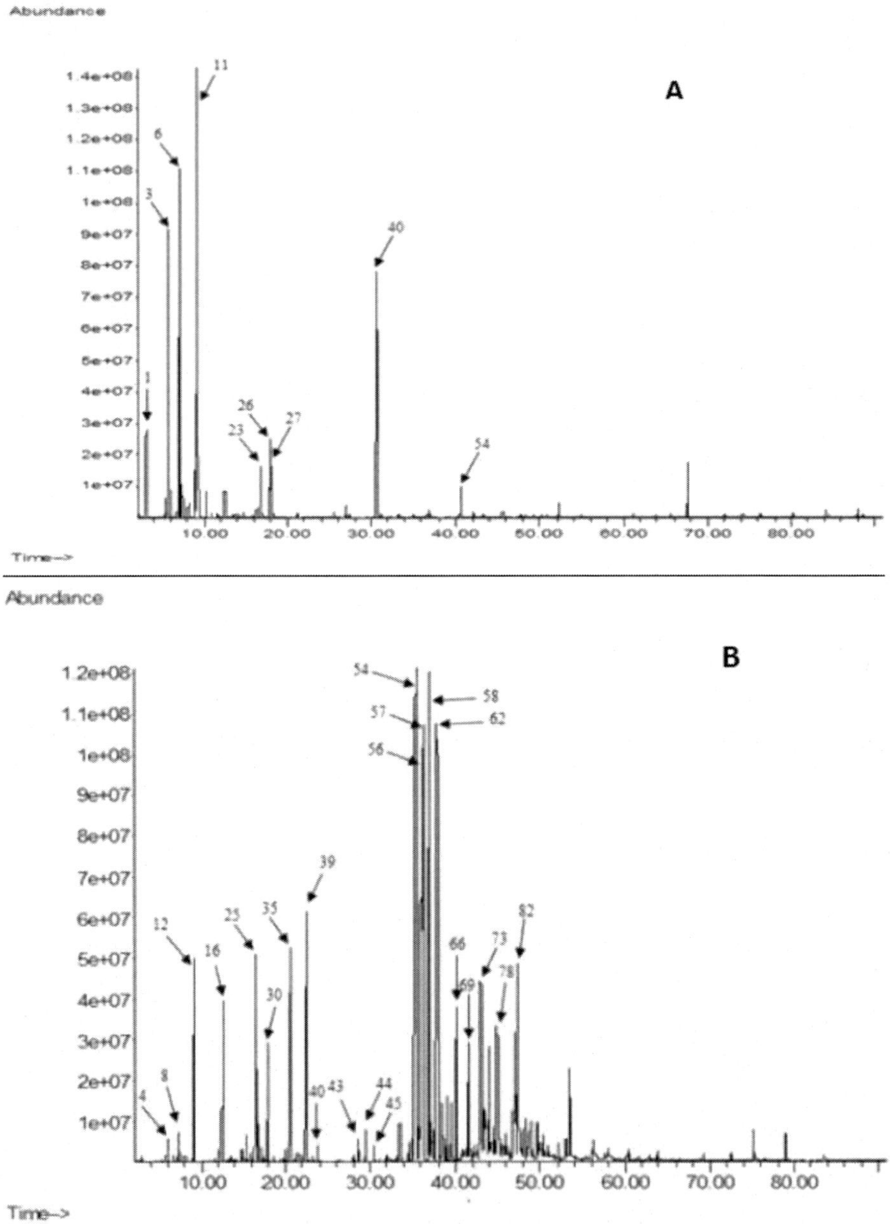

Figure 2. Analytical gaseous chromatogram of the essential oils of ginger understudy. A: Sweet ginger. B: Spicy ginger.

The components detected in both essential oils are presented in Table 5.

The alcoholic extracts of the two species were elaborated from the vegetable rhizomes, and the physical-chemical parameters are presented in Table 6.

These extracts were also subjected to phytochemical screening, and the results are presented in Table 7.

Table 5. Components found in both essential oils

No	Compound	Relative abundance %	
		Sweet Ginger	Spicy Ginger
1.	α-pinene	5.66	0.03
2.	Camphene	0.51	0.11
3.	β-pinene	13.55	0.01
4.	Myrcene	0.63	0.15
5.	α-phellandrene	0.22	0.04
6.	o-cymene	2.54	0.03
7.	1,8-Cineol	34.4	1.43
8.	Terpinolene	0.12	0.02
9.	Linalool	0.72	1.55
10.	Trans-p-menth-2-en-1-ol	0.06	0.05
11.	Borneol	0.41	3.05
12.	4-terpineol	1.72	0.35
13.	p-cymene-8-ol	0.02	0.07
14.	Myrtenal	0.01	0.10
15.	α-terpineol	3.13	1.29
16.	Caryophyllene	0.25	0.04
17.	α-selinene	0.08	0.11
18.	δ-selinene	0.02	0.59
19.	δ-cadinene	0.02	0.28
20.	Caryophyllene oxide	1.23	0.13

Table 6. Quality control parameters of sweet and spicy ginger extracts

Parameter	Sweet Ginger	Spicy Ginger
Density g/ml	0.9224	0.8331
Refractive Index	1.3840 a 25°C	1.3840 a 25°C
pH	6	7
Total Solids (%)	2.2193	1.4526
Taste	Spicy	Very Spicy

Table 7. Phytochemical screening of the alcoholic extracts of the ginger species studied

Metabolites	Sweet Ginger	Spicy Ginger
Resins	(+) Precipitate	(+) Precipitate
Saponins	(+)	(+)
Flavonoids	(-)	(-)
Phenols And Tannins	(++) red wine	(++) red wine
Lactones	(-)	(-)
Reducing Compounds	(+)Precipitate	(-)
Triterpenes-Steroids	(-)	(+) bright green
Quinones	(-)	(-)
Anthocyanidins	(+)	(+)

DISCUSSION

In the physicochemical analysis of the rhizomes was observed that the total ash presented a slightly higher value for the sweet ginger, while in the case of the water-soluble ones, it was much smaller. The acid-insoluble ashes for sweet ginger were markedly superior to spicy ginger. These results suggest that in the sweet species, the alkali metal content (groups 1 and 2) is lower than that of the spicy species, while heavy metals are more abundant in the latter. However, the values obtained for both species are within the range reported for plant species (WHO 2011).

The residual moisture, determined by the azeotropic method to the rhizomes of the species studied, was higher for sweet ginger (24.96%), about spicy ginger (18.624%). Although roots and rhizomes accept a higher water content than other plant organs, it is considered that the values obtained were a little high and that, therefore, the rhizomes should be used in a short time to avoid possible microbial contamination. These values could have been influenced by the fact that the plants were dried at 30°C, to prevent the loss of essential oil. Additionally, it is necessary to take into account that the rhizome of sweet ginger presented a more exceptional thickness than that of spicy ginger.

Regarding soluble substances, differences between species were also observed. Sweet ginger presented values of water-soluble substances superior to those soluble in alcohol, contrary to what happens for spicy ginger, also highlighting the fact that the values obtained for both extracts were much higher in sweet ginger in comparison to spicy ginger. These results point to the fact that there are marked differences in the chemical composition of the species studied.

In the qualitative chemical composition of both species in general, no differences were observed. The metabolites detected were oils and fats, reducing compounds, phenols, and tannins, triterpenes, and steroids, lactones, and saponins.

As for the yield of essential oil, a higher value was obtained for sweet ginger, which yielded 0.5%, while for spicy ginger, the value obtained was 0.2%. In both cases, the yields obtained were low in comparison with those reported, which may influence, among other factors, the place and time of collection, the climate, and the type of soil (Ospina, Orozco, and Correa 2016).

In the chromatographic analysis of the essential oils, differences were observed in the profiles of the essential oils obtained. For the sweet ginger essential oil, structures could be assigned to a total of 62 compounds, highlighting 1,8-cineol (peak 11), as the primary component with 34.4% relative abundance, followed by methyl -eugenol (peak 40) with 18.21%; β -pinene (peak 6) with 13.55% and α -pinene 5.66% (peak 3). The rest of the identified components presented abundances of 1% and lower (Table 3).

Among the components that had the highest abundance in the spicy ginger essential oil, we can point out: sesquiphellandrene (peak 62), 8.53%; zingiberene (peak 57) 8.18%; farnesene (peak 58) 7.99%; citral (peak 39) 6.69%. With relative abundance, we can point out the muruulene (peak 56) 4.35%; geraniol (peak 35) 3.88% and borneol (peak 25) 3.05%. The rest of the components had percentages of an abundance of 1% or less (Table 4).

It should be noted that around 20 components present in both essential oils are similar, but the concentration was different. It should be emphasized the presence of a higher percentage of terpinen-4-ol for the sweet variety so it can be presumed that it must have higher anti-inflammatory activity.

In regards to the physicochemical parameters of the extracts, it was observed that except for the refractive index, there were differences in the rest of the parameters analyzed. Spicy ginger had lower density and total solids content than sweet ginger, and the pH value was in the neutral range, while for sweet it was in the acid range, which may be due to a more significant amount of compounds of phenolic nature.

Regarding the flavor, the sweet ginger presented spicy flavor, characteristic of the species; however, the spicy ginger presented an extraordinarily spicy flavor, causing eye irritation and burning in the mouth. These extracts were also subjected to phytochemical screening, and it is worth noting once again the differences in the metabolites present in both extracts, as well as some differences between the results of the alcoholic extract concerning the vegetable rhizome.

Among the extracts, the following metabolites showed differences: reducing compounds that were positive in the sweet ginger and negative in the spicy and triterpenes and steroids that were positive for spicy ginger and negative for sweet. Concerning plant drugs, compounds such as resins and anthocyanidins tested negative for the drug plant, were positive for the extracts.

Conclusion

The taxonomic classification, as well as the determination of the physicochemical parameters of plant drugs, enabled us to establish that the species called sweet ginger has differences in these parameters in respect to spicy ginger, so it is either one variety or another species, which should be demonstrated through genetic studies. The essential oils of both species showed a different chemical composition, being able to identify 62 compounds for sweet ginger and 92 for spicy ginger. In the alcoholic extracts, there were also differences in the physicochemical parameters and the qualitative chemical composition.

References

Baliga, Manjeshwar Shrinath, Raghavendra Haniadka, Manisha Maria Pereira, Jason Jerome D'Souza, Princy Louis Pallaty, Harshith P Bhat & Sandhya Popuri. (2011). "Update on the chemopreventive effects of ginger and its phytochemicals." *Critical Reviews in Food Science and Nutrition*, *51* (6), 499-523. doi: 10.1080/10408391003698669.

Benavides Manzano, Aida, Carmen Cabadiana Guaman & Cinthya Cordova Tay Hing. (2010). "*Elaboración de un proyecto para la comercialización del aceite de jengibre y su uso en la elaboración de pasteles en la ciudad de Guayaquil*. [*Preparation of a project for the commercialization of ginger oil and its use in the preparation of cakes in the city of Guayaquil*]." Escuela Superior Politécnica del Litoral. [Polytechnic Superior School of the Coast.]

Brahma Naidu, Parim, V. V. Sathibabu Uddandrao, Ramavat Ravindar Naik, Pothani Suresh, Balaji Meriga, Mustapha Shabana Begum, Rajesh Pandiyan & Ganapathy Saravanan. (2016). "Ameliorative potential of gingerol: Promising modulation of inflammatory factors and lipid marker enzymes expressions in HFD induced obesity in rats." *Molecular and Cellular Endocrinology*, *419*, 139-147. doi: 10.1016/j.mce.2015.10.007.

Butt, Masood Sadiq & Tauseef Sultan, M. (2011). "Ginger and its Health Claims: Molecular Aspects." *Critical Reviews in Food Science and Nutrition*, *51* (5), 383-393. doi: 10.1080/10408391003624848.

Ebrahimzadeh Attari, Vahideh, Mohammad Asghari Jafarabadi, Maryam Zemestani & Alireza Ostadrahimi. (2015). "Effect of Zingiber officinale Supplementation on Obesity Management with Respect to the Uncoupling Protein 1 -3826A>G and ß3-adrenergic Receptor Trp64Arg Polymorphism." *Phytotherapy Research*, *29* (7), 1032-1039. doi: 10.1002/ptr.5343.

Ebrahimzadeh Attari, Vahideh, Alireza Ostadrahimi, Mohammad Asghari Jafarabadi, Sajjad Mehralizadeh & Sepideh Mahluji. (2016). "Changes of serum adipocytokines and body weight following Zingiber officinale supplementation in obese women: a RCT." *European Journal of Nutrition*, *55* (6), 2129-2136. doi: 10.1007/s00394-015-1027-6.

Geiger, James L. (2005). "The essential oil of ginger, *Zingiber officinale*, and anaesthesia." *International Journal of Aromatherapy*, *15* (1), 7-14. doi: 10.1016/j.ijat.2004.12.002.

Green, Aliza. (2007). *El Libro de las especias: hierbas aromáticas y especias. [The Spice Book: aromatic herbs and spices]*: Ediciones Robinbook.

Kizhakkayil, Jaleel & Bhaskaran Sasikumar. (2011). "Diversity, characterization and utilization of ginger: a review." *Plant Genetic Resources*, *9* (3), 464-477. doi: 10.1017/ S1479262111000670.

Lee, Jung Ok, Nami Kim, Hye Jeong Lee, Ji Wook Moon, Soo Kyung Lee, Su Jin Kim, Joong Kwan Kim, Sun Hwa Park & Hyeon Soo Kim. (2015). "[6]-Gingerol Affects Glucose Metabolism by Dual Regulation via the AMPKα2-Mediated AS160–Rab5 Pathway and AMPK-Mediated Insulin Sensitizing Effects." *Journal of Cellular Biochemistry*, *116* (7), 1401-1410. doi: 10.1002/jcb.25100.

Li, Chunbo & Lin Zhou. (2015). "Inhibitory effect 6-gingerol on adipogenesis through activation of the Wnt/β-catenin signaling pathway in 3T3-L1 adipocytes." *Toxicology in Vitro*, *30*, (1, Part B), 394-401. doi: 10.1002/jcb.25100.

Mao, Qian-Qian, Xiao-Yu Xu, Shi-Yu Cao, Ren-You Gan, Harold Corke, Trust Beta & Hua-Bin Li. (2019). "Bioactive Compounds and Bioactivities of Ginger (*Zingiber officinale* Roscoe)." *Foods (Basel, Switzerland)*, *8* (6), 185. doi: 10.3390/foods8060185.

Miranda, M. & Cuellar, A. (2000). "*Manual de prácticas de laboratorio: Farmacognosia y productos naturales*." [*Manual of laboratory practices: Pharmacognosy and natural products*]. Ciudad Habana: Universidad de la Habana. [Havana City: University of Havana.]

Misawa, Koichi, Kojiro Hashizume, Masaki Yamamoto, Yoshihiko Minegishi, Tadashi Hase & Akira Shimotoyodome. (2015). "Ginger extract prevents high-fat diet-induced obesity in mice via activation of the peroxisome proliferator-activated receptor δ pathway." *The Journal of Nutritional Biochemistry*, *26* (10), 1058-1067. doi: 10.1016 / j.jnutbio.2015.04.014.

Nammi, S., Sreemantula, S. & Roufogalis, B. D. (2009). "Protective effects of ethanolic extract of Zingiber officinale rhizome on the development of metabolic syndrome in high-fat diet-fed rats." *Basic & Clinical Pharmacology & Toxicology*, *104* (5), 366-73. doi: 10.1111/j.1742-7843.2008.00362.x.

Ospina, Johannes Delgado, Manuel Salvador Sánchez Orozco & Carmen Rosa Bonilla Correa. (2016). "Efecto del secado y la edad de las plantas en la composición de los aceites esenciales de *Lippia alba* (Mill.) NE Br. ex Britton & P. Wilson y *Lippia origanoides* Kunth. [Effect of drying and plant age on the composition of the essential oils of *Lippia alba* (Mill.) N.E.Br. former Britton & P. Wilson and *Lippia origanoides* Kunth]." *Acta Agronómica*, *65* (2), 170-175.

Ravindran, P. N., Nirmal Babu, K. & Shiva, K. N. (2016). "Botany and crop improvement of ginger." In *Ginger*, 35-106. CRC Press.

Roufogalis, Basil D. (2014). "Zingiber officinale (Ginger): a future outlook on its potential in prevention and treatment of diabetes and prediabetic states." *New Journal of Science*, 2014. doi: 10.1155/2014/674684.

Salgado, F. (2011). "El jengibre (*Zingiber officinale*). [Ginger (*Zingiber officinale*)]." *Revista Internacional de Acupuntura*, *5* (4), 167-173. doi: 10.1016/S1887-8369(11)70041-2.

Saravanan, Ganapathy, Ponnusamy Ponmurugan, Machampalayam Arumugam Deepa & Balasubramanian Senthilkumar. (2014). "Anti-obesity action of gingerol: effect on lipid profile, insulin, leptin, amylase and lipase in male obese rats induced by a high-fat diet." *Journal of the Science of Food and Agriculture*, *94* (14), 2972-2977. doi: 10.1002/ jsfa.6642.

Sasidharan, Indu, Venugopal, V. V. & Nirmala Menon, A. (2012). "Essential oil composition of two unique ginger (*Zingiber officinale* Roscoe) cultivars from Sikkim." *Natural Product Research*, *26* (19), 1759-1764. doi: 10.1080/14786419.2011.571215.

Sharma, Gurumayum Jitendra, Pukhrambam Chirangini & Rajkumar Kishor. (2011). "Gingers of Manipur: diversity and potentials as bioresources." *Genetic Resources and Crop Evolution*, *58* (5), 753-767. doi: 10.1007/ s10722-011-9678-5.

Shirin, A. P. R. & Prakash, J. (2010). "Chemical composition and antioxidant properties of ginger root (*Zingiber officinale*)." *Journal of Medicinal Plant Research*, *4* (24), 2674-2679. doi: 10.5897/JMPR09.464.

Shukla, Yogeshwer & Madhulika Singh. (2007). "Cancer preventive properties of ginger: A brief review." *Food and Chemical Toxicology*, *45* (5), 683-690. doi: 10.1016/ j.fct.2006.11.002.

Srinivasan, Krishnapura. (2017). "Ginger rhizomes (*Zingiber officinale*): A spice with multiple health beneficial potentials." *PharmaNutrition*, *5* (1), 18-28. doi: 10.1016/ j.phanu.2017.01.001.

Stoilova, I., Krastanov, A., Stoyanova, A., Denev, P. & Gargova, S. (2007). "Antioxidant activity of a ginger extract (*Zingiber officinale*)." *Food Chemistry*, *102* (3), 764-770. doi: 10.1016/j.foodchem.2006.06.023.

Suk, Sujin, Sang Gwon Seo, Jae Gak Yu, Hee Yang, Eunsun Jeong, Young Jin Jang, Soonham Sami Yaghmoor, Youssri Ahmed, Jehad Mustafa Yousef & Khalid Omer Abualnaja. (2016). "A Bioactive Constituent of Ginger, 6-Shogaol, Prevents Adipogenesis and Stimulates Lipolysis in 3 T 3-L 1 Adipocytes." *Journal of Food Biochemistry*, *40* (1), 84-90. doi: 10.1111/ jfbc.12191.

Tripathi, Pramila, Dubey, N. K. & Shukla, A. K. (2008). "Use of some essential oils as post-harvest botanical fungicides in the management of grey mould of grapes caused by *Botrytis cinerea*." *World Journal of Microbiology and Biotechnology*, *24* (1), 39-46. doi: 10.1007/s11274-007-9435-2.

Tzeng, Thing-Fong & I-Min Liu. (2013). "6-Gingerol prevents adipogenesis and the accumulation of cytoplasmic lipid droplets in 3T3-L1 cells." *Phytomedicine*, *20* (6), 481-487. doi: 10.1016/j.phymed.2012.12.006.

Vásquez, O., Alva, A. & Marreros, J. (2001). "Extracción y caracterización del aceite esencial de jengibre (*Zingiber officinale*). [Extraction and characterization of the essential oil of ginger (*Zingiber officinale*)]." *Revista Amazónica de Investigación Alimentaria*, *1* (1), 38-42.

Wang, Jing, Weixin Ke, Rui Bao, Xiaosong Hu & Fang Chen. (2017). "Beneficial effects of ginger *Zingiber officinale* Roscoe on obesity and metabolic syndrome: a review." *Annals of the New York Academy of Sciences*, *1398* (1), 83-98. doi: 10.1111/nyas.13375.

WHO. (2011). *Quality control methods for herbal materials*. World Health Organization.

In: Medicinal Plants ...
Editors: A. Cardador Martínez et al.
ISBN: 978-1-53618-061-9

Chapter 9

NEW HORIZONS IN THE DIAGNOSIS AND TREATMENT OF PARKINSON'S DISEASE

*María Goretti Arvizu-Espinosa**
Bioengineering Department, Tecnologico de Monterrey,
Querétaro, México

ABSTRACT

In this chapter, we will address Parkinson's disease, one of the neurodegenerative diseases whose incidence and prevalence has increased in recent decades. Different hypotheses about its origin - from age to the intestinal microbiota - will be addressed, accompanied by different advances in their diagnosis. Besides, the symptomatology of the disease is thoroughly reviewed since we are increasingly aware that Parkinson's is not only linked to tremors, 4 out of 10 patients do not present them, so the correct identification of the typical and atypical symptomatology is a cornerstone in the early detection of the disease. Lastly, we develop topics related to the detection, prevention, and therapeutics of the disease, taking into account the patient's quality of life, traditional medicine remedies, and even nutritional and occupational, which makes Parkinson's a disease that must be treated in an individual and multidisciplinary way. Indeed, so far, Parkinson's has no cure or apparent cause, but we must take into account that even when it doesn't kill, it still takes away your life. This condition must be accepted, treated, and be given visibility. The patients with Parkinson's disease and their families are not alone but rather are

* Corresponding Author's Email: goretti@tec.mx.

accompanied by an army of people working so they can have the best life despite having it as a constant companion.

Keywords: Parkinson's disease, dopamine, levodopa, neuroprotection, treatment for Parkinson's disease

ABBREVIATIONS

α-syn	(alpha-Synuclein)
(BDNF)	Brain-derived neurotrophic factor
(COMT)	Catechol-O-methyltransferase
(COX-2)	Cyclooxygenase 2
(DBS)	Deep brain stimulation
DNA	(Deoxyribonucleic acid)
(DA)	Dopamine
(GDNF)	Glial cell-derived neurotrophic factor
(HSPs)	Heat shock proteins
(PD)	Parkinson's disease
(MAO)	Monoamine oxidase
(MAO-B)	Monoamine oxidase B
MPTP	(1-methyl-4-phenyl-1,2,3,6-tetrahydropyridine)
(OECD)	Organization for Economic Co-operation and Development
(SIBO)	Small intestinal bacterial overgrowth
(THC)	Tetrahydrocannabinol

INTRODUCTION

In this day and age, degenerative diseases are a major health problem given the increase in its incidence in the population and, although they are thought to be a problem that occurs only in older people, they may also occur in young people between 20 and 40 years of age.

There are several different approaches regarding the timely diagnosis of degenerative diseases, but in many cases, work is being done to find the root cause of them, as is the case with Parkinson's disease (Parkinson's Disease Research Group 1993).

Parkinson's disease (PD) is a progressive degenerative disease of the nervous system that mainly affects the brain structures responsible for coordinated movement, balance, and posture. Alterations in cognitive function, generalized pain, alterations of the autonomic nervous system, and depression can also be triggered by it (Beitz 2014).

THEORETICAL PERSPECTIVES

Parkinson's Disease Before J. Parkinson

The first reference to Parkinson's disease (PD) can be found in the ayurvedic texts from 2500 a. C, where different types of tremors are described, sometimes with additional manifestations such as excessive saliva, somnolence, and reptilian look, calling it *kampavata* (kampa: tremor), treating it with a set of herbal remedies among which were seeds of plants of the genus Mucuna (Katzenschlager et al. 2004).

In his medical compendiums, the last master of the classical era, Galen (129-199 AD) makes a clear reference to posture changes and the tremor of Parkinson's *"A type of paralysis that prevents walking straight. The tremor is an unfortunate disease; the movement is unstable and without control."*

After the classical Greek, there are no known references until the 17th century, probably due to the drop in life expectancy of the inhabitants caused by the numerous territorial battles.

Subsequently, in 1641, Nicolaes Pietersz Tulp resumed the use of the term tremor and the sufferings related to it.

Franciscus Sylvius de la Boë began evaluating what is now known as tremor disorders, identifying and differentiating between those tremors produced by attempts at voluntary movement, and those that occur while the body was at rest (*Tremor coactus*). This is still an important component of the patients' medical history in use nowadays.

Over time many notable figures from different fields referenced the symptoms of tremors and various motor disorders until finally in 1812 "An essay on the shaking palsy" was published, by James Parkinson, where for the first time the symptoms of the disease were detailed, thanks to the observation of six London patients between 50 and 72 years old, where bradykinesia and postural instability stood out due to their importance (Stern 1989).

James Parkinson stated in his publication that it was a disease that progressed so slowly that patients in the study did not remember when they had presented the first symptoms, although these could start with a certain weakness and a tendency for their hands to tremble. (Kempster et al. 2007)

The symptoms began with progressive tremors; subsequently, the patient had difficulty initiating a movement, and their walk had short steps and with a particular swing of their arms. The symptoms worsened until they disabled the patients, an important consideration to denominate it as a new type of disease (Garcia Ruiz 2004).

Unfortunately, he could not perform any autopsies. However, due to his experience as a scientist and his good clinical eye, he asserted that it was a problem of the central nervous system and not of the peripheral nerves.

Six decades later, Jean-Martin Charcot resumed the studies of J. Parkinson, describing the symptomatology of the disease in further detail, paying more attention when differentiating the types of tremors that the patients showed, especially in states of stillness. Later on, he discovered sclerosis plaques in the brain in patients with a tremor in motion, which were not found in patients with tremor at rest, managing to differentiate between multiple sclerosis disease and the other condition that he named "Parkinson's maladies" in honor of its predecessor (Goetz 1986).

History

Paul Blocq and Georges Marinesco identified cases with parkinsonian tremors due to a tumor in the substantia nigra.

In 1894, Edouard Brissaud said that the location of Parkinson's disease was thalamic, leaning towards the hypothesis of its cerebral origin and therefore rejecting the idea that it was a neurotic or muscular disorder; for him, it was a central alteration of muscle tone.

Later on, around 1913, the German pathologist Friederich Lewy described cytoplasmic inclusions in neurons of the black substance and proposed that they were a marker of the disease. Nowadays, these structures are known as Lewy bodies (Parkinson 1817).

Between the years of 1915 and 1925, Constantine Von Economo was in charge of identifying a disease that became a pandemic, what years later, we would know as the Spanish flu (Spanish influenza). This global epidemic caused a high number of deaths, around 500,000 on the European continent, and with unique sequelae in those who survived, in particular, encephalic manifestations, including Parkinsonian symptoms after suffering. These symptoms were accompanied by a dyskinetic-dystonic crisis, oculogyric crises, bilateral akinetic rigid predominance with some symmetry (Birkmayer et al. 1961).

In 1919, Konstantin Tretiakoff described the loss of neurons in the midbrain area in idiopathic Parkinson's disease and also in post-encephalic Parkinson's (Lange et al. 1994).

By the 1940s, treatments for Parkinson's disease were surgical, such as the works of Spiegel and Wycis, by causing a lesion in the thalamus and subthalamic region, to later be modified by Cooper who used the globus pallidus as a target.

Around 1957, Arvid Carlsson developed a method to measure the accumulation of dopamine in brain tissues, and it was there that he found that dopamine levels in the basal ganglia were very high, a vital brain area for motor functions, he then demonstrated that by decreasing dopamine levels there was a loss in movement control. These effects were very similar to the symptoms of Parkinson's disease. So when levodopa (precursor of dopamine) was administered to animals, which had been used as models, the symptoms improved. These findings meant a change in approach to the disease, and they began to treat patients with different precursors of dopamine, which until now remains as the main treatment (Clarke 1995).

In 1960, Hornikyewicz and Birkmayer, following the path set by Carlsson, were able to demonstrate that the brains of patients with Parkinson's disease presented dopamine levels up to 90% lower than what they usually had, concluding that if the said substance was administered the improvement was notorious and could relieve the patient.

In the decade of the 1960s, a distinctive defect of the disease was irrefutably identified: the selective loss of dopamine-producing neurons, which are a key piece for the control of movement and different motor functions of the body (Watts 1997).

Unfortunately, although it was believed that the problem was solved by administering the missing substance, the eradication of the disease was still far from being achieved since the chronic treatment of the drug brought not only resistance but also some undesirable side effects.

In the 1980s, Birkmayer and his research group found increased odds of survival in patients with Parkinson's disease treated with selegiline. This observation opened a new line of research to treat the disease by focusing on the neuroprotective effect of drugs and to not only counteract the amount of dopamine in the brain (Pearce 1989).

After this and armed with a better comprehension of the pathogenesis, later efforts have been directed not only to the surgical approach in the basal ganglia through tissue implants but also to nuclei stimulation, the use of radiosurgery, and others (Calne et al. 1978).

By the end of the 20th century and with the help of genetic engineering, a new strategy was proposed to attack Parkinson's disease which was cell therapy. Dopamine producing cells from fetuses and also from genetically modified nerve cells were used to produce dopamine. Researchers in different countries managed to perform the transplants, and the patients showed some degree of progress.

In 1997 the World Health Organization established that on April 11 World Parkinson's Day, corresponding to the date of birth of James Parkinson, would be celebrated, with the aim of not only commemorating the British doctor but also of raising awareness amongst the general population of the needs of people suffering from this disease (Kempster et al. 2007).

In 2014, experiments in rat models of Parkinson's disease were performed using embryonic stem cells, which are transformed into dopaminergic neurons and thus restore motor function.

Among the recent clinical trials are those of the research carried out at the University Hospital of Kyoto, Japan, led by neurosurgeon Takayuki Kikuchi and his team, which have implanted around two and a half million precursor cells of dopaminergic neurons in different centers of dopamine activity in a 50-year-old patient. These precursor cells were the result of reprogramming a donor's skin cells. If this trial is successful, it could mean new treatment for patients with this disease (López-González et al. 2018).

General Description

The anatomopathological basis in Parkinson's disease is the progressive destruction of dopaminergic neurons that are in a region of the brain called the basal ganglia; these circuits are involved in the control of movements within the central nervous system. But to understand the above, it is necessary to analyze how of the communication between neurons using the involved neurotransmitters and what happens during the PD (Hurtado et al. 2016).

Structure of the Synapse

The majority of the communication between neurons occurs through the synapse, mediated by peptide and small molecule neurotransmitters.

The small molecule neurotransmitters are usually synthesized in the cytoplasm of the terminal boutons and are introduced into synaptic vesicles;

These are then released from the boutons by exocytosis, because the neuron was stimulated by action potentials, which causes the calcium channels, activated by voltage, to open and the calcium ions enter the bouton, causing the vesicles to fuse with the presynaptic membrane and empty their contents into the synaptic cleft, where they produce postsynaptic potentials in other neurons due to the union of said neurotransmitters with their corresponding subtypes of membrane receptors.

Small molecule neurotransmitters tend to be released at the targeted synapse and activate receptors that act directly on ion channels since they transmit rapid, brief, excitatory, or inhibitory signals to adjacent cells (Pinel 2003).

The monoamines constitute a class of small neurotransmitters and are synthesized from a single amino acid, hence the name of monoamine (Figure 1). These tend to produce diffuse effects, thus regulating the level of alertness, attention, appetite, and other global functions related to balance and motor functions.

The monoamines are present in small groups of neurons whose cell bodies are mostly located in the brainstem. Often, these neurons have very branched axons with many varicosities that release the monoamines to the extracellular fluid.

There are four main monoamines: dopamine, noradrenaline, adrenaline, and serotonin. They are subdivided into two broad groups, catecholamines and indoleamines, depending on their structure.

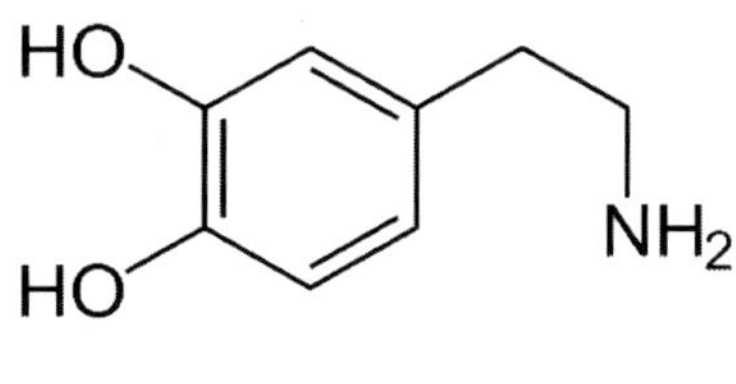

Figure 1. Chemical structure of dopamine (DA), 4-(2-aminoethyl) benzene-1,2-diol.

What happens after the transmission of the message can follow two mechanisms that end it and prevent the communication channel from being obstructed. These two mechanisms of completion are reuptake and enzymatic degradation.

Reuptake is the most common mechanism of neurotransmitters deactivation. Most neurotransmitters, once released, recede almost immediately to presynaptic boutons where they are packaged back into vesicles for reuse.

The other mechanism is degradation, which is performed by specific enzymes for each type of neurotransmitter.

Monoamine oxidase (MAO) and catechol-O-methyltransferase are the main enzymes that metabolize dopamine.

Dopamine serves multiple purposes in the brain, including its participation in behavior, cognition, motor activity, sleep regulation, mood, attention, and learning (Garcia Ruiz 1996).

The neurons whose primary neurotransmitter is dopamine are known as dopaminergic neurons and are found mostly in the ventral tegmental area in the midbrain and the compact part of the substantia nigra, the latter being a heterogeneous portion of the mesencephalon and is one of the fundamental element that helps in connection with the basal ganglia composed of corpus striatum, subthalamic nucleus and the pale external and internal globules (Figure 2) (Obeso et al. 2002).

The striatum is composed of two main nuclei, the caudate nucleus, and the lentiform nucleus.

The striatum has an important role in the motor circuits, specifically in the so-called extrapyramidal circuits, which regulate voluntary movement.

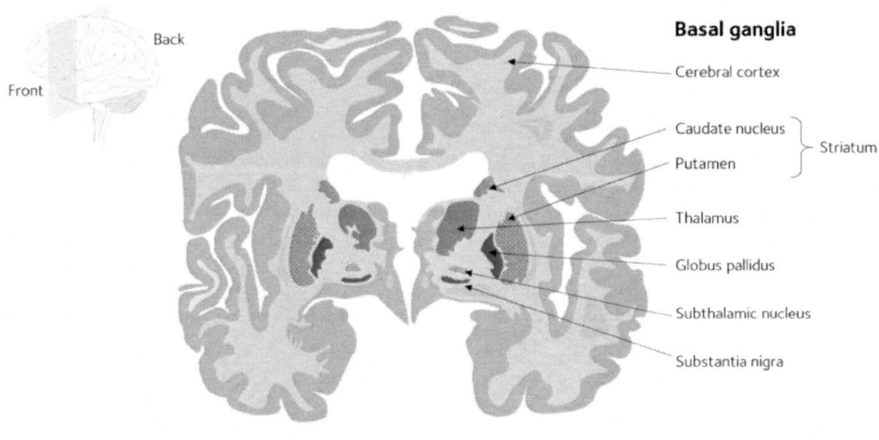

Figure 2. Basal ganglia (by Beckie Port).

The caudate nucleus is involved in cognitive functions since it participates in the connections with the association areas of the cortex and sends them to the prefrontal cortex (Chase et al. 1993).

Among the neurological diseases called synucleinopathies, we can find Parkinson's disease, which is characterized in part by the presence of α-synuclein protein aggregates, which increases intracellular calcium levels causing an increase in calcineurin enzyme activity which in turn affects the function of other proteins and this results in the activation of a toxic program that leads to cell death (Brissaud 1895).

Dopaminergic neuronal destruction causes damages to the substantia nigra, provoking alterations in the activity of the basal ganglia, causing mainly motor disorders and other cardinal symptoms of the disease, among these non-motor symptoms, are sleep disorders and related to mood, dysfunction of autonomous organic systems and cognitive symptoms (Rajput et al. 1997).

Besides, the lack of dopamine produces a tendency for the neurons in the basal ganglia to discharge in an oscillatory manner instead of the physiological tonic activation.

The etiology is unknown, and in general terms, the exact cause of this neuronal loss is unknown, but there may be different environmental or genetic factors or the combination of these that lead to the development of this disease (Braak et al. 2008).

Risk Factors

Advanced age is one of the higher risk factors since it is in these ages where Parkinson's disease most commonly occurs.

The incidence of PD is slightly higher in men than in women.

Family history is another factor that must be taken into account since it is estimated that individuals with one or several first-degree relatives with PD have twice the risk of developing the disease, and it is due to the combination of genetic factors coupled with the environmental ones (Collier et al. 2011)

Genetic Factors

Only 15% of people with PD have a family history of this condition, which can be caused by different mutations in various genes, for example, PARK2, PARK7, PINK1, among others and there are also alterations in genes such as GBA and UCHL1 that seem to modify the risk of developing the disease for some families.

Some gene mutations seem to disrupt the machinery of dopaminergic neurons, and as a result, some proteins do not degrade and accumulate, leading to neuronal inefficiency or death. The above, together with mutations that could affect the mitochondria, causes an increase in the production of free radicals that are also toxic for the cells.

The PARK2 gene encodes the parkin protein, which plays the role of cell degradation by marking damaged proteins and excess ubiquitin molecules, the latter acts as a signal to move proteins that are not needed to proteasomes where they are subsequently degraded. Parkin also seems to be involved in the maintenance of mitochondria since they participate in the process of destroying them when they are not working correctly.

The PARK7 gene encodes the DJ-1 protein, which has different functions, including oxidative stress cell protection, especially in brain cells, as well as serving as a chaperone molecule that helps fold the proteins properly. Several mutations in this gene have been identified that are associated with the early onset of Parkinson's disease, for example, abnormalities in the synthesis of DJ-1 protein cause it to be unstable and therefore its functioning is damaged and is not able to carry out its fusion, increasing oxidative stress and consequently neuronal damage.

The PINK1 gene is responsible for encoding the PTEN protein, which is found in cells throughout the body. Within the cells, the protein can be found in the mitochondria and is thought to function as a protector during periods of cellular stress, especially when there is an unusual demand for high energy. The mutations associated with this protein are related to the early onset of PD. The mutations cause the protein's function to be lost so that the functioning of the mitochondria is affected, resulting in oxidative stress cells and, therefore, their death. The losses of the cells weaken the communication between the brain and the muscles, which causes an inability of the brain to control motor functions (Pickrell and Youle 2015).

The UCHL1 gene is the one that codes for ubiquitin carboxyl-terminal esterase enzyme L1 found in neurons. Ubiquitin serves as a signal to differentiate the proteins that must be displaced to the proteasome to be degraded. The ubiquitin-proteasome system acts as a quality system for the cells because it allows the elimination of proteins that are damaged or in excess. Mutations lead to the reduction of hydrolase activity, which can alter the ubiquitin-proteasome system and instead of degrading unnecessary proteins they could accumulate and therefore be toxic, damaging and even leading to the death of brain nerve cells, which translates into the different symptoms that PD can present (Polymeropoulos et al. 1997; Maraganore et al. 2004).

As for the SNCA gene, it is the one that codes for the α-synuclein protein. This protein is abundant in the brain, being found mainly in presynaptic endings. They interact with lipids and proteins within the structures of α-synuclein. The presynaptic terminations release neurotransmitters that are recognized by their respective receptors. Mutations in α-synuclein cause the formation of aggregates, which causes the presence of Lewy bodies. Other types of alterations related to the SNCA gene cause the synthesis of α-synuclein to double or even triple, which then impairs the functioning of neurons in specific regions (Killinger et al. 2019).

The GBA gene encodes the β-glucocerebrosidase enzyme, which is in charge of activating the lysosomes responsible for breaking down toxic substances and recycling cellular components, helping to break down the glucocerebrosidase molecule into glucose and ceramide. If this enzyme is modified due to a mutation in the GBA gene, toxic substances or protein deposits could accumulate and kill the dopaminergic cells. (Sidransky and López 2012). Most cases of patients with PD occur in people with no family history, which could be the result of some unknown hereditary pattern.

Oxidative Stress

Oxidation-reduction reactions are essential for biological processes; these reactions are mainly based on the transfer of electrons, which in turn generates free radicals and reactive oxygen species.

There must be a balance in the body between the pro-oxidants and antioxidant mechanisms since without such a control the free radicals and reactive oxygen species, what is known as oxidative stress, can cause damage to different structures such as mitochondrial DNA, protein oxidation and therefore the denaturation of these, reactions of lipid peroxidation which would result in the alteration of cell membranes, among others and this would eventually trigger cell damage or even their death. (Ding et al. 2019)

Although there is no direct evidence that oxidative stress is responsible for Parkinson's disease, there are multiple data that implicate the oxidative mechanisms in this condition, such as (Hwang 2013; Obeso et al. 2002):

- Decreased reduced glutathione in the substantia nigra
- Increased iron in the substantia nigra
- Decreased glutathione peroxidase
- Increased activity of peroxide dismutase
- Increased products derived from lipid peroxidation
- Decreased polyunsaturated fatty acids in the substantia nigra

- Alteration of mitochondrial complex I
- Alteration of mitochondrial α-ketoglutarate dehydrogenase.

Proteasome Dysfunction in Parkinson's Disease

Lewy bodies, rich in α-synuclein, are the result of the inefficient removal of α-synuclein. These bodies depend on the balance between the aggregation of α-synuclein and the ability of cells to remove those proteins before a critical concentration level is reached.

It should be considered that Lewy bodies could even be a defensive response of the body itself to avoid the cytotoxicity of aggregate compounds, which could make it part of the pathological process of a neurodegenerative disease such as PD. (Wang et al. 2019).

Under normal physiological conditions, when cellular proteins are no longer used or when they are misfolded or excessively folded, they can be rapidly degraded by different systems, although two pathways are mainly presented, the first being by chaperone heat shock proteins, also known as HSPs or ubiquitin-proteasome.

The union of the HSPs directs the proteins to be degraded by two routes, the lysosomal and the proteasomal; The ubiquitin destines them to the proteasomal path.

The ubiquitination process must be balanced precisely, where ubiquitins bind to the lysine residues of the protein that are meant to be degraded (Ding et al. 2019).

In Parkinson's disease, proteasome activity is decreased in the central nervous system since an increased aggregation of α-synuclein inhibits this activity because the proteasome is dependent on protein concentration.

This could mean that when an altered ubiquitin-proteasome system is present, it can cause oxidative stress, which would then lead to cell death.

On the other hand, the alteration in protein folding could indicate a poorly regulated system at the endoplasmic reticulum level that would also lead to cell death.

By not having an adequate proteasome function, many cellular functions would be affected. Also, since the increased amount of α-synuclein cannot be degraded, this breaks with homeostasis in dopaminergic neurons, further increasing oxidative stress and thus feeding the cycle of degradation and dopamine neuronal loss (Malik et al. 2019).

Other Risk Factors

Neuroinflammation

When referring to inflammation, it is in its conventional definition, with four parameters: heat pain, blushing and swelling; This is because of mediators found in local blood vessels. On the other hand, this type of process can also include the accumulation of fluids, plasma proteins, and white cell cells (Hirsch et al. 2009).

Inflammation of the brain can be neuroprotective since sometimes it benefits from it by promoting homeostasis and repair, but it can also be neuro-destructive because it can favor the action of inflammatory mediators (Michel et al. 2016).

Among the failures associated with neuroinflammation is the overexpression of the major histocompatibility complex molecules, which in turn translates as an increase in the proinflammatory response. Another of the abnormalities that also occur is the formation of autoantibodies against neural structures and the synthesis of pro-apoptotic proteins (Tansey et al. 2010).

The inflammatory pathway of cyclooxygenase 2 (COX-2) has also been implicated in neurodegeneration. COX-2 is expressed and regulated in glial cells by cytokines and lipopolysaccharides catalyzing the formation of prostaglandins, which promote the reduction of levels of oxidizing agents, however, when lesions, synaptic excitation, neuronal death by apoptosis and cerebral ischemia occurs, COX-2 is expressed mainly in neurons (McGeer et al. 1988; Bauer et al. 2007; McGeer and McGeer 2008)

Lewy Bodies

The formation of Lewy bodies with an affectation of the trunk may occur in some cases. These intracellular inclusions, which appear in the substantia nigra, form insoluble aggregates of abnormally folded α-synuclein protein, causing an alteration in the normal cellular physiology resulting in the cognitive damage of the patient and causing dementia at a later stage (Shimoji et al. 2005)

Environmental

Regarding the role of environmental factors, epidemiological studies have identified various environmental factors related to the risk of suffering from neurodegenerative diseases to a certain degree. As for the most important for PD, we have the following:

Pesticides

Parkinsonism was common in the 1980s due to the use of pesticides with opioid components such as MPTP, which is a selective toxic of the substantia nigra. In addition to this component, some pesticides also induce the degeneration of neuronal dopaminergic (Ritz et al. 2009).

Metals

In patients with PD, a greater amount of iron, copper, and zinc have been found compared to those of healthy people. These metals participate in the formation of senile plaques in addition to promoting oxidation processes and interfering with the neuronal homeostasis of important ions such as calcium, which can lead to cell death.

Also, the presence of parkinsonism has been linked to the high exposure of manganese and lead (Bjorklund et al. 2018).

Dissolvent

When working with dissolvent or being exposed to them, they can cause neuropsychiatric symptoms, sometimes even neuronal damage, especially in patients with high exposure to hydrocarbon dissolvents, although they have not been identified as directly related to a predisposition or risk to suffer PD (Dick 2006).

Nutrition

The diet components could play an important part because even though the norms and regulations related to the possible environmental agents involved in PD have been hardened, the prevalence of this disease has not changed; therefore, nutrition is gaining relevance as a disease modifier.

For men, in particular, the consumption of dairy products may be related to PD due to the presence of dopaminergic neurotoxins such as pesticides and polychlorinated biphenyls in these types of products.

As for the excessive consumption of iron, it could be related to a risk factor since it accumulates more in the substantia nigra than in other regions of the brain, induces the release of free radicals such as hydroxyl and is also present in Lewy bodies, plus it favors the accumulation of α-synuclein. The above must also go hand in hand with a genetic predisposition regarding iron regulation (Killinger et al. 2019).

The Gut Microbiota

Trillions of microbial cells colonize the human body; this is literally ten times more than the cells that form the body itself, so its complexity and physiological behavior must be related to the microbiota.

The interactions between the microbiota and the human being influence biological events and processes of health and disease, including those related to the central nervous system that had previously been separated from this complex system (Almaguer et al. 2017).

The intestinal microbiota could even modulate the clinical presentation of neurodegenerative diseases caused by the relationship in the microbiota-intestine-brain axis, due to the influence on cerebral neurochemistry.

The intestinal epithelium is a barrier against pathogens, but since there is an imbalance in the microbiota, damage can significantly alter its permeability and produce oxidative stress, The increase in intestinal permeability is often found in patients with PD, and this is accompanied by a greater accumulation of oxidative stress in the tissues, including some modifications in the morphology of intestinal epithelial barriers. There are even studies that assume that patients with inflammatory bowel disease have a higher risk of developing PD (Hertel et al. 2019).

Several studies mention four primary mediators of inflammation that relate to the central nervous system, enteric nervous system, and Parkinson's disease.

Lymphatic System

This is about a possible way of communication between the gastrointestinal tract and the central nervous system: the lymphatic system. The sinuses of the dura will drain to the brain so that the fluid continues through the body, and both the cerebrospinal fluid and the immune cells can be in contact between these two systems.

In the case of PD, one of the key pathological characteristics is the accumulation of α-synuclein protein, and some studies in animal models have shown that the forms of α-synuclein propagate from the gastrointestinal tract to the brain (Bjarnason et al. 2005).

Toll-Like Receivers

The ability to delimit tolerogenic responses in the intestine while allowing certain inflammatory responses requires communication between the immune cells themselves with intestinal epithelial cells and commensal bacteria of the microbiota. If there is inadequate signaling between any of the factors, it can lead to uncontrolled inflammation.

Toll-like receptors recognize molecular indicators conserved in the microbiota but can also interact with α-synuclein by activating microglial responses that increase the deposition of α-synuclein which would result in more significant dopaminergic degeneration (Streit 2002).

Molecular Mimicry

Molecular mimicry refers to the common elements of different structures that developed in response to evolutionary pressures. In the case of the microbiota, they produce amyloid proteins that can produce oxidative stress, an altered proteostasis, and even activate the innate immune system, and therefore, a pro-inflammatory response that is directly related to PD. (González-Torres et al. 2005)

Aging and Alteration of the Microbiota

The aging process affects the composition of the intestinal microbiota, and this, in turn, modifies the interaction of the immune system, which triggers an increase in chronic inflammation, increasing the levels of inflammatory markers that can be related to PD.

On the other hand, the first studies of the relationship of the microbiota with PD are those that evaluated the association between *Helicobacter pylori* infestation and disease.

In patients over 80 years old, and with parkinsonian manifestations, an increase in the level of *H. pylori* antibodies was observed. On the other hand, it was shown that pathologies, such as gastritis or chronic infections caused by said bacteria, were related to PD. In addition to this, the relationship between the eradication of this bacterium and the decrease in PD symptoms has also been shown (Biagi et al. 2013).

This has suggested that *H. pylori* could influence PD through the activation of microglia, either by the production of neurotoxic substances that could be transmitted and affect brain stem neurons or due to the diffusion of proinflammatory leukocytes or cytokines that could cross the blood-brain barrier.

As for small intestinal bacterial overgrowth (SIBO), it was also associated with PD, since almost a quarter of patients suffer from it. SIBO is directly related to bodily motor deficiencies, and by eradicating it, this results in an improvement of physical motor symptoms; also, this disease can affect absorption due to inflammation of the intestinal mucosa and altered metabolism of bacteria. For example, in patients with PD, there is a decrease in Prevotella enterobacteria, which is responsible for the production of short-chain neuroactive fatty acids and the biosynthesis of folate and thiamine that have a neuroactive health-promoting function. This same bacterium is related to the abundance of the hormone ghrelin, and its secretion is altered in patients with PD and who may be involved in the protection of the normal function of dopamine.

So far, it cannot be entirely determined if the changes in the microbiota are causal or effect of PD, but it can be said that it plays a key point in the promotion of inflammatory cascades, and also of oxidative stress in the brain (Yang et al. 2019).

All of those mentioned above serve to show us that Parkinson's disease has different hypotheses of its pathogenesis, as shown in Figure 3.

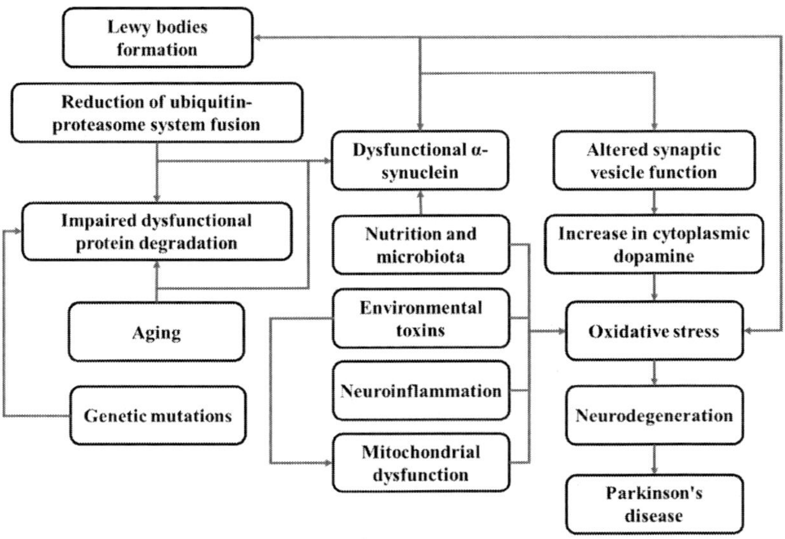

Figure 3. Parkinson's disease pathogenesis hypotheses.

Conditions Associated with Parkinson's Disease

There are different pre-existing conditions in patients that can influence the presence of neurodegenerative diseases such as PD, including diabetes mellitus and hyperhomocysteinemia.

As for diabetes mellitus, the hyperglycemic toxic effects on neurons or even insulin resistance may have a vasoactive effect that affects the metabolism of β-amyloid (Sulzer 2007; Sergi et al. 2019).

As for the increase in homocysteine, it is a neurotoxic substance since it induces motor alterations, causes an imbalance in calcium concentrations due to increasing the flow of said intracellular ion, also generates reactive oxygen species, activates microglia, increases β-amyloid in the plasma and brain. The role that this substance plays in PD is uncertain because some treatments with certain medications increase its level (Siriam et al. 2002; Olanow et al. 2009).

Epidemiology

Parkinson's disease affects 1 in 100 people over 60 years of age, meaning that about 6.2 million people in the world suffer from this disease, and it is estimated that by the year 2030, this figure could be doubled, leading to a public health problem. Nowadays, PD is the second most frequent neurodegenerative disease in the world after Alzheimer's, and that is before taking into account that the global aging of the population will cause that the number of people who will suffer this pathology also increases (Ascherio and Schwarzschild 2019).

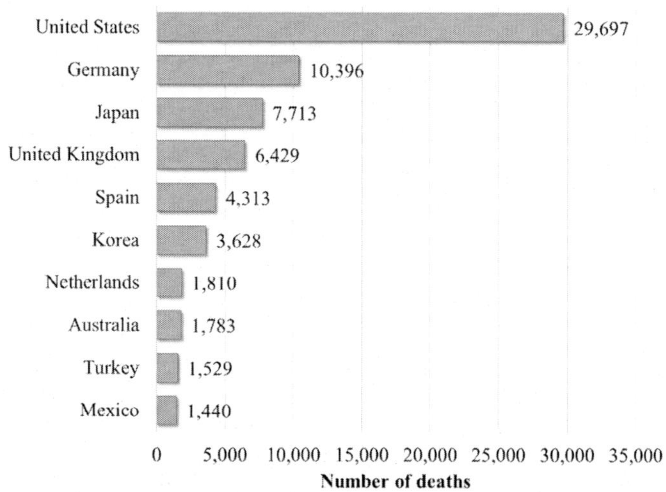

Figure 4. The top 10 countries of the OECD with the highest number of deaths attributed to Parkinson's disease in the year 2015 (Organization for Economic Co-operation and Development, 2019).

It has been estimated that the incidence of this disease in people over 60 is 13.4 per 100,000 inhabitants/year in the United States. In Mexico, the estimated prevalence is between 40 to 50 cases per 100,000 inhabitants/year. In the

National Institute of Neurobiology and Neurosciences, it is the fourth cause of consultation (Parkinson's Disease Research Group 1993). The prevalence of PD has been estimated to be 0.3% and close to 2% in people over 60 years of age. Some studies report a higher incidence in men than in women; this could be explained due to the neuroprotective factors of estrogen, although this is still not proven and is controversial.

The average age of onset is 55 years, and the mean duration of the disease has been calculated to be between 10 to 13 years.

Figure 4 shows the ranking of the countries of the Organization for Economic Co-operation and Development (OECD) with the highest number of deaths recorded due to Parkinson's disease.

Parkinson's Disease Symptomatology

Symptomatology in PD varies in each person; in fact, the first signs can be mild and go unnoticed. The preclinical latency period has been estimated to be from five to ten years, but it can vary. Symptoms might even begin on one side of the body or both. These manifestations are mainly motor-related but may also be non-motor. (Davie 2008)

Motor Manifestations

The patient with PD typically exhibits slow and rhythmic tremors. In 70% of the cases, they occur in a resting state and decrease when performing some voluntary movement. The frequencies revolve around 5Hz.

Muscular rigidity is also present and is known as plastic hypertonia or cogwheel stiffness because, although the limb has resistance to being moved, after a certain point, the resistance disappears, and the movement is easily performed. This is due to the lack of dopamine, causing acetylcholine to stimulate the muscles and, in turn, making it difficult to move.

Postural disturbances occur when the person is standing yet seems tilted, their elbows and knees are bent, which can make it more challenging to maintain balance in the long term (Dauer et al. 2003).

As for the movement disorders that may occur, these include walking with alternating short and fast steps (festinating gait), slow marching, and sometimes it becomes difficult to stop. Episodes may happen where the person with PD locks their feet because they feel like they are stuck to the ground.

Besides, bradykinesia and hypokinesia, which include both the difficulty to start and complete movements, as well as slow voluntary and autonomous movements, cause the simplest tasks to be complicated, severely hindering the quality of life of the patient (Dauer et al. 2003).

Non-Motor Manifestations

The impact that the non-motor manifestations of people with PD have may be greater than that of the motor ones since the negative effect on the quality of life of patients is even greater.

Amongst the consequences caused by motor manifestations that translate into non-motor, we can find sleep disorders since stiffness and hypokinesia can hinder the sleep at night due to the difficulty of turning, changing posture, or getting up, causing in turn daytime drowsiness. When sleep disorder escalates, hallucinations can occur.

Also present are sensory disorders, which can affect up to 50% of patients, manifesting as pain, numbness, and tingling.

Depression and anxiety are diagnosed in almost 30% of people with PD, not only because of the diagnosis of their disease but also as a consequence of the deregulation of the dopaminergic synapse due to neuronal death or alteration.

Cognitive disorders are another manifestation that the patient may present, starting with some confusion, difficulty concentrating, memory loss, and even dementia in very advanced stages (Wider and Wszolek 2008).

In older people, complications of sleep disorder coupled with dementia can trigger the development of psychosis (Sánchez-Martínez et al. 2019).

Clinical Forms

Different classifications are depending on the stages observed or about age or symptoms that occur. Up next, two different ratings are shown; the first related to the age and predominant symptom (Table 1) and the second related to the progression of the symptoms of the disease following the Hoehn & Yahr stages (Table 2) (Bjarnason et al. 2005; Hughes et al. 1992; Lange 1998; Mínguez-Castellanos et al. 2007; Zhao et al. 2010; DeMaagd and Philip 2015).

Table 1. Classification by stages of the disease that are related to the age at which the disease or the most predominant symptom occurs

Name	Features
Tremors	High amplitude tremors predominate, while the rest of the Parkinson's signs are subtle
Rigid akinetic	It is more disabling than Tremoric. There is a higher prevalence of non-motor manifestations, such as depression, sleep disturbances, and dementia.
Juvenile	It occurs in people under 50 years of age; of a more aggressive course, motor abnormalities develop, especially over abnormal and involuntary movements.
Late start	It originates in people from 70 to 90 years. The tremor is not very pronounced, and disturbances of balance or gait disorders evolve faster. The development of dementia in this classification is more common.

Table 2. Classification of patients with Parkinson's disease according to the Hoehn & Yahr stages

Classification	Stage	Symptoms
Recently diagnosed patients	Stage I Unilateral affectation	-Disease onset -Erect posture -Normal facial expression -Slight symptoms of the parkinsonian triad (stiffness, tremor, and bradykinesia) begin
	Stage II Bilateral affectation, normal balance	-There is an asymmetry in the intensity of the symptoms, with the initial side being the most affected. -Presence of first postural disorders. -Start of the adduction of the upper limbs. -Depression symptoms
Moderately affected patients	Stage III Bilateral involvement, with impaired balance	-The emergence of balance disorders. -The affection of postural reflexes-Spontaneous falls -Festinating gait -Freezing of gait
	Stage IV Increase in the degree of dependency	- Major bilateral affectation and increased postural instability. -Inability to stay upright unless helped -Cognitive Difficulties -Behavioral problems
Severely affected patients	Stage V Severe and severely developed disease.	-Not all patients reach this stage -Complete dependant - Accentuated language disorders -Development of contractures -Possibility of ulcers and infections -Confinement to bed or wheelchair

There are other types of Parkinson's, but they are as a consequence of other neuropathological alterations that also affect the substantia nigra and the striate body projections; these should be ruled out for the differential diagnosis of the disease, for example (Hughes et al. 1992).

Natural aging: In old age, slow movements, modified posture, instability, and muscle stiffness are normal and can be differentiated from PD since in the latter the progression of the signs is accelerated in addition to the resting tremor usually present.

Progressive supranuclear paralysis: Also known as Steel-Richardson-Olszewski disease, where oculomotor disorders predominate and are generated from the deterioration of cells in areas of the brain that control body movements and reasoning, it can cause life-threatening complications such as swallowing problems.

Post-encephalic parkinsonism: This disease represents the classic sequelae of lethargic encephalitis due to a condition of different neurotropic viruses (Toledo-Aral et al. 2002).

Diagnosis of Parkinson's Disease

Currently, there is no specific test to diagnose PD, but the neurologist will diagnose the disease based on the person's medical history, review of signs and symptoms, as well as physical and neurological exams.

Between 20% and 40% of people with Parkinson's disease show signs of depression since the onset of the disease and, in some cases, even a few years earlier. Slowness and clumsiness, which can be caused by PD, are frequently associated with effects related to depression, causing a significant delay in diagnosis.

On the other hand, morphological and functional neuroimaging techniques such as computed tomography by monophotonic emission or dopamine transporter scan can help support the suspected diagnosis (Olanow et al. 2001; Mínguez-Castellanos et al. 2007)

There is a proposal for selective diagnostic criteria to increase its safety, which is the following (Radhakrishnan et al. 2018).

Step I: There must be bradykinesia and at least one of the following symptoms: muscle stiffness, posture instability, or resting tremor between 4 to 6Hz.

Step II: Criteria for exclusion of PD, where diseases, symptoms, intoxications, drug treatments or sequelae that could present Parkinsonian syndromes are eliminated.

Step III: Prospective support criteria: These are the positive support data during the follow-up of the disease. Three or more of the following signs must be present: unilateral onset, presence of tremor at rest, progressive course, persistent asymmetry with a more significant effect of the side where symptoms or alterations began to be noticed, 70% improvement in response when provided antiparkinsonian treatments, response to levodopa for at least five years.

As for genetic studies, they are only recommended in cases with a clear family transmission with several first-degree relatives affected by this pathology (Orayj et al. 2019)

Finally, the post-mortem diagnosis is the only one with certainty where depigmentation and degeneration of the substantia nigra with Lewy bodies are conclusive (Hughes et al. 1992)

Prediction and Prevention

There are no simple and non-invasive techniques that can identify or quantify the neurodegenerative changes that the brain is beginning to suffer and that are related to Parkinson's.

For that reason, the development of techniques that allow diagnosing patients in the prodromal stage is essential, considering that the success of many therapies to slow down or stop the neurodegenerative process depends entirely on its early application.

Researchers are working on the identification of biomarkers, that is, a substance that can be used as an indicator of biological status. The criteria proposed must be linked to the fundamental characteristics of the neuropathology of PD and its neurodegeneration mechanisms, as well as to the relationship of the disease progression evaluated by different clinical classifications. (Olanow and Kordower 2009)

Currently, there is no well-identified biomarker, but there are some substances that could become good study options such as pathological forms of α-synuclein, some patterns of genetic expression, protein profiles, among others (Caraceni et al. 1991).

On the other hand, magnetic resonance imaging in its diffusion resonance modality, using a procedure called tractography, allows us to identify how different areas of the brain are connected between themselves, which lets us elaborate a "road map" with increased or reduced communication capacity, enabling us to know thus how and with whom the neurons connect, obtaining an automatic learning algorithm that can then differentiate between healthy people and people with Parkinson's disease, as well as in people susceptible to having prodromal Parkinson's (Jellinger 1999).

Treatment

Although Parkinson's disease has no cure, medications could significantly improve symptoms, always accompanied by an interdisciplinary team.

The purpose of treatment is to control and relieve symptoms, which improves the patient's quality of life for as long as possible. These treatments range from physical exercise, diet, complementary therapies such as speech therapy, emotional support to the ideal drug treatment for the stage of the disease, or even, in some cases, surgical treatment (Grandas et al. 1998).

There are preventive treatments that are mainly aimed at neuroprotection since they interfere with the cause of death of dopaminergic neurons to try to prevent or slow the progression of the condition, although, for this treatment to be applicable, the diagnosis is necessarily required very early (Lange 1998).

Another therapy under investigation is the use of anti-inflammatory agents of which COX-2 inhibitors have given good results in animals, although this does not precisely reflect the entire cascade of processes that are not resolved by a single therapy.

Regarding pharmacological treatments against PD, three categories can be observed. The first, where medications are aimed at increasing levels of dopamine in the brain. The second, where the medications are specifically to treat Parkinson's disease, affecting the other neurotransmitters, but relieving some symptoms of the disease. And finally, the third category is those prescribed to control the non-motor symptoms of the disease.

Medicines that Increase Dopamine Levels in the Brain

The drugs that are commonly used for PD and that are precursors of dopamine usually first cross the blood-brain barrier and then are biochemically modified to become dopamine, the most frequently used is levodopa (Figure 5) (Cotzias 1968).

Levodopa

Levodopa is the most effective medication for the treatment of PD since it is decarboxylated and transformed into dopamine. The reason why levodopa is administered instead of dopamine is that the former can cross the blood-brain barrier, and the latter cannot. The levodopa takes advantage of the membrane transporters of aromatic amino acids of the central nervous system; later it is transformed into dopamine and transported inside the presynaptic or postsynaptic dopaminergic terminals where they can be stored again or metabolized because the nitric and striated body cells have not decreased and they retain their receptivity to the dopamine that is given (Carlsson et al. 1957; Markham and Diamond 1981).

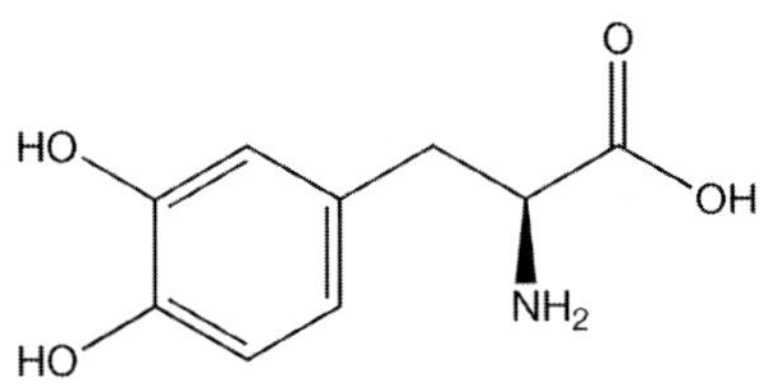

Figure 5. Levodopa (L-3,4 dihydroxyphenylalanine).

Often levodopa is so effective that some people may not show symptoms during the early stages of the disease as long as they take the medication properly. However, levodopa is not a cure. Although it can reduce symptoms over time, the ability to transform levodopa into dopamine is lost, as well as the loss of its receptivity, which leads to a decrease in the response of the medication (Marsden and Parkes 1977; Fahn et al. 1984).

Usually, levodopa is normally administered together with carbidopa or benserazide since this is a dopa decarboxylase inhibitor and enzyme inhibition does not occur; levodopa decarboxylates into the periphery transforming into dopamine which due to its nature it is not possible to enter the central nervous system. When decarboxylase is inhibited, the fraction of the levodopa that remains without metabolism increases (almost 80%), crossing the blood-brain barrier (Block et al. 1997, Quinn et al. 1986).

There are short- and long-term side effects when using levodopa, and these are: (Marsden 1994).

- In the short term: The person may have orthostatic hypotension, nausea, vomiting, sleep disturbances.
- In the long term: after three to five years of maintaining treatment with levodopa, more than 60% of patients will present with chronic levodopa therapy syndrome, which consists of fluctuations in mobility and presence of dyskinesias, not only due to progressive nigrostriatal degeneration but also for the chronic administration of levodopa (Clarke 1995).

Dopamine Agonist Medications

Unlike levodopa, dopamine agonist medications are not transformed into dopamine, but they do mimic the effects of this catecholamine in the brain, and although they are not as effective as levodopa, your period of duration is longer.

Many potential side effects are similar to those caused by levodopa since the neurological effect is the same; these are among them:

- Sleep disorders such as drowsiness, sudden onset of sleep, nightmares, among others.
- Confusion
- Dyskinesias
- Vomit

Some examples of dopamine agonist medications are pramipexole, ropinirole, cabergoline, fenoldopam, among others, and their presentations vary according to the needs, since they range from injectables for rapid relief such as apomorphine, to patch administration such as rotigotine (Figure 6) (Defer 1999).

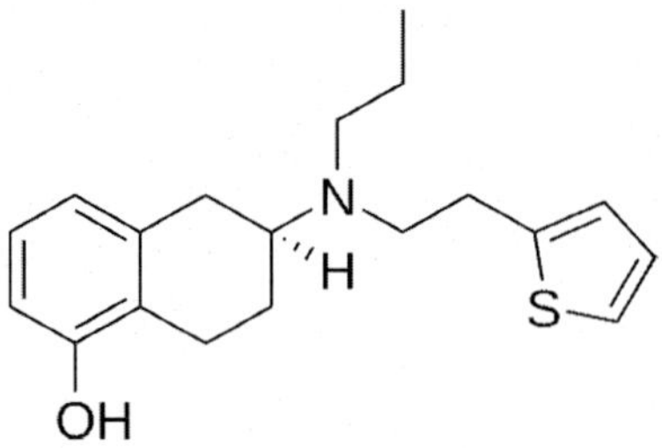

Figure 6. Rotigotine, dopamine agonist medication.

Medicines That Inhibit the Degradation of Dopamine

Within this category of drugs, we find two main groups of enzyme inhibitors that participate in the degradation of catecholamine, which are:

Monoamine Oxidase B (MAO-B) Inhibitors

These medications inhibit the MAO-B enzyme, which causes dopamine not to degrade and increase its amount, accumulating it in the surviving neurons and therefore reducing the symptoms of PD.

One of the most commonly used MAO-B inhibitors in selegiline (Figure 7), which is a substituted phenethylamine. This medicine binds to plasma proteins at a rate of 94%, thus crossing the blood-brain barrier and reaching where the dopaminergic neuron is found and thus inhibiting MAO.

Generally, medications such as selegiline, are administered with levodopa, and this seems to increase and prolong the response of this second drug.

As for the side effects of MAO-B inhibitors, they may include nausea, orthostatic hypotension, or insomnia, although they are usually well-tolerated (Larsen et al. 1999; Przuntek et al. 1999).

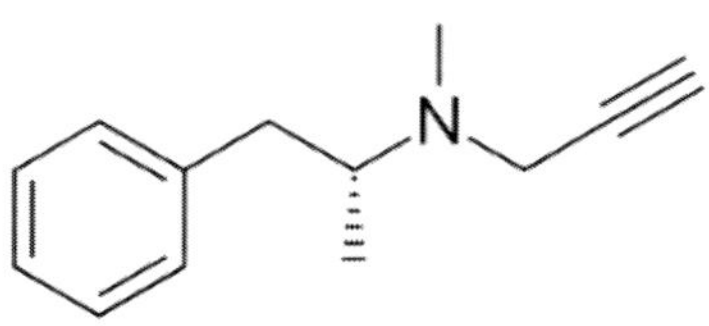

Figure 7. Selegiline, MAO-B inhibitor.

Catechol-O-methyltransferase (COMT) Inhibitors

This class of drugs inhibits the enzymatic activity of catechol-*O*-methyltransferase (COMT) that participates in the degradation of dopamine.

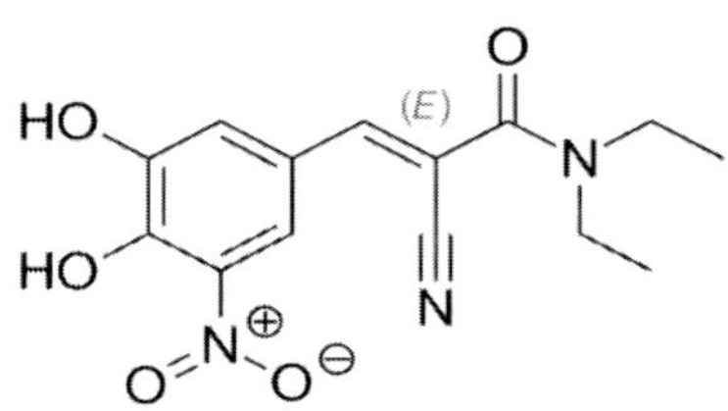

Figure 8. Entacapone, COMT inhibitor.

Among the most commonly used COMT inhibitors drugs are entacapone (Figure 8) and tolcapone, which also not only prevent dopamine from degrading, but also prolong the effects of levodopa, as it increases the chemical stability of the latter in the plasma, so it causes to increase the amount of levodopa available to cross the blood-brain barrier, and therefore the amount that reaches the brain is greater.

Among the most common side effects of this type of medication are diarrhea, although they can also cause nausea, dizziness, change in urine color, abdominal pain and some sleep disorders (Orayj and Lane 2019; Van Kessel and El Aidy 2019).

Central Anticholinergics

By decreasing dopamine due to the death of dopaminergic neurons, acetylcholine, a dopamine antagonist neurotransmitter, produces more intense effects and interacts with their respective receptors more easily, which causes some effects such as stiffness to intensify and also trembling at rest. The above does not refer to the fact that there is an increase in the synthesis of acetylcholine but that the effect on its receptors is increased (Trousseau 1861; Jenner 1995).

Anticholinergic drugs act on the action of acetylcholine by decreasing the action of this neurotransmitter and therefore decreasing the effects of overstimulation of its receptors.

Some of the drugs found in this classification are trihexyphenidyl, benztropine, and ethopropazine, having efficacy particularly on tremors.

However, the benefits of this type of medication are usually counteracted by their side effects, since sometimes they tend to affect the patient's quality of life more often, including loss of memory, confusion, hallucinations, urination problems, among others.

Other Drugs: Amantadine

This drug is an antiviral specifically developed to treat type A influenza in children but is currently not recommended for that use. It is currently used in the early stages of PD, and although it is not known how it works exactly, it is assumed that it has an anticholinergic effect, in addition to participating in the increase of releasing dopamine and in the inhibition of its reuptake.

Among the side effects of amantadine is difficulty concentrating, anxiety, gastrointestinal intolerance, and intoxication causing in some cases renal failure (Orayj et al. 2019; García-Revilla et al. 2019; Gazerani 2019).

Pharmacological Treatments of Non-Motor Manifestations

In addition to most motor manifestations, attention should also be paid to non-motor symptoms, which usually have pharmacological treatment options, which, although sometimes limited, can usually improve the quality of life of patients by counteracting said types of symptoms (Schapira 2009).

Table 3 shows some of the non-motor symptoms and the drugs used to keep them under control.

Table 3. Pharmacological treatments for non-motor symptoms of PD

Non-motor symptom	Drug	Type of drug
Dementia	Rivastigmine	Acetylcholinesterase Inhibitor
Depression	Pramipexole	Dopamine Agonists
	Citalopram, escitalopram	Serotonin reuptake inhibitors
	Desipramine	Tricyclic antidepressants
	Nortriptyline	Tricyclic antidepressants
Psychosis	Clozapine	Atypical antipsychotics
	Rivastigmine	Acetylcholinesterase Inhibitor
Rapid eye movement behavior disorder	Clonazepam	Benzodiazepine
Constipation	Polyethylene glycol	Osmotic laxatives
	Lubiprostone	Chloride Channel Activator
Gastrointestinal motility	Domperidone	Peripheral Dopamine Antagonist
Orthostatic hypotension	Domperidone	Peripheral Dopamine Antagonist
	Fludrocortisone	Mineralocorticoids
Sialorrhea	Atropinics	Anticholinergic
Chronic fatigue	Methylphenidate	Dopamine and norepinephrine reuptake inhibitor

Surgical Treatments

Surgical treatment is proposed to improve symptomatic control in patients that drug therapy is no longer sufficient or due to the appearance of limiting side effects, which some surgical treatments imply in the destruction of specific areas of the brain and contributes to the improvement of the symptoms of the disease (Jellinger 1999).

The surgical procedure for injury is pallidotomy, which consists of selectively destroying a portion of the brain known as a pale balloon causing a scar and reducing brain activity in the area, which helps relieve motor symptoms such as tremor and stiffness, slow movement, and even in some cases, balance and speech are improved. (Samii et al. 1999).

On the other hand, there is thalamotomy, which is the invasive surgical procedure, which aims to remove or excise a small part of the thalamus, found near the base of the brain, which is responsible for controlling some involuntary movements, and, therefore, after the extraction, it is intended to reduce the tremor in PD. (Krack et al. 1998)

Currently, the surgical treatment is based on deep brain stimulation; this method is based on implanting an electrode in the brain, usually in the subthalamus or pale globule. This electrode is similar to a pacemaker that generates the pulse, through the use of a battery, which is implanted in the thorax under the clavicle and sends small and controlled electrical signals through a cable placed under the skin. (Benbid et al. 1996) The pulse generator and electrodes stimulate the brain painlessly to help block the signals that cause disease symptoms (Limousin et al. 1998) (Table 4).

Table 4. General effects of deep brain stimulation (DBS) on brain nuclei

Nucleus	Effect of DBS
Subthalamic	Improves the processing of sensory signals, movement initiation, verbal abilities, visual memory and face recognition.
Internal pale globule	Improves swallowing, balance, and gait, as well as inhibiting dystonia.
Intermediate ventral nucleus of the thalamus	Decreases essential tremor and tremor refractory to therapy.

The pulse generator can be programmed externally, and a manual device can also be used. The battery can last between 3 and 5 years (Hassler et al. 1958; Limousin et al. 1995).

Patients who can benefit from deep brain stimulation are those with motor complications or dyskinesias due to drug treatment, or in those who do not have improvements in their symptoms.

Deep brain stimulation is not a total cure against PD, since continuous degeneration and symptoms can return gradually, and like any brain surgery, this technique presents atypical but potential complications, such as cardiovascular accidents, cerebral hemorrhages, as well as the risk of infection, among others (Freeman et al. 2006).

Complementary Therapies

As for chronic and degenerative diseases, there is a wide and variable class of complementary therapies, including physiotherapy, occupational, and language therapies, as well as psychological therapy to cope with the disease. Without forgetting that nutrition, mentioned above as a risk factor, is also a great tool to be able to counteract the effects of the disease (Donate et al. 2007).

Physical Exercise

In recent times, physical exercise has shown beneficial effects in patients with PD. These effects can be observed in the control of blood pressure in patients, improvement in mobility and balance, increase in gait speed, control over bodyweight and, therefore, physical endurance and muscle strength.

The psychological benefits such as increased self-esteem and well-being are also significant, which leads to a reduction in stress, it also improves the social behavior of patients since it avoids social isolation.

Due to those above, patients with PD must carry out rehabilitation therapies to obtain better results in symptom control processes and help their functional recovery; however minor it may be (Palasz et al. 2019).

Nutrition as Supportive Therapy

Part of the involvement and origin of neuronal death is related to oxidative mechanisms, so antioxidant therapy can result in effective treatment. These types of compounds are acquired naturally from the diet, so this type of supportive therapy is gaining more and more relevance.

Microbiota Restorers

The influence of the intestinal microbiota on the functioning of the central nervous system, and the relationship between its changes and the clinical severity or presentation of PD, concludes that a therapeutic strategy that should be used is prebiotics and probiotics in affected patients.

Some specific probiotics can restore the microbiota and thus maintain immune homeostasis, as well as modulate brain function, and improve symptoms of anxiety and depression, which are psychological effects that frequently occur in patients with PD.

By improving intestinal function, the associated neuroinflammation decreases, and even the absorption of medications is improved. (Hirsch et al. 2009).

On the other hand, by supplementing with prebiotics, such as galactooligosaccharides and fructooligosaccharides, the proliferation of pathogenic bacteria can be antagonized, balancing, and improving homeostasis.

The bacteria of the microbiota, when in equilibrium, can produce short-chain fatty acids that improve immune function and promote neuroprotection, in addition to promoting the integrity of the intestinal epithelium (González-Torres et al. 2005).

Another of the properties that some probiotic strains possess is antioxidant since they produce enzymes such as superoxide dismutase and, therefore, could limit the effects of prooxidant substances.

Flavonoids

Flavonoids are a family of polyphenolic compounds, products of the secondary metabolism of plants, which are found abundantly in fruits, seeds, and leaves. These metabolites participate in the protection against UV light, cold, different pathogens, among others.

The flavonoids family is heterogeneous and can have various beneficial effects for different diseases, depending on the type of structure they possess.

One of the most studied benefits, and perhaps one of the most prominent, is its antioxidant activity since it has been shown that they trap free radicals and are even chelators of metal ions; they also can act as indirect antioxidants and interact with antioxidant enzymes.

Different mechanisms have been proposed to explain the neuroprotective action of this class of metabolites; for example, flavonoids capable of activating endogenous antioxidant pathways of neurons have been reported, which as a consequence results in an action against their degeneration. (Larit et al. 2018).

Baicalein, a flavonol, is effective for reducing the production of hydrogen peroxide, thus preventing damage to dopaminergic neurons.

There are also different flavonoids, such as quercetin, rutin, and isoquercetin, that increase the expression of antioxidant enzymes, such as glutathione peroxidase, catalase, and superoxide dismutase in PC3 cells.

Also, flavonoids have been found to attenuate the JNK, ERK5, and p38 signaling pathways, which cause neuroinflammation processes to be negatively regulated. (Hirsch et al. 2012)

PHYTOCHEMICAL NEUROPROTECTIVE COMPONENTS

In the last decade, an exhaustive investigation has been carried out on the discovery of candidates for new neuroprotective drugs based on natural products such as plant extracts to treat PD.

A summary of some of these molecules that are under clinical investigation to be used as potential neuroprotective agents in PD can be seen in Table 5.

Table 5. Phytochemical neuroprotective components

Bioactive compound	Biological Effect
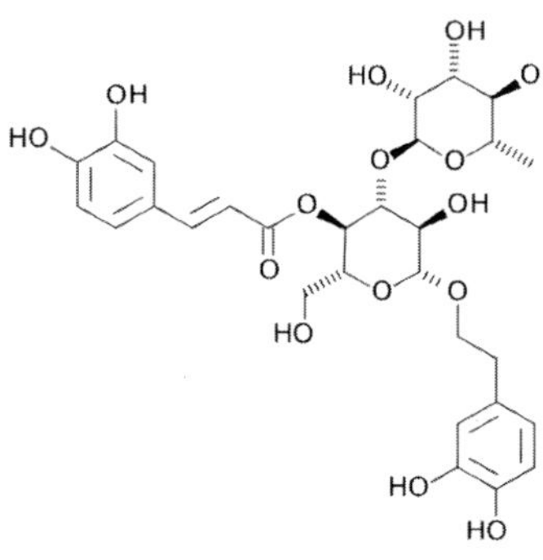 Acteoside	- Reduces the excision of parkin protein. - Inhibits the expression of α-syn - Increases content of DA. (Gao and Pu 2007; Lee et al. 2005; Zhao and Pu 2006)
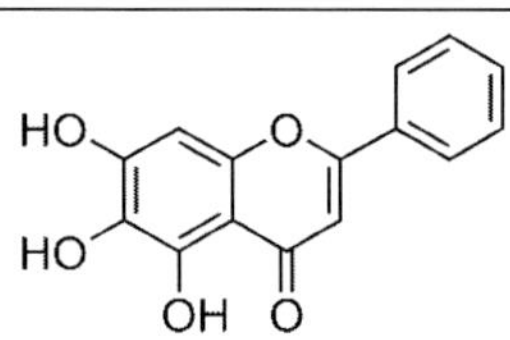 Baicalein	- It improves mitochondrial functioning and prevents the production and accumulation of reactive oxygen species. - Attenuates muscle tremors in rats. - Improves impaired spontaneous motor activity. - Increases the count of dopaminergic neurons. (Mu et al. 2011; Cheng et al. 2008; Lu et al. 2011)

Table 5. (Continued)

Bioactive compound	Biological Effect
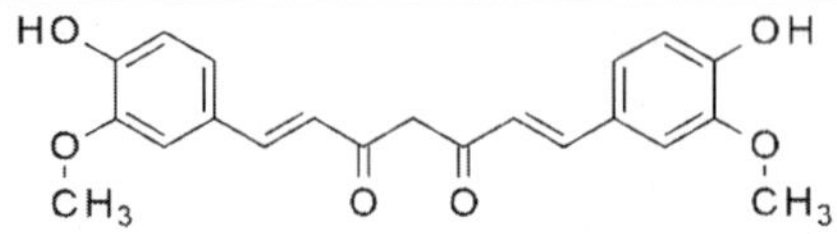 Curcumin (Keto form)	- Decreases: - Loss of dopamine axons. - The disappearance of dopaminergic neurons. - The cytokinins. - Total nitrite generation. - The expression of inflammatory protein markers. (Gupta et al. 2012; Jiang et al. 2013; Wang et al. 2010; Tripanichkul and Jaroensuppaperch 2012)
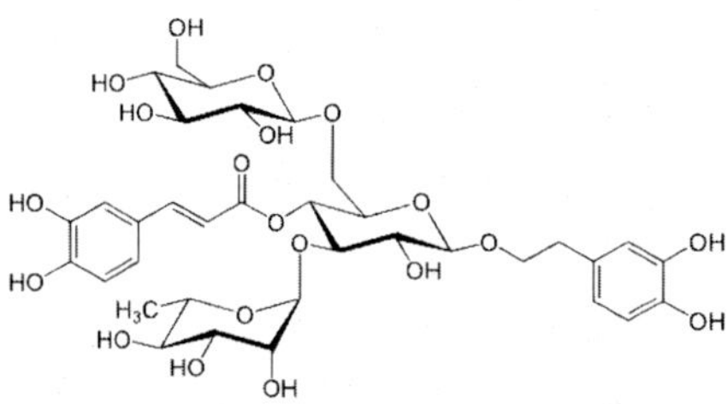 Echinacoside	- Active inhibitor of oral apoptosis. - The inductor of neurotrophic factors. (Zhao et al. 2010)
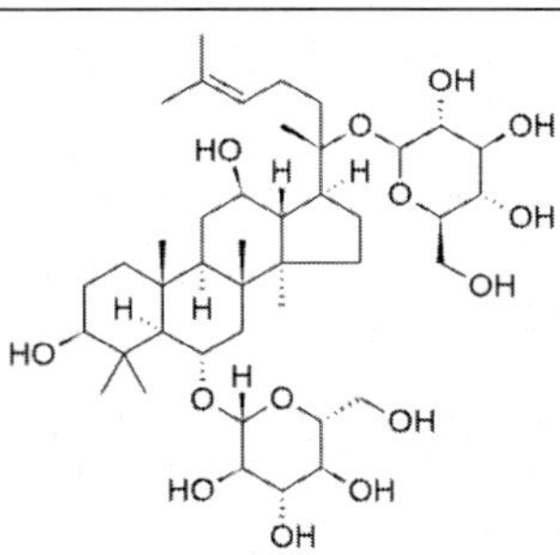 Ginsenoside Rg1	- Decreases the overproduction of reactive oxygen species. - Presents neuroprotective effects in dopaminergic neurons. (Hu et al. 2011; Xu et al. 2009)
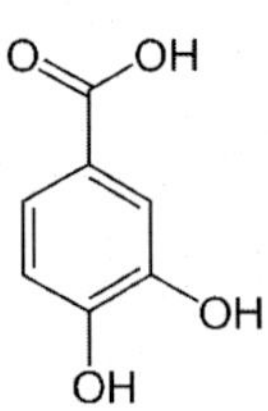 Protocatechuic acid	- Decreases: - Apoptotic morphology. - Cytotoxicity. - Mitochondrial dysfunction. - The abnormal entanglement of α-syn. (Guan et al. 2006; Zhang et al. 2009; Zhang et al. 2010)

Bioactive compound	Biological Effect
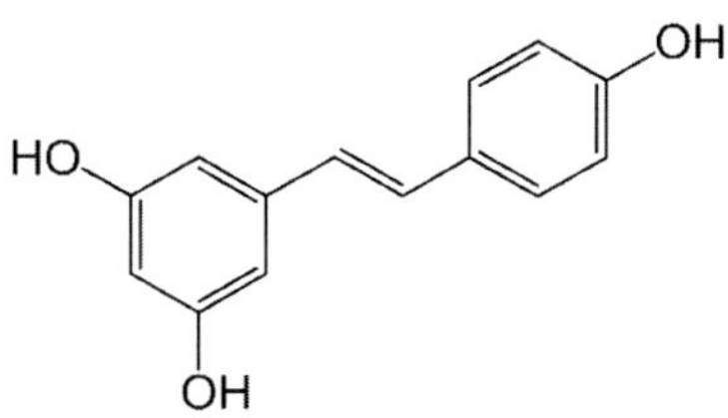 Resveratrol	- Attenuates induced dopaminergic cell death. - Modulate myeloperoxidase levels. - Improves degradation of α-syn. (Wu et al. 2011; Khan et al. 2010; Wang et al. 2011; Chao et al. 2010)

Vitamins

Since oxidative stress plays an important role in the mechanism of dopaminergic neuron death in PD, vitamins are valuable antioxidant agents that can counteract some of the effects of the pathophysiological mechanisms of the disease (Yang et al. 2019).

Vitamins are essential nutrients that the body is not able to synthesize, so they must be present in the diet. Vitamins can be classified as fat-soluble such as A, D, and E, and water-soluble such as B and C.

The action of vitamin A in Parkinson's disease is related to the inhibition of the formation of α-synuclein fibrils that are the main component of Lewy's bodies.

Within the vitamin B complex, activities related to the decrease in homocysteine levels have been found, which is a metabolite that participates in the induction processes of neuronal apoptosis.

Vitamin E supplementation has shown protective effects against striatal damage, it also protects neurons against the neurotoxic effects caused by glutamate and also, together with vitamin C, increase the dosage intervals of levodopa.

The diet pattern could provide more information because individual eating habits and interaction with nutrients can serve as a protective factor since not only can the antioxidant activity be promoted but also anti-inflammatory, which would be useful for the treatment of the illness (Fabbrini et al. 1987; Van Laar et al. 2019; Gazerani 2019).

Restorative Therapies and Neurotrophic Factors

Neurotrophic factors or neurotrophins are a family of proteins that belong to the family of growth factors; they can bind to receptors of certain cells such as neurons and stimulate their survival. Among them, we can find the brain-derived neurotrophic factor (BDNF), which acts on different types of neurons such as the hippocampal, neocortical, cholinergic septal, basal neurons of the anterior brain and dopaminergic neurons of the substantia nigra, the latter being the most affected by PD.

Related to restorative therapies, we have the techniques that are aimed at causing higher dopaminergic function, but these are not yet fully developed compared to the surgical procedures mentioned before, and some are even still in the experimental phase (Rangasamy et al. 2010).

The transplantation of fetal cells to the brains of people with PD has improved the motor symptoms of the disease. For this type of treatment, micro-injections of dopaminergic cells obtained from fetuses have been used, providing the function of releasing dopamine from neurons affected by the disease, making it possible for several patients undergoing this experimental biological treatment to leave their medications. These types of treatments are not yet conclusive, but they give new impetus to biological therapies, although this also opens the way to different bioethical debates.

Taking into account the low availability of human fetal mesencephalic cells in addition to the ethical dilemmas that this represents, it has been decided to test the transplantation of porcine fetal mesencephalic cells, although this leads to issues such as immunological rejection or possible sources of infections (Pardo et al. 1995).

Medicinal Plants for the Treatment of Parkinson's Disease

Pharmacological research of medicinal plants, as well as natural products against PD, is aimed at potential targets that produce or favor neuroprotection such as those that have a specific antioxidant effect on neuronal tissue (Ding et al. 2018), that also participate in the reduction of anti-inflammatory processes cerebral, in addition to those that neutralize the mediators identified in the pathogenesis of the disease such as those that act on the dopaminergic system as agonists or those that prevent the degradation of dopamine (Javed et al. 2019).

Mucuna pruriens (L.) DC.

Mucuna pruriens, also known as velvet bean (Figure 9), is a vigorous climbing plant with stems that can reach up to 18m long. Its leaves are trifoliate with white or purple flowers. The pods are produced in groups of 10 to 14 and measure between 0.5 to 2 cm wide, and 4 to 13 cm long, and are covered with fine white or light brown hairs, hence the name velvet. Each pod contains between 2 and 7 seeds; these can be black, white, reddish, brown, or mottled (Brunner et al. 2011). It can grow in a wide variety of habitats, although it is native to India and Southeast Asia, especially in humid tropical areas, such as tropical rainforests; it is also found in grasslands and thickets.

This velvet bean or kapikachu with a unique appearance has been used since ancient times, mainly in Ayurvedic medicine as a tonic for aphrodisiac purposes, due to increasing the libido, in addition to being used to treat nervousness.

This legume has a high protein content (between 20 to 35%), which is why it is considered a rich source of food protein comparable to beans and soybeans.

The powder of the seeds of *Mucuna pruriens* contains concentrations of up to 7% of levodopa, so in large concentrations (up to 30g/dose) it has shown an effect comparable to that of Parkinson's medication, suggesting that it could be a sustainable alternative to the commercialized levodopa. (Katzenschlager et al. 2004; Johnson et al. 2018)

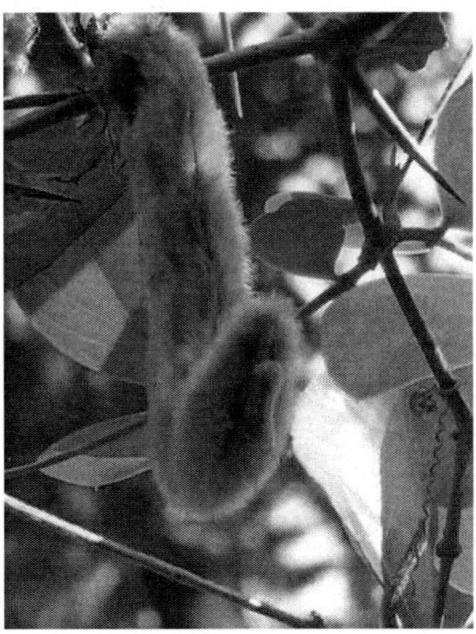

Figure 9. Mucuna pruriens in their habitat. (By Shobha R).

Withania somnifera

Withania somnifera is a plant of the Solanaceae family; it is commonly known as Ashwagandha, which means "horse aroma" due to the particular smell that emerges from it.

It is an erect shrub, with a greenish flower, it can reach a height of 1.5m. Its fruit can be round, yellow, and small; its berry is also small and orange in color. It is native to India, Pakistan, and Sri Lanka. It grows in temperate climates (Dutta et al. 2019).

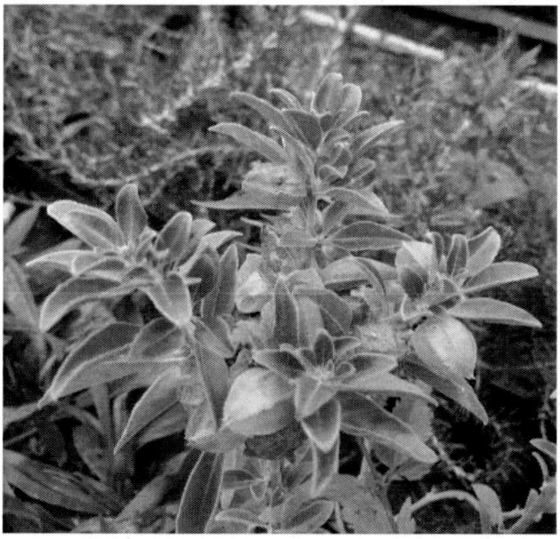

Figure 10. *Withania somnifera*.

In Ayurvedic medicine, it is known as an adaptogen because it acts as a general tonic, especially in cases of physical and mental stress, it also favors the processes of repair and rest. Adaptogens are equilibrating plants because they help the body regain its natural form.

Withania somnifera leaf extracts decreased the activity of superoxide dismutase, catalase and glutathione peroxidase enzymes in the rat model of PD, in addition to an improvement in all physiological abnormalities presented in the model, such as stride length and gait defects, which suggests that leaf extracts of this plant species may become a potential natural source to treat Parkinson's disease (RajaSankar et al. 2009).

Centella asiatica (L). Urb

Centella asiatica is identified by different common names, such as Gotu Kola, Taquibsuso or Asiatic pennywort.

It belongs to the Apiaceae family, usually develops creeping or climbing stems, which are cream-colored and covered with root hairs. It can reach up to a meter and a half high. Its leaves are fan-shaped, orbicular, and peltada and with closed margins. Its flowers have a pinkish to red color, small and rounded (Alonso 2009).

It is native to India, although it is also present in the southern African continent, in Indonesia, and the south of the United States. It is found mainly in cloud forests and riparian spaces, usually near some source of fresh water.

It has been used in traditional Indian medicine for centuries to combat lepra, blood stagnation, dysentery, digestive, and respiratory disorders. It is also widely used as an aid in skin health, as a sexual stimulant, fertility aid, among others.

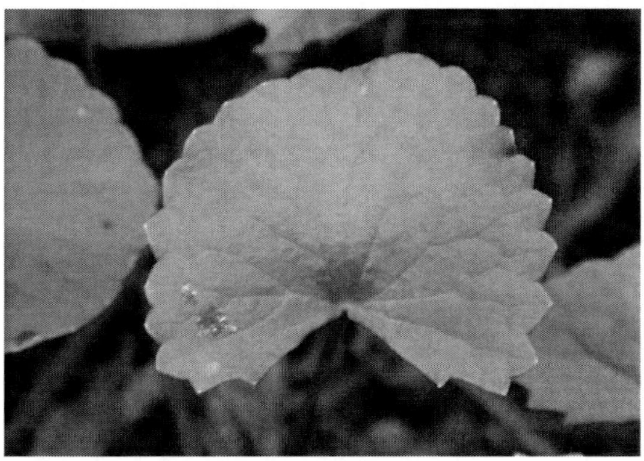

Figure 11. *Centella asiatica* (By Forest & Kim Starr).

The fresh plant and its extracts have different properties that include healing, antioxidants, anti-inflammatory, anti-proliferative, anti-microbial, immunomodulatory, and anti-mutagenic (Gohil et al. 2010).

As for its relationship with the approach to treat PD, this plant has a neuroprotective effect, since extracts of *Centella asiatica* presented a significant decrease in oxidants such as superoxide dismutase, glutathione peroxidase, and catalase, all of which are enzymes marking an effect of peroxidation and related to diseases (More et al. 2013; Lokanathan et al. 2016; Javed et al. 2019).

Sida cordifolia

Sida cordifolia is also known as bala. It is an evergreen shrub that reaches a height of up to one and a half meters. Its roots and stems are dense. Its green leaves have heart shapes serrated and truncated. Its flowers are small, with yellow and white colors. Its seeds are known as bijabanda and are gray to black in color (Ferrer-Gallego et al. 2015).

This species is native to India, but has been naturalized around the world considered as a weed or invasive.

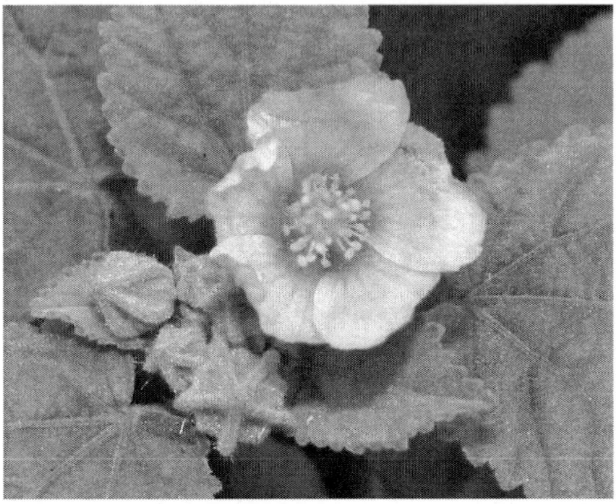

Figure 12. *Sida cordifolia*, (By J. M. Garg).

It is used in traditional Indian medicine in inflammatory processes. For example, it is used to massage patients who have paralysis, diseases that affect joints, their oils are used to soothe pain and inflammation, as well as in eye wounds.

It is also used in traditional African medicine to treat various diseases such as bronchitis, asthma, nasal congestion, stomatitis, etc. (Galai et al. 2015).

As for the physiological effects reported, these include: a depressive effect on the central nervous system, can lower blood pressure as well as heart rate, and it also has hypoglycemic, anti-inflammatory and antioxidant effects.

Regarding the activity related to PD, ethanolic extracts of the root of *Sida cordifolia* in rat brain models treated with quinolinic acid decrease the products of lipid peroxidation as well as the activity of oxidizing enzymes, which indicates that they have antioxidant activity in the brain, in addition to the fact that inflammatory markers such as cyclooxygenase and lipoxygenase decreased significantly, the above being comparable with the results shown by selegiline, a drug commonly used in Parkinson's disease (Swathy et al. 2010).

Bacopa monnieri

Bacopa monnieri, known in Mexico as Baraima, is one of the most appreciated plants of Indian Ayurvedic medicine, known there as Brahmi. It is a plant that has been so exploited as a resource in some countries that it is considered threatened.

It is a small herb of herbaceous shape, perennial, and succulent, with roots in its nodes and of the thin stem. Its size ranges between 5 to 50cm tall. Its leaves are a light green color, oval, spatulated, fleshy, with a rounded apex, petioles generally from the same side as the leaves. Its fruit comes in the form of an ovoid capsule, and its seeds are ellipsoid of a pale color between yellow and brown (Jain 1994).

This plant is an aquatic or underwater species, typically found in a tropical, subtropical or temperate climate. It can be found in mangroves, in cenotes, swampy zones, lakeshore, and streams as well as in coastal dunes. It sometimes forms small thickets.

It is a very adaptable plant easy to care for, as long as it has medium to high lighting.

It is native to tropical Asia but nowadays it can be found in almost all tropical and subtropical regions of the world (Mathur et al. 2016).

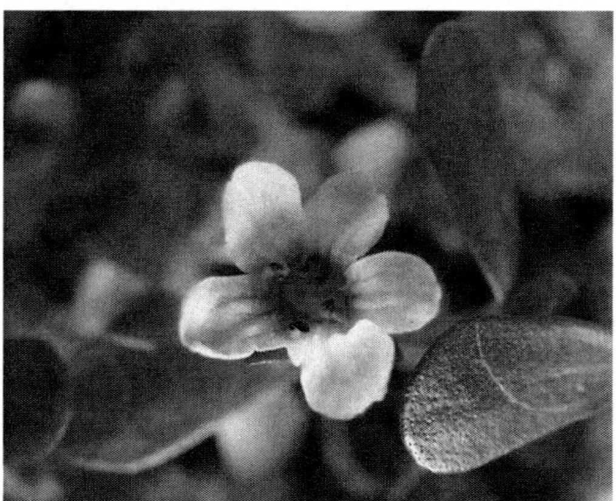

Figure 13. *Bacopa monnieri*, (By David Eickhoff).

In Ayurvedic medicine, it lists this species as one of the rayanas and celestial medicines, since they increase the maximum lifespan, promote a lack of diseases, foster intellect and memory. It is also used in a tonic to improve mental clarity, control nerves, and in combination with other plants, it is used to treat epilepsy, hysteria and mental disorders. (Manap et al. 2019).

In addition, the *B. monnieri* species presents antiparkinsonian activities in the *Caenorhabditis elegans* model where it can be observed that it reduces aggregation of α-synuclein, prevents dopaminergic neurodegeneration, as well as restoring the lipid content in the nematode (Singh et al. 2019).

Camellia sinensis

This species is known as camellia or the tea plant since its leaves and buds are used to make tea.

It is a small tree, it can reach a height between 1 to 9 meters, although it is usually trimmed so that it does not exceed two meters when grown for tea making. Its leaves are glabrous and have serrated edges. The flowers are axillary and solitary, although they can sometimes be found in groups of three, their color ranges from white to yellow. The seeds of this species are measured in the order of centimeters and are brownish in color.

It is an herbaceous plant native to China and Southeast Asia, although it is currently widely cultivated worldwide, mainly in tropical and subtropical areas, as long as rainfall can reach up to 2000 mm^3 per year, and the height is around 2500 m. It prefers acid and permeable soils. The ideal temperature for this plant ranges from 10 to 30°C.

Buddhist monks were the main promoters of tea as they adopted it as a ritual and tonic drink, but it was during the Song dynasty that Chinese tea art reached its maximum sophistication, it was during this period that it extended to Japan. (Liu et al. 2013).

Whereas Europe is concerned, tea became popular for the first time in France and the Netherlands. Tea suddenly became a popular drink in the United Kingdom. The British East India Company began to import it starting from 1669, and during the following century, tea became the most important element in English traffic with the East.

Infusions of *C. sinensis* were used in treatments for various conditions such as tumors, abscesses, and fatigue, as well as for bladder related problems. It was indicated for diarrhea, bronchitis, and asthma, in addition to being used as an adjunct in treatments for weight loss and arteriosclerosis. Tonics were used to make creams and gels to reduce local adiposities (Bhattacharjee 2015; Gupta and Kumar 2016).

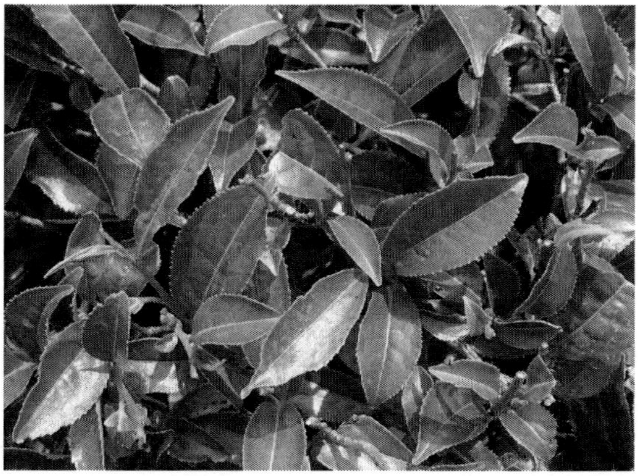

Figure 14. *Camellia sinensis* (By Axel Boldt).

This species has polyphenols such as catechins, which have shown, in animal models, an improvement in reference and working memory, as well as antidepressant effects, which indicates that they could be beneficial for neurodegenerative disorders such as Parkinson's disease.

Extracts from *C. sinensis* significantly reversed the decreases in striatal content of dopamine, 3,4-dihydroxyphenylacetic acid, and homovanillic acid (metabolites of the neurotransmitter dopamine), in models of injured animals where PD was simulated (Ittiyavirah and Ruby 2014; Mirza et al. 2019).

Hypericum perforatum

Hypericum perforatum is known mainly as hypericum or St. John's Wort.

It is a perennial plant, slightly aromatic, whose height ranges from 20 cm to 1 meter. The stem is erect and then branches off at the top. Its leaves are small, very abundant and numerous, opposite, oval or oblong. Its flowers are numerous and of a characteristic golden yellow color, with black or purple spots. The fruit is a capsule that contains small, rounded seeds of black color.

This species is native to Europe, but it can be found in North and South Africa, it is also found in South America, in Australia and New Zealand. This species grows in low and medium height terrains, especially on the sidelines of the roads, under bushes and in wooded areas, as long as they are not too densely populated, with mostly semi-dry soils (Borrás et al. 2001).

The Greeks used the hypericum as an anti-inflammatory and refreshing remedy.

In the Middle Ages, it was believed the aroma of this plant drove away from the evil spirits and that, to get these properties, it had to be collected at dawn on June 24, the day of St. John, which coincides with the date of its flowering.

It was used as an external tonic for the treatment of pain caused by bruises and wounds, as well as nerve pain.

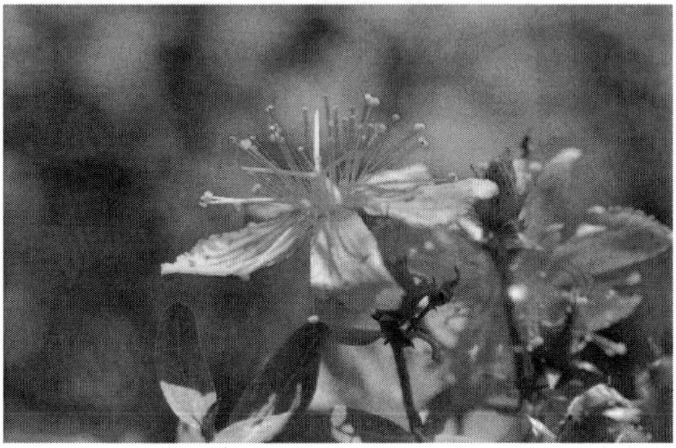

Figure 15. *Hypericum perforatum* (By Aiwok).

Other uses in traditional medicine that are given to this species are against insomnia, anxiety, and nocturnal enuresis; In addition, the oil extract of *H. perforatum* has been used topically in the treatment of sores, wounds, and burns. (Henderson et al. 2002).

Hypericum extracts are well known for their antidepressant properties, but only recently have their nootropic effects against various neurodegenerative disorders been demonstrated.

The hypericum has phloroglucinols such as hyperforin that not only shows inhibition of the monoamine oxidase enzyme but also decreases the dopaminergic cell death of the substantia nigra in rat models with brain damage, which gives it a neuroprotective effect (Hostanska 2003).

Also, hydroethanolic extracts of this species have shown a significant increase in the release of dopamine in *in vivo* models.

This demonstrates that it could be a good option as an adjunctive treatment in PD (Vecchia et al. 2015; Rabiei et al. 2019).

Rehmannia glutinosa

Rehmannia glutinosa is known as rehmania, and in traditional Chinese medicine, it is known as dihuáng.

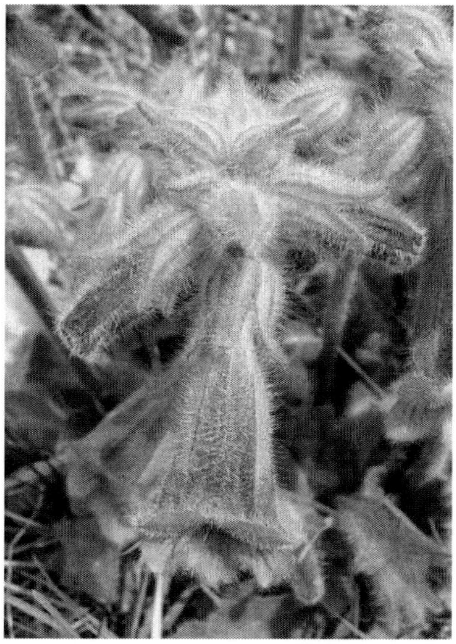

Figure 16. *Rehmannia glutinosa*, (By Shizhao).

This is species is an herb, phanerogam, perene and hairy, belonging to the family Phrymaceae. It can reach a height of up to 40 cm. It has tubular flowers of a purple to light red color, it has a tuberous root of the orange and thick color.

It is a plant native to China, but it can also be found in Korea and Japan.

In traditional Chinese medicine, it was used to stimulate the functioning of the heart, for its diuretic properties, laxatives, to reduce blood glucose levels, as well as for dementia (Zhang et al. 2008).

It was found that Rehmannia induces the gene expression of glial cell-derived neurotrophic factor (GDNF) *in vitro*, this growth factor promotes survival and neurons in the central nervous system. (Yu et al. 2006).

It has also been found that catalpol, present in this plant, demonstrates neuroprotective activity due to its activity against oxidative stress and the presence of neurotoxins (Jiang et al. 2008).

In addition, formulations with Rehmannia root relieve symptoms of dyskinesia in rats with Parkinson's disease, modulating neurotransmitter signaling in the striatum (Teng et al. 2014; Choi et al. 2018).

Ligusticum striatum

This species belongs to the Apiaceae family and is usually known as chuanxiong.

It is an herbaceous plant that reaches a height of 30 to 120cm. The root is cylindrical. The stem is unbranched and straightforward, normally its base is covered in remanent pods. The leaves are generally oval. It has leaves with white petals, and its fruits are ovoid.

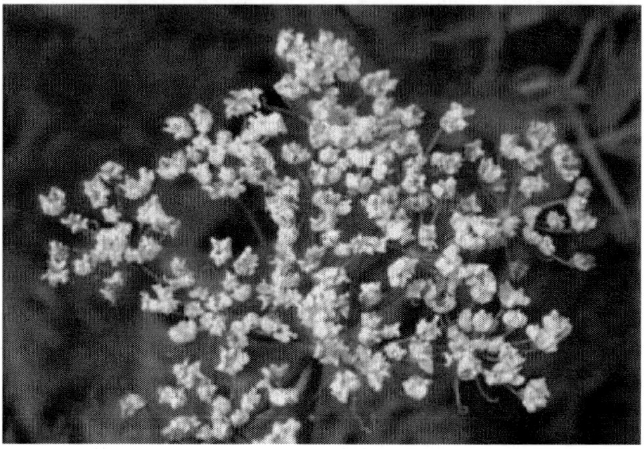

Figure 17. *Ligusticum striatum*.

Chuanxiong is a species native to China, but it can also be found in India, Kashmir, and Nepal. It is usually located in forests at an altitude of 1599 to 3700m.

In traditional Chinese medicine, it is used to combat menstrual cycle disorders such as menstrual pain and absence of menstruation, as well as limb numbness, joint pain, headache, among others (Wang et al. 2013).

Tetramethylpyrazine is one of the main bioactive components of this plant, which has anti-apoptotic, anti-inflammatory, and antioxidant effects, suggesting that it can prevent neurobiological and behavioral deficits of PD (Lu et al. 2014; Wang et al. 2014; Jin et al. 2019).

Cannabis sativa

Also known as marijuana, it is an herbaceous species native to the Himalayan mountain ranges.

It belongs to the Cannabaceae family, has opposite leaves, palamdas and its leaves have a serrated margin. It presents curved tector hairs.

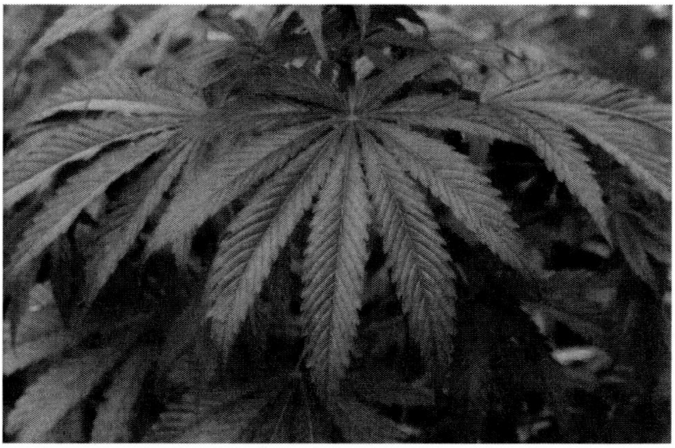

Figure 18. *Cannabis sativa* (By Lode Van de Velde).

The human's relationship with this species dates back to prehistoric times, its fibers have been used as textiles for clothing, to obtaining pulp for paper, extracting seed oil as fuel and human, pet, and livestock food (Shah 2004).

As it presents psychoactive properties, it has been used as a mystical and spiritual tool.

Also, positive effects have been observed in patients with PD when using marijuana as it improves motor and non-motor symptoms such as tremor, stiffness, insomnia, and pain. In particular, bradykinesia, it is the symptom with the most relief in cannabis users. (Sánchez-Martínez Sánchez-Martínez et al. 2019; Patel et al. 2019).

Tetrahydrocannabinol (THC) has shown improvement in hand-eye coordination in animal models with PD. Other factors, such as mood, memory, and fatigue, were also improved with cannabis use (Babayeva et al. 2016).

Marijuana can, therefore, be used as an alternative or complementary option in adults with PD to help improve the quality of life of patients with PD.

CONCLUSION

Parkinson's disease is complex in its diagnosis, clinical, and treatment, but by accepting it as multifactorial and not only as a progressive neurodegenerative condition, it opens the doors to different targets of action.

As time passes, we will have to wait for more knowledge of molecular pathways, timely initial diagnoses, and more personalized and effective treatments or combinations that not only focus on the symptoms but also cover the problems associated with the disease.

Parkinson's disease is not a deadly disease, so one must learn to accept it, treat it, and live with it.

REFERENCES

Almaguer, Luis E., Martínez, Wilmer and Guach, David. 2017. Implicaciones de la microbiota intestinal en la etiología y terapéutica de la enfermedad de Parkinson. [Implications of the intestinal microbiota in the etiology and therapeutics of Parkinson's disease]. *Revista Habanera de Ciencias Médicas*, 17:48-57 http://www.revhabanera.sld.cu/index.php/rhab/article/view/2094/1987.

Alonso, J. M. 2009. *Centella asiática* una planta con historia e interesantes propiedades. [*Centella asiatica* a plant with history and interesting properties] *Ámbito farmacéutico Fitoterapia* 28:98-104. https://www.elsevier.es/es-revista-offarm-4-pdf-13139754.

Ascherio, A. and Schwarzschild, M. A. 2019. The epidemiology of Parkinson's disease: risk factors and prevention. *The Lancet Neurology* 15: 1257-1272. doi: 10.1016/S1474-4422(16)30230-7.

Babayeva, Mariana, Assefa, Haregewein, Basu, Paramita, Chumki, Sanjeda, and Loewy, Zvi. 2016. Marijuana Compounds: A Nonconventional Approach to Parkinson's Disease Therapy. *Parkinson's Disease*. 2016:1-19. doi: 10.1155/2016/1279042.

Bauer, Sylvian, Kerr, Bradley J. and Patterson, Paul H. 2007. The neuropoietic cytokine family in development, plasticity, disease and injury. *Nature Reviews Neuroscience* 8:221-232. doi:10.1038/nrn2054.

Beitz, Janice M. 2014. Parkinson's disease: a review. *Frontiers in Bioscience* 6:65-74 doi: 10.2741/s415.

Benbid, Alim L., Pollak, Pierre, Gao, Dongming, Hoffman Dominique, Limousin, Patricia, Gay, Emmanuel, Payen, Isabelle, and Benazzouz, Abdhelhamid. 1996. Chronic electrical stimulation of the ventralis intermedius nucleus of the thalamus as a treatment of movement disorders. *Journal of Neurosurgery* 84:203-214. doi: 10.3171/jns.1996.84.2.0203.

Bhattacharjee, J. 2015. A Study on the Benefits of Tea. *International Journal of Humanities & Social Science Studies* 2:109-121 https://www.ijhsss.com/files/Jayeeta-Bhattacharjee_69b015ze.pdf.

Biagi, Elena, Candela, Marco, Turroni, Silvia, Garagnani, Paolo, Franceschi, Claudio, and Brigidi, Patrizia. 2013. "Ageing and gut microbes: Perspectives for health maintenance and longevity." *Pharmacological Research* 69: 11-20. doi: 10.1016/j.phrs.2012.10.005.

Birkmayer, W. and Hornykiewicz, O. 1961. The L-3,4-dioxyphenylalanine (DOPA)-effect in Parkinson-akinesia. *Wien Klin Wochenschr* 73:787-788. doi: 10.1016/s1353-8020(98)00013-3.

Bjarnason, Inguar T., Charlett, André, Dobbs, R. John, Dobbs, Sylvia M., Ibrahim, Mohammad A. A., Kerwin, Robert W., Mahler, Robert F., Oxlade, Norman L., Peterson, Dale W., Plant, J. Malcolm, Price, Ashley B., and Weller, Clive. 2005. Role of chronic infection and inflammation in the gastrointestinal tract in the etiology and pathogenesis of idiopathic parkinsonism. Part 2: response of facets of clinical idiopathic parkinsonism to *Helicobacter pylori* eradication. A randomized, double-blind, placebo-controlled efficacy study" *Helicobacter* 10:276-287. doi: 0.1111/j.1523-5378.2005.00330.x.

Bjorklund, G., Stejskal, V., Urbina, M. A., Dadar, M., Chirumbolo, S. and Mutter, J. 2018. "Metals and Parkinson's Disease: Mechanisms and Biochemical Processes." *Current Medicinal Chemistry* 25:2198-2214. doi: 10.2174/0929867325666171129124616.

Block, G., Liss, C., Reines, S., Irr J. and Nibbelink D. C. 1997. "The FIRST Study Group, comparison of immediate release and controlled release carbidopa/levodopa in Parkinson's disease. A multicenter 5-year study." *European Neurology* 37:23-27. doi: 10.1159/000117399.

Borrás-Blasco, J., Navarro-Ruiz, A. and González-Delgado M. 2001. "Hierba de San Juan (*Hypericum perforatum* sp)" Farmacia *Hospitalaria (Madrid)* Vol. 25: 356-362 https://www.sefh.es/fh/2001/n6/6.pdf.

Braak, Heiko and Del Tredici, Kelly. 2008. "Invited Article: Nervous system pathology in sporadic Parkinson disease." *Neurology* 70:1916-1925. doi: 10.1212/01.wnl.0000312279.49272.9f.

Brissaud, E. 1895. Vingt-deuxième Leçon: Pathologie et symptômes de la maladie de Parkinson. [Twenty-second Lesson: Pathology and Symptoms of Parkinson's Disease]. In: H, M. (ed.) *Leçons sur les maladies nerveuses.* [*Lessons about nerve diseases*] Paris: Masson, Salpêtrière 1893-1894.

Brudek, T. 2019. Inflammatory Bowel Diseases and Parkinson's Disease. *Journal of Parkinson's Disease* 9:331-344 doi: 10.3233/JPD-191729.

Calne, D. B., Plotkin, C., Williams, A. C., Nutt, J. G., Neophytides, A. and Teychenne, P. F. 1978. Long-term treatment of parkinsonism with bromocriptine. *The Lancet* 1:735-738. doi: 10.1136/jnnp.42.2.143.

Caraceni, Tommaso, Scigliao, Giulio and Musicco, Massimo. 1991. "The occurrence of motor fluctuations in parkinsonian patients treated long term with levodopa: role of early treatment and disease progression." *Neurology* 41:380-384. doi: 10.1212/wnl.41.3.380.

Carlsson, A., Lindqvist, M. and Magnusson, T. 1957. "3,4-Dihydroxyphenylalanine and 5-hydroxytryptophan as reserpine antagonists." *Nature* 180:1200. doi: 10.1038/1801200a0

Chao J., Li H., Cheng K. W., Yu M. S., Chang R. C. and Wang M. 2010. Protective effects of pinostilbene, a resveratrol methylated derivative, against 6-hydroxydopamine-induced neurotoxicity in SH-SY5Y cells. *Journal of Nutritional Biochemistry* 21:482–489. doi:10.1016/j.jnutbio.2009.02.004.

Chase, T. N., Mouradian, M. M and Engber, T. M. 1993. Motor response complications and the function of striatal efferent systems (Review). *Neurology*. 43:23-27.

Cheng Y., He G., Mu X., Zhang T., Li X., Hu J., Xu B. and Du G. 2008. "Neuroprotective effect of baicalein against MPTP neurotoxicity: behavioral, biochemical and immunohistochemical profile." *Neuroscience Letters* 441:16–20. doi: 10.1016/j.neulet.2008.05.116.

Choi, J. H., Jang, M., Lee, J. I., Chung, W. S. and Cho, I. H. 2018. Neuroprotective Effects of a Traditional Multi-Herbal Medicine Kyung-Ok-Ko in an Animal Model of Parkinson's Disease: Inhibition of MAPKs and NF-κB Pathways and Activation of Keap1-Nrf2 Pathway. *Frontiers Pharmacology* 9:1-15 doi: 10.3389/fphar.2018.01444.

Clarke, C. E. 1995. Does levodopa therapy delay death in Parkinson´s disease? A review of the evidence. *Movement Disorders*. 10:250-256. doi: 10.1002/mds.870100303.

Collier, Timithy J., Kanaan, Nicholas M. and Kordower, Jeffrey H. 2011. Ageing as a primary risk factor for Parkinson's disease: evidence from studies of non-human primates. *Nature Reviews Neuroscience* 12;359-366. doi: 10.1038/nrn3039.

Cotzias, G. C. 1968. L-Dopa for Parkinsonism. *The New England Journal of Medicine* 278:630. https://www.ncbi.nlm.nih.gov/pmc/articles/PMC1946468/pdf/canmedaj01334-0061.pdf.

Dauer, William, and Przedborski, Sege. 2003. Parkinson's disease: mechanisms and models. *Neuron*, 39: 196-221 doi: 10.1016/s0896-6273(03)00568-3.

Davie, C. A. 2008. A review of Parkinson´s disease. *British Medical Bulletin* 86: 109-127. doi: 10.1093/bmb/ldn013.

Defer, G. L. 1999. "Controverse sur le traitement initial de la maladie de Parkinson: L-dopa ou agonistas dopaminergiques?. [Controversy over initial treatment for Parkinson's disease: L-dopa or dopaminergic agonists?] *Revue Neurologique* 155:43-45.

DeMaagd, G. and Philip, A. 2015. *Parkinson's Disease and Its Management. Part 1: Disease Entity, Risk Factors, Pathophysiology, Clinical Presentation, and Diagnosis Pharmacy and Therapeutics* Aug; 40:504-532. https://www.ncbi.nlm.nih.gov/pmc/articles/PMC4517533/.

Dick, F. D. 2006. Solvent neurotoxicity. *Occupational and Environmental Medicine* 63:221–226. doi: 10.1136/oem.2005.022400.

Ding, D., Ao, X., Liu, Y., Wang, Y. Y., Fa, H. G., Wang, M. Y., He, Y. Q. and Wang, J. X. 2019. Post-translational modification of Parkin and its research progress in cancer. *Cancer Communications (Lond).* 39:77. doi: 10.1186/s40880-019-0421-5.

Ding, Y., Xin, C., Zhang, C. W., Lim, K. L., Zhang, H., Fu, Z., Li, L. and Huang, W. 2018. Natural Molecules From Chinese Herbs Protecting Against Parkinson's Disease via Anti-oxidative Stress. *Frontiers in Aging Neuroscience*. 10:246. doi: 10.3389/fnagi.2018.00246.

Donate, Susana and Carrasco, Laura. 2007. Cuidarse para cuidar mejor en la enfermedad de Parkinson. [Take care of yourself to take better care of Parkinson's disease]. *Asociación Parkinson Madrid* 15-44.

Dutta, R., Khalil, R., Green, R., Mohapatra, S. S. and Mohapatra, S. 2019. *Withania Somnifera* (Ashwagandha) and Withaferin A: Potential in Integrative Oncology. *International Journal of Molecular Sciences* 20:1-19 doi: 10.3390/ijms20215310.

Fabbrini, G., Juncos, J., Mouradian, M. M., Serrati, C. and Chase, T. N. 1987. Levodopa pharmacokinetic mechanisms and motor fluctuations in Parkinson's disease. *Annals of Neurology*. 21:370-376. doi: 10.1002/ana.410210409.

Fahn, S. and Bressman, S. B. 1984. Should levodopa therapy for parkinsonism be started early or late? Evidence against early treatment. *Canadian Journal of Neurological Sciences* 11:200-206. doi: 10.1017/s0317167100046412.

Ferrer-Gallego, P. P., Ferrando, I. and Laguna-Lumbreras, E. 2015. *Sida cordifolia* L. (Malvaceae), nuevo polizón para la flora valenciana. [*Sida cordifolia* L. (Malvaceae), new stowaway for the Valencian flora]. *Bouteloua* 21:49-51.

Freeman, Thomas B. and Brundin, Patrik. 2006. Important Aspects of Surgical Methodology for Transplantation in Parkinson's disease. In *Restorative*

Therapies in Parkinson's Disease, edited by Springer, 131-165, Boston, MA doi: 10.1007/0-387-32823-2_8.

Galal, A., Raman, V and Khan, I. A. 2015. *Sida cordifolia*, a Traditional Herb in Modern Perspective – A Review. *Current Traditional Medicine*, 1, 5-17 doi: 10.2174/2215083801666141226215639.

Gao, Y. and Pu, X. P. 2007. Neuroprotective effect of acteoside against rotenone-induced damage of SH-SY5Y cells and its possible mechanism. *Chinese Pharmacological Bulletin* 23:161–165.

García Ruiz, P. J. 1996. Neurología bíblica. [Biblical neurology]. *Revista Neurología* 24:580-581. doi: 10.33588/rn.24129.96574.

García Ruiz, P. J. 2004. Prehistory of Parkinson's disease. *Neurologia,* 19:735-7.

García-Revilla, J., Alonso-Bellido, I. M., Burguillos, M. A., Herrera, A. J., Espinosa-Oliva, A. M., Ruiz, R., Cruz-Hernández, L., García-Domínguez, I., Roca-Ceballos, M. A., Santiago, M., Rodríguez-Gómez, J. A., Soto, M. S., Venero, J. L. and de Pablos, R. M. 2019. Reformulating Pro-Oxidant Microglia in Neurodegeneration. *Journal of Clinical Medicine* 8:1719. doi: 10.3390/jcm8101719.

Gazerani, P. 2019. Probiotics for Parkinson's Disease. *International Journal of Molecular Sciences* 20:1-26. doi: 10.3390/ijms20174121.

Goetz, C. G. 1986. Charcot on Parkinson's disease. *Movement Disorders* 1:27-32. doi: 10.1002/mds.870010104.

Gohil, K. J., Patel, J. A. and Gajjar, A. K. 2010. "Pharmacological Review on *Centella asiatica*: A Potential Herbal Cure-all" *Indian Journal of Pharmaceutical Sciences* 72:546–556. doi: 10.4103/0250-474X.78519.

González-Torres, Laura, and Armendáriz-Borunda, Juan. 2005. Aspectos inmunológicos en la enfermedad de Parkinson. [Immunological aspects in Parkinson's disease]. *Archivos de Neurociencias* 3:168-174.

Grandas, F., Martínez-Martín, P. and Linazasoro, G. 1998. Quality of life in patients with Parkinson´s disease who transfer from standard levodopa to Sinemet CR: the STAR study. *The Journal of Neurology* 245:31-33. doi: 10.1007/pl00007736.

Guan S., Jiang B., Bao Y. M. and An L. J. 2006. Protocatechuic acid suppresses MPP+ -induced mitochondrial dysfunction and apoptotic cell death in PC12 cells. *Food and Chemical Toxicology* 44:1659–1666. doi: 10.1016/j.fct. 2006.05.004.

Gupta S. C., Patchva S., Koh W. and Aggarwal B. B. 2012. Discovery of curcumin, a component of golden spice, and its miraculous biological activities. *Clinical and Experimental Pharmacology and Physiology* 39:283–299. doi: 10.1111/j.1440-1681.2011.05648.x.

Gupta, D. and Kumar, M. 2016. Evaluation of *in vitro* antimicrobial potential and GC-MS analysis of *Camellia sinensis* and *Terminalia arjuna*. *Biotechnology Reports* 13:19-25. doi: 10.1016/j.btre.2016.11.002.

Hassler, R. and Riechert, T. 1958. Symptomatology & surgery of extrapyramidal movement disorders. *Med Klin*, 53:817-24.

Henderson, L., Yue, Q. Y., Bergquist, C., Gerden, B. and Arlett, P. 2002. St John's wort (*Hypericum perforatum*): drug interactions and clinical outcomes. *The British Journal of Clinical Pharmacology* 54:349-356. doi: 10.1046/j.1365-2125.2002.01683.x.

Hertel, J., Harms, A. C., Heinken, A., Baldini, F., Thinnes, C. C., Glaab, E., Vasco, D. A., Pietzner, M., Stewart, I. D., Wareham, N. J., Langenberg, C., Trenkwalder, C., Krüger, R., Hankemeier, T., Fleming RMT, Mollenhauer, B. and Thiele, I. 2019. Integrated Analyses of Microbiome and Longitudinal Metabolome Data Reveal Microbial-Host Interactions on Sulfur Metabolism in Parkinson's Disease. *Cell Reports* 29:1767-1777 doi: 10.1016/j.celrep.2019.10.035.

Hirsch, Etienne C. and Hunot, Stéphane. 2009. Neuroinflammation in Parkinson's disease: a target for neuroprotection?. *The Lancet Neurology* 8:382–397. doi: 10.1016/S1474-4422(09)70062-6.

Hirsch, Etienne C., Vyas, Sheela and Hunot, Stéphane. 2012. Neuroinflammation in Parkinson's disease. *Parkinsonism & related disorders* 18:210–212. doi: 10.1016/S1474-4422(09)70062-6.

Hoehn, M. M. and Yahr, M. D. 1967. Parkinsonism: onset, progression and mortality. *Neurology* 17:427-442. doi: 10.1212/wnl.17.5.427.

Hostanska, K., Reichling, J., Bommer, S., Weber, M. and Saller, R. 2003. Hyperforin a constituent of St John's wort (*Hypericum perforatum* L.) extract induces apoptosis by triggering activation of caspases and with hypericin synergistically exerts cytotoxicity towards human malignant cell lines. *The European Journal of Pharmaceutics and Biopharmaceutics* 56:121-132. doi:10.1016/s0939-6411(03)00046-8.

Hu, S. Han, R., Mak, S. and Han, Y. 2011. Protection against 1-methyl-4-phenylpyridinium ion (MPP+)-induced apoptosis by water extract of ginseng (*Panax ginseng* C. A. Meyer) in SH-SY5Y cells. *Journal of Ethnopharmacology* 135:34–42. doi: 10.1016/j.jep.2011. 02. 017.

Hughes, Andrew J., Daniel, Susan E., Kilford, Linda and Lees Andrew J.1992. Accuracy of clinical diagnosis of idiopathic Parkinson's disease: a clinicopathological study of 100 cases. *Journal of Neurology, Neurosurgery & Psychiatry* 55:181-184. doi: 10.1136/jnnp.55.3.181.

Hurtado,F., Cardenas, Melissa A. N., Cardenas, Fernando and León, Laura A. 2016. La Enfermedad de Parkinson: Etiología, Tratamientos y Factores Preventivos. [Parkinson's Disease: Etiology, Treatments and Preventive Factors]. *Universitas Psychologica* 15:1-26 doi: 10.11144/Javeriana. upsy15-5.epet.

Hwang, O. 2013. Role of oxidative stress in Parkinson's disease. *Experimental Neurobiology* 22:11-17. doi: 10.3233/JPD-130230.

Ittiyavirah, S. P. and Ruby, R. 2014. Effect of hydro-alcoholic root extract of *Plumbago zeylanica* L. alone and its combination with aqueous leaf extract of *Camellia sinensis* on haloperidol induced parkinsonism in wistar rats. *Annals of Neurosciences* 21:47-50. doi: 10.5214/ans.0972.7531.210204.

Jain, S. K. 1994. Ethnobotany and research on medicinal plants in India. *Ciba Foundation symposium*. 185:153-164.

Javed, H., Nagoor Meeran, M. F., Azimullah, S., Adem, A., Sadek, B. and Ojha, S. K. 2019. Plant Extracts and Phytochemicals Targeting α-Synuclein Aggregation in Parkinson's Disease Models. *Frontiers in Pharmacology* 9:1555. doi: 10.3389/fphar.2018.01555.

Jellinger, K. A. 1999. Post mortem studies in Parkinson's disease--is it possible to detect brain areas for specific symptoms?. *Journal of Neural Transmission* 56:1-29. doi: 10.1007/978-3-7091-6360-3_1.

Jenner, P. 1995. The rationale for the use of dopamine agonists in Parkinson's disease. *Neurology* 45:6-12. doi: 10.1212/wnl.45.3_suppl_3.s6.

Jiang, B., Zhang, H., Bi, J. and Zhang, X. L. 2008. Neuroprotective activities of catalpol on MPP+/MPTP-induced neurotoxicity. *Neurological Research* 30:639-44. doi: 10.1179/174313208X289543.

Jiang T. F., Zhang Y. J., Zhou H. Y., Wang H. M., Tian L. P., Liu J., Ding J. Q. and Chen S. D. 2013. Curcumin ameliorates the neurodegenerative pathology in A53T alpha-synuclein cell model of Parkinson's disease through the downregulation ofmTOR/p70S6K signaling and the recovery of macroautophagy. *Journal of Neuroimmune Pharmacology* 8:356–369. doi: 10.1007/s11481-012-9431-7.

Jin, X. C., Zhang, L., Wang, Y., Cai, H. B., Bao, X. J., Jin, Y. Y. and Zheng, G. Q. 2019. An Overview of Systematic Reviews of Chinese Herbal Medicine for Parkinson's Disease. *Frontiers in Pharmacology* 10:155. doi: 10.3389/fphar.2019.00155.

Johnson, S. L., Park, H. Y., DaSilva, N. A., Vattem, D. A., Ma, H. and Seeram, N. P. 2018. Levodopa-Reduced *Mucuna pruriens* Seed Extract Shows

Neuroprotective Effects against Parkinson's Disease in Murine Microglia and Human Neuroblastoma Cells, *Caenorhabditis elegans*, and *Drosophila melanogaster*. *Nutrients* 10:1139. doi: 10.3390/nu10091139.

Katzenschlager, R., Manson, A. Patsalos, P. N., Ratnaraj, N., Watt, H. Timmermann, L., Van der Giessen, R., and Lees, A. J. 2004. *Mucuna pruriensin* Parkinson's disease: a double blind clinical and pharmacological study. *Journal of Neurology, Neurosurgery, and Psychiatry* 75:1672-1677. doi: 10.1136/jnnp.2003.028761.

Kempster, P. A., Hurwitz, B. and Lees, A. J. 2007. A new look at James Parkinson's Essay on the Shaking Palsy. *Neurology* 69:482-5.

Killinger, Bryan A., Melki, Ronald, Brundin, Patrik, and Kordower, Jeffrey H. 2019. Endogenous alpha-synuclein monomers, oligomers and resulting pathology: let's talk about the lipids in the room. *NPJ Parkinsons Disease* 5:1-8. doi: 10.1038/s41531-019-0095-3.

Khan M. M., Ahmad A., Ishrat T., Khan M. B., Hoda M. N., Khuwaja G., Raza S. S., Khan A., Javed H., Vaibhav K. and Islam F. 2010. Resveratrol attenuates 6-hydroxydopamine-induced oxidative damage and dopamine depletion in rat model of Parkinson's disease. *Brain Research* 1328:139–151. doi: 10.1016/j.brainres.2010.02.031.

Krack, P., Pollak, P., Limousin, P., Hoffman, D., Xie, J., Benazzouz, A., and Benabid, A. L. 1998. Subthalamic nucleus or internal pallidal stimulation in young onset Parkinson's disease. *Brain* 121:451-457. doi: 10.1093/brain/121.3.451.

Lange, K. W. 1998. Clinical pharmacology of dopamine agonists in Parkinson's disease. *Drugs & Aging* 13:381-389. doi: 10.2165/00002512-199813050-00004.

Lange, K. W., Rausch, W. D., Gsell W., Naumann M., Oestreicher E. and Riederer P. 1994. Neuroprotection by dopamine agonists. *Journal of Neural Transmission* 43:183-201.

Larit, F., Elokely, K. M., Chaurasiya, N. D., Benyahia, S., Nael, M. A., León, F., Abu-Darwish, M. S., Efferth, T., Wang, Y. H., Belouahem-Abed, D., Benayache, S., Tekwani, B. L. and Cutler, S. J. 2018. Inhibition of human monoamine oxidase A and B by flavonoids isolated from two Algerian medicinal plants. *Phytomedicine* 40:27-36. doi: 10.1016/j.phymed.2017.12.032.

Larsen, Jan P., Boas, Jette, Erdal, John E., and the Norwegian-Danish Study Group. 1999. Does selegiline modify the progression of early Parkinson's disease? Results from a five-year study." *European Journal of Neurology* 6:539-547 doi:10.1046/j.1468-1331.1999.650539.x.

Lee J. Y., Woo E. R. and Kang K. W. 2005. Inhibition of lipopolysaccharide-inducible nitric oxide synthase expression by acteoside through blocking of AP-1 activation. *Journal of Ethnopharmacology* 97:561–566 doi: 10.1016/j.jep.2005.01.005.

Lees, A. J., Selikhova, M., Andrade, L. A. and Duyckaerts, C. 2008. The black stuff and Konstantin Nikolaevich Tretiakoff. *Movement Disorders* 23:777-783. doi: 10.1002/mds.21855.

Limousin, P., Pollak, P., Benazzouz, A., Hoffmann, D., Le Bas, J. F., Broussolle, E., Perret, J. E. and Benabid, A. L. 1995. Effect of parkinsonian signs and symptoms of bilateral subthalamic nucleus stimulation. *The Lancet* 345:91-95. doi: 10.1016/s0140-6736(95)90062-4.

Limousin, Patricia, Krack, Paul, Pollak, Pierre, Benazzouz, Abdelhamid, Ardouin, Claire, Hoffman, Dominique, and Benabid, Alim-Lois. 1998. Electrical stimulation of the subthalamic nucleus in advanced Parkinson´s disease. *The New England Journal of Medicine*, 339:1105-1111 doi: 10.1056/NEJM199810153391603.

Liu, Y., Ahmed, S. and Long, C. 2013. Ethnobotanical survey of cooling herbal drinks from southern China. *Journal of Ethnobiology and Ethnomedicine* 9:82. doi: 10.1186/1746-4269-9-82.

Lokanathan, Y., Omar, N., Ahmad Puzi, N. N., Saim, A. and Hj Idrus, R. 2016. Recent Updates in Neuroprotective and Neuroregenerative Potential of *Centella asiatica*. *Malaysian Journal of Medical Sciences* 23:4-14.

López-González, Natalia, Quiroga-Varela, Ana, Garbayo, Elisa, Carballo-Carbajal, Iria, Fernández-Santiago, Rubén, Monje, Mariana H. G., Trigo-Damas, Inés, Blanco-Prieto, María J. and Blesa, Javier. 2018. Advances in Parkinson's Disease: 200 Years Later. *Frontiers in Neuroanatomy* 12:1-14. doi: 10.3389/fnana.2018.00113.

Lu J. H., Ardah M. T., Durairajan S. S., Liu L. F., Xie L. X., Fong W. F., Hasan M. Y., Huang J. D., El-Agnaf O. M. and Li M 2011. Baicalein inhibits formation of alpha-synuclein oligomers within living cells and prevents Abeta peptide fibrillation and oligomerisation. *ChemBioChem*, 12:615–624. doi: 10.1002/cbic.201000604.

Lu, C., Zhang, J., Shi, X., Miao, S., Bi, L., Zhang, S., Yang, Q., Zhou, X., Zhang, M., Xie, Y., Miao, Q. and Wang, S. 2014. Neuroprotective effects of tetramethylpyrazine against dopaminergic neuron injury in a rat model of Parkinson's disease induced by MPTP. *International Journal of Biological Sciences* 10:350-357. doi: 10.7150/ijbs.8366.

Malik, B. R., Maddison, D. C., Smith, G. A. and Peters, O. M. 2019. Autophagic and endo-lysosomal dysfunction in neurodegenerative disease. *Molecular Brain* 12:100. doi: 10.1186/s13041-019-0504-x.

Manap, A. S. A., Vijayabalan, S., Madhavan, P., Chia, Y. Y., Arya, A., Wong, E. H., Rizwan, F., Bindal, U. and Koshy, S. 2019. *Bacopa monnieri*, a Neuroprotective Lead in Alzheimer Disease: A Review on Its Properties, Mechanisms of Action, and Preclinical and Clinical Studies. *Drug Target Insights* 13:1-13. doi: 10.1177/1177392819866412.

Maraganore, D. M., Lesnick, T. G., Elbaz, A., Chartier-Harlin, M. C., Gasser, T., Krüger, R., Hattori, N., Mellick, G. D., Quattrone, A., Satoh, J., Toda, T., Wang, J., Ioannidis, J. P., de Andrade, M., Rocca, W. A. and UCHL Global Genetics Consortium. 2004. UCHL1 is a Parkinson's disease susceptibility gene. *Annals of Neurology* 55 4: 512-21. doi: 10.1002/ana. 20017.

Markham, Charles H. and Diamond, Shirley G. 1981. Evidence to support early levodopa therapy in Parkinson's disease. *Neurology*, 31:125-131. doi: 10.1212/wnl.31.2.125.

Marsden, C. D. 1994. Parkinson's disease. *Journal of Neurology Neurosurgery & Psychiatry* 57:672-681. doi: 10.1136/jnnp.57.6.672.

Marsden, C. D. and Parkes J. D. 1977. Success and problems of long-term levodopa therapy in Parkinson's disease. *The Lancet* 1:345-349. doi: 10.1016/s0140-6736(77)91146-1.

Mathur, D., Goyal, K., Koul, V. and Anand, A. 2016. The Molecular Links of Re-Emerging Therapy: A Review of Evidence of Brahmi (*Bacopa monniera*). *Frontiers in Pharmacology* 4:7:44. doi: 10.3389/fphar. 2016.00044.

McGeer, Patrick L. and McGeer, Edith G. 2008. Glial reaction in Parkinson's disease. *Movement Disorders* 23:474-483. doi:10.1002/mds.21751.

McGeer, Patrick L., Itagaki, Shigeru, Akiyama, Haruhiko and McGeer, Edith G. 1988. Rate of cell death in parkinsonism indicates active neuropathological process. *Annals of Neurolgy* 24:574-576. doi:10.1002/ ana.410240415.

Michel, Haidy E., Tadros, Mariane G., Esmat, Ahmed, Khalifa, Amani E. and Abdel-Tawab, Ahmed M. 2016. Tetramethylpyrazine Ameliorates Rotenone-Induced Parkinson's Disease in Rats: Involvement of Its Anti-Inflammatory and Anti-Apoptotic Actions. *Molecular Neurobiology*, 54:4866-4878. doi: 10.1007/s12035-016-0028-7.

Mínguez-Castellanos, Adolfo, Escamilla-Sevilla, Francisco, Hotton, Gary R, Toledo-Aral, Juan J., Ortega-Moreno, Ángel, Méndez-Ferrer, Simón,

Martín-Linares, José M., Katati, Majed J., Mir, Pablo, Villadiego, Javier, Meersmans, Miguel, Pérez-García, Miguel, Brooks, David J., Arjona, Ventura, and López-Barneo, José. 2007. Carotid body autotransplantation in Parkinson's disease: a clinical and positron emission tomography study. *Journal of Neurology, Neurosurgery & Psychiatry* 78:825-831. doi: 10.1136/jnnp.2006.106021.

Mirza, B., Ikram, H., Bilgrami, S., Haleem, D. J. and Haleem, M. A. 2013. Neurochemical and behavioral effects of green tea (*Camellia sinensis*): a model study. *Pakistan Journal of Pharmaceutical Sciences* 26:511-6.

More, S. V., Kumar, H., Kang, S. M., Song, S. Y., Lee, K. and Choi, D. K. 2013. Advances in neuroprotective ingredients of medicinal herbs by using cellular and animal models of Parkinson's disease. *Evidence-Based Complementary* and *Alternative Medicine* 2013:957875. doi: 10.1155/2013/957875.

Mu X., He G. R., Yuan X., Li X. X. and Du G. H. 2011. Baicalein protects the brain against neuron impairments induced by MPTP in C57BL/6 mice. *Pharmacology Biochemistry and Behavior* 98:286–291. doi: 10.1016/j.pbb.2011.01.011.

Obeso, José A., Rodríguez-Oroz, María C., Rodríguez, Manuel, Arbizu, Javier and Giménez-Amaya, José M. 2002. The basal ganglia and disorders of movement: pathophysiological mechanisms. *News in Physiological Sciences* 17:51-55. doi: 10.1152/nips.01363.2001.

Olanow, C. W., Kordower, J. H., Lang, A. E. and Obeso, J. A. 2009. Dopaminergic transplantation for Parkinson's disease: current status and future prospects. *Annals of Neurology* 66:591-6. doi: 10.1002/ana.21778.

Olanow, C. W. and Kordower, J. H. 2009. Modeling Parkinson's disease. *Annals of Neurology* 66:432-436. doi: 10.1002/ana.21832.

Olanow, Warren, Watts, Ray L., and Koller, William C. 2001. An algorithm (decision tree) for the management of Parkinson's disease. *Neurology* 56:1-88. doi: 10.1212/wnl.56.suppl_5.s1.

Orayj, Khalid, and Lane, Emma. 2019. Patterns and Determinants of Prescribing for Parkinson's Disease: A Systematic Literature Review. *Hindawi Parkinson's Disease* 2019:1-40. doi: 10.1155/2019/9237181.

Organisation for Economic Co-operation and Development. 2019. *Health Status: Causes of mortality.* Accessed December 2019. https://stats.oecd.org/Index.aspx?QueryId=30115.

Palasz, Ewelina, Niewiadomski, Wiktor, Gasiorowska, Anna, Wysocka, Adrianna, Stepniewska, Anna and Niewiadomska, Grazyna. 2019. Exercise-Induced Neuroprotection and Recovery of Motor Function in

Animal Models of Parkinson's Disease. *Frontiers in Neurology* 10:1-15. doi: 10.3389/fneur.2019.01143.

Pardo, B., Mena, M. A., Casarejos, M. J., Paino, C. L. and De Yébenes, J. G. 1995. Toxic effects of L-dopa on mesencephalic cells cultures: protection with antioxidants. *Brain Research.* 682:133-143. doi: 10.1016/0006-8993(95)00341-m.

Parkinson, J. 1817. An essay on the shaking palsy. *The Journal of Neuropsychiatry and Clinical Neurosciences* 14: 223-236. doi: 10.1176/jnp.14.2.223.

Parkinson's Disease Research Group. 1993. Comparisons of therapeutic effects of levodopa, levodopa and selegilina, and bromocriptine in patients with early, mild Parkinson's disease: three-year interim report. *The BMJ.* 307:469-472. doi: 10.1136/bmj.307.6902.469.

Patel, R. S., Kamil, S., Shah, M. R., Bhimanadham, N. N. and Imran, S. 2019. Pros and Cons of Marijuana in Treatment of Parkinson's Disease. *Cureus* 11:4813. doi: 10.7759/cureus.4813.

Pearce, J. M. 1989. Aspects of the history of Parkinson's disease. *Journal of Neurology, Neurosurgery, and Psychiatry* 52:6-10. doi: 10.1136/jnnp.52.suppl.6.

Pickrell, A. M. and Youle, R. J. 2015. The Roles of PINK1, Parkin and Mitochondrial Fidelity in Parkinson's Disease. *Neuron* 85:257–273. doi: 10.1016/j.neuron.2014.12.007

Pinel, John P. J. 2007. *Biopsicología.* Pearson Educación. Cap. III.

Polymeropoulos, M. H., Lavedan, C., Leroy, E., Ide, S. E., Dehejia, A., Dutra, A., Pike, B., Root, H., Rubenstein, J., Boyer, R., Stenroos, E. S., Chandrasekharappa, S., Athanassiadou, A., Papapetropoulos, T., Johnson, W. G., Lazzarini, A. M., Duvoisin, R. C., Di Iorio, G., Golbe, L. I. and Nussbaum, R. L. 1997. Mutation in the alpha-synuclein gene identified in families with Parkinson's disease. *Science* 276:2045-2047. doi: 10.1126/science.276.5321.2045.

Przuntek, H., Conrad, B., Dichgans, J., Kraus, P. H., Krauseneck, P., Pergande, G., Rinne, U., Schimrigk, K., Schnitker, J. and Vogel H. P. 1999. SELEDO: a 5-year long-term trial on the effect of selegiline in early parkinsonian patients treated with levodopa. *European Journal of Neurology* 6: 141-150. doi: 10.1111/j.1468-1331.1999.tb00007.x.

Quinn, N., Parkes, D., Janota, I. and Marsden, C. D. 1986. Preservation of the substantia nigra and locus coeruleus in a patient receiving levodopa (2 Kg) plus decarboxylase inhibitor over a 4-year period. *Movement Disorders* 1:65-68. doi: 10.1002/mds.870010109.

Rabiei, Z., Solati, K. and Amini-Khoei, H. 2019. Phytotherapy in treatment of Parkinson's disease: a review. *Pharmaceutical Biology* 57:355-362. doi: 10.1080/13880209.2019.1618344.

Radhakrishnan, Divya M. and Goyal, Vinay. 2018. Parkinson´s: a review. *Neurology India* 66:26-35. doi: 10.4103/0028-3886.226451.

RajaSankar, Srinivasagam, Manivasagam, Thamilarasan, and Surendran, Sankar. 2009. Ashwagandha leaf extract: A potential agent in treating oxidative damage and physiological abnormalities seen in a mouse model of Parkinson's disease. *Neuroscience Letters* 454:11-15. doi: 10.1016/j.neulet.2009.02.044.

Rajput, A. H., Fenton, M. E., Birdi, S. and Macaulay, R. 1997. Is levodopa toxic to substantia nigra? *Movement Disorders* 12:634-638. doi: 10.1002/mds.870120503.

Rangasamy, Suresh B., Soderstrom, Katherine, Bakay, Roy A. and Kordower, Jeffrey H. 2010. Neurotrophic factor therapy for Parkinson's disease. *Progress in Brain Research* 184:237-264. doi: 10.1016/S0079-6123(10)84013-0.

Ritz, B. R., Manthripragada, A. D., Costello, S., Lincoln, S. J., Farrer, M. J., Cockburn, M. and Bronstein, J. 2009. Dopamine transporter genetic variants and pesticides in Parkinson's disease. *Environmental Health Perspectives* 117:964-969. doi: 10.1289/ehp.0800277.

Samii, A., Turnbull, I. M., Kishore, A., Schulzer, M., Mak, E., Yardley, S. and Calne, D. B. 1999. Reassessment of unilateral pallidotomy in Parkinson´s disease. *Brain*. 122:417-425. doi: 10.1093/brain/122.3.417.

Sánchez-Martínez, C. M., Choreño-Parra, J. A., Placencia-Álvarez, N., Nuñez-Orozco, L. and Guadarrama-Ortiz, P. 2019. Frequency and Dynamics of Non-motor Symptoms Presentation in Hispanic Patients With Parkinson Disease. *Frontiers in Neurology* 10:1197. doi: 10.3389/fneur.2019.01197.

Schapira, Anthony H. 2009. Neurobiology and treatment of Parkinson's disease. *Trends in Pharmacological Sciences* 30:41-47. doi: 10.1016/j.tips.2008.10.005.

Sergi, D., Renaud, J., Simola, N. and Martinoli, M. G. 2019. Diabetes, a Contemporary Risk for Parkinson's Disease: Epidemiological and Cellular Evidences. *Frontiers in Aging Neuroscience* 11:302. doi: 10.3389/fnagi.2019.00302.

Shah, N. C. 2004. Indigenous Uses and Ethnobotany of *Cannabis sativa* L. (Hemp) in Uttaranchal (India). *Journal of Industrial Hemp* 9:69-77. doi: 10.1300/J237v09n01_07.

Shimoji, Mika, Zhang, Li, Mandir, Allen S., Dawson, Valina L. and Dawson, Ted M. 2005. Absence of inclusion body formation in the MPTP mouse model of Parkinson's disease. *Molecular Brain Research* 134:103-108. doi: 10.1016/j.molbrainres.2005.01.012.

Sidransky, E. and Lopez, G. 2012. The link between the GBA gene and parkinsonism. *The Lancet Neuroly* 11:986-98. doi: 10.1016/S1474-4422(12)70190-4.

Singh, B., Pandey, S., Rumman, M. and Mahdi, A. A. 2019. Neuroprotective effects of Bacopa monnieri in Parkinson's disease model. *Metabolic Brain Disease* 34:1-9. doi: 10.1007/s11011-019-00526-w.

Sriram, Krishnan, Matheson, Joanna M., Benkovic, Stanley A., Miller, Diane B., Luster, Michael I. and O'Callaghan, James P. 2002. Mice deficient in TNF receptors are protected against dopaminergic neurotoxicity: implications for Parkinson's disease. *The FASEB Journal* 16:1474-1476. doi: 10.1096/fj.02-0216fje.

Stern, G. 1989. Did parkinsonism occur before 1817?. *Journal of Neurology, Neurosurgery, and Psychiatry* 52:11-12. doi: 10.1136/jnnp.52.suppl.11.

Streit, Wolfgang J. 2002. Microglia as neuroprotective, immunocompetent cells of the CNS. *Glia* 40:133-139. doi: 10.1002/glia.10154.

Sulzer, David. 2007. Multiple hit hypotheses for dopamine neuron loss in Parkinson's disease. *Trends Neurosciences* 30:244-250. doi: 10.1016/j.tins.2007.03.009.

Swathy, S. S., Panicker, S., Nithya, R. S., Anuja, M. M., Rejitha, S. and Indira, M. 2010. Antiperoxidative and antiinflammatory effect of *Sida cordifolia* Linn. on quinolinic acid induced neurotoxicity. *Neurochemical Research* 35:1361-7. doi: 10.1007/s11064-010-0192-5.

Tansey, Malú G. and Goldberg, Matthew S. 2010. Neuroinflammation in Parkinson's disease: its role in neuronal death and implications for therapeutic intervention. *Neurobiology of Disease* 37:510-8. doi: 10.1016/j.nbd.2009.11.004.

Teng, L., Hong, F., Zhang, C., He, J. and Wang, H. 2014. Compound Formula Rehmannia alleviates levodopa-induced dyskinesia in Parkinson's disease. *Neural Regeneration Research* 9:407-12. doi: 10.4103/1673-5374.128246.

Toledo-Aral, Juan J., Mendez-Ferrer, Simón, Pardal, Ricardo and Lopez-Barneo, José. 2002. Dopaminergic cells of the carotid body: physiological significance and possible therapeutic applications in Parkinson's disease. *Brain Research Bullettin* 57:847-853. doi: 10.1016/s0361-9230(01)00771-7.

Tripanichkul W. and Jaroensuppaperch E. O. 2012. Curcumin protects nigrostriatal dopaminergic neurons and reduces glial activation in 6-hydroxydopamine hemiparkinsonian mice model. *International Journal of Neuroscience* 122:263–270. doi: 10.3109/00207454.2011.648760.

Trousseau, A. 1861. Lecture XV. *Senile trembling and paralysis agitans.* Lectures on Clinical Medicine Delivered at the Hotel Dieu. Paris.

van Kessel, S. P. and El Aidy, S. 2019. Contributions of Gut Bacteria and Diet to Drug Pharmacokinetics in the Treatment of Parkinson's Disease. *Frontiers in Neurology* 15;10:1087. doi: 10.3389/fneur.2019.01087.

Van Laar, T., Boertien, J. M. and Herranz, A. H. 2019. Faecal Transplantation, Pro- and Prebiotics in Parkinson's Disease; Hope or Hype?. *Journal of Parkinson's Disease* 9:371-379. doi: 10.3233/JPD-191802.

Vecchia, D. D., Schamne, M. G., Ferro, M. M., Santos AFCd, Latyki, C. L., Lara, D. V., Ben, J., Moreira, E. L., Prediger, R. D. and Miyoshi, E. 2015. Effects of *Hypericum perforatum* on turning behavior in an animal model of Parkinson's disease. *Brazilian Journal of Pharmaceutical Sciences* 51:111-115. doi: 10.1590/S1984-82502015000100012.

Wang M. S., Boddapati S., Emadi S. and Sierks M. R. 2010. Curcumin reduces alpha-synuclein induced cytotoxicity in Parkinson's disease cell model. *BMC Neuroscience* 11:57. doi: 10.1186/1471-2202-11-57.

Wang Y., Xu H., Fu Q., Ma R. and Xiang J. 2011. Protective effect of resveratrol derived from *Polygonum cuspidatum* and its liposomal form on nigral cells in parkinsonian rats. *Journal of theNeurological Sciences* 304:29–34.doi: 10.1016/j.jns.2011.02.025.

Wang, L., Zhang, J., Hong, Y., Feng, Y., Chen, M. and Wang, Y. 2013. Phytochemical and pharmacological review of da chuanxiong formula: a famous herb pair composed of chuanxiong rhizoma and gastrodiae rhizoma for headache. *Evidence-Based Complementary* and *Alternative Medicine* 2013:425369. doi: 10.1155/2013/425369.

Wang, Q., Zhang, Y., Wang, M., Song, W. M., Shen, Q., McKenzie, A., Choi, I., Zhou, X., Pan, P. Y., Yue, Z. and Zhang, B. 2019. The landscape of multiscale transcriptomic networks and key regulators in Parkinson's disease. *Nature Communications* 10:5234. doi: 10.1038/s41467-019-13144-y.

Watts, R. L. 1997. The role of dopamine agonists in early Parkinson's disease. *Neurology* 49:34-48. doi: 10.1212/wnl.49.1_suppl_1.s34.

Wider, Christian and Wszolek, Zbigniew K. 2008. Etiology and pathophysiology of frontotemporal dementia, Parkinson disease and

Alzheimer disease: lessons from genetic studies. *Neurodegener Diseases* 5:122-125. doi: 10.1159/000113680.

Wu Y., Li X., Zhu J. X., Xie W., Le W., Fan Z., Jankovic J. and Pan T. 2011. Resveratrol-activated AMPK/SIRT1/autophagy in cellular models of Parkinson's disease. *NeuroSignals* 19:163–174. doi: 10.1159/000328516.

Xu, L., Chen, W. F. and Wong, M. S. 2009. Ginsenoside Rg1 protects dopaminergic neurons in a rat model of Parkinson's disease through the IGF-I receptor signalling pathway. *British Journal of Pharmacology* 158:738–748. doi: 10.1111/j.1476-5381.2009. 00361. X.

Yahr, M. D., Duvoisin, R. C., Schear, M. J., Barrett, R. E. and Hoehn, M. M. 1969. Treatment of parkinsonism with levodopa. *Archives of Neurology* 21:343-54. doi: 10.1001/archneur.1969.00480160015001.

Yang, Dongming, Zhao, Deming, Ali Shah, Syed Z., Wu, Wei, Lai, Mengyu, Zhang, Xixi, Li, Jie, Guan, Zhiling, Zhao, Huafen, Li, Wen, Gao, Hongli, Zhou, Xiangmei and Yang, Lifeng. 2019. The Role of the Gut Microbiota in the Pathogenesis of Parkinson's Disease. *Frontiers in Neurology* 10:1155. doi: 10.3389/fneur.2019.01155.

Yu, H., Oh-Hashi, K., Tanaka, T., Sai, A., Inoue, M., Hirata, Y. and Kiuchi, K. 2006. *Rehmannia glutinosa* induces glial cell line-derived neurotrophic factor gene expression in astroglial cells via cPKC and ERK1/2 pathways independently. *Pharmacological Research* 54:39-45. doi: 10.1016/j.phrs.2006.01.014.

Zhang, R. X., Li, M. X. and Jia, Z. P. 2008. *Rehmannia glutinosa*: review of botany, chemistry and pharmacology. *Journal of Ethnopharmacology* 117:199-214. doi: 10.1016/j.jep.2008.02.018.

Zhang H. N., An C. N., Xu M., Guo D. A., Li M. and Pu X. P. 2009. Protocatechuic acid inhibits rat pheochromocytoma cell damage induced by a dopaminergic neurotoxin. *Biological and Pharmaceutical Bulletin* 32:1866–1869. doi: 10.1248/bpb.32.1866.

Zhang H. N., An C. N., Zhang H. N. and Pu X. P. 2010. Protocatechuic acid inhibits neurotoxicity induced by MPTP *in vivo*. *Neuroscience Letters*, 474: 99–103. doi: 10.1016/j.neulet.2010.03.016.

Zhao, L. and Pu, X 2006. Neuroprotective effect of acteoside against MPTP-induced mouse model of Parkinson's disease. *Chinese Pharmacological Bulletin* 23:42–46.

Zhao Q., Gao J., Li W. and Cai D. 2010. Neurotrophic and neurorescue effects of Echinacoside in the subacute MPTP mouse model of Parkinson's disease. *Brain Research* 1346:224–236. doi: 10.1016/j.brainres.2010.05.018.

Zhao, Y. J., Wee, H. L., Chan, Y. H., Seah, S. H., Au, W. L., Lau, P. N., Pica, E. C., Li, S. C., Luo, N. and Tan, L. C. 2010. Progression of Parkinson's disease as evaluated by Hoehn and Yahr stage transition times. *Movement Disorders* 25:710-6. doi: 10.1002/mds.22875.

About the Editors

Anaberta Cardador Martínez

Research Professor

Tecnologico de Moterrey, Escuela de Ingeniería y Ciencias.

Dra. Anaberta Cardador is a professor at Tecnologico de Monterrey (Mexico) since 2007. Her research projects are focused on the identifications and use of compounds from crops and food by-products to develop nutraceuticals products. Also, to study biological activities of such compounds, for instance, antioxidant, antihypertensive, hypocholesterolemic, antimicrobial and anti-inflammatory.

Víctor M. Rodríguez García

Research Professor

Tecnologico de Moterrey, Escuela de Ingeniería y Ciencias.

Dr. Victor Rodriguez is a research professor at the ITESM (Mexico) since 2013, collaborating in the Department of Bioengineering. His current research projects are focused on the genetic background for metabolic conditions in Mexican populations, medicinal plant's bioprospecting and molecular ecology of endemic plant species used as raw materials for the production and extraction of medicinal compounds.

Patricia Manzano

Professor
ESPOL Polythecnic University, Escuela Superior Politécnica del Litoral,
ESPOL, Centro de Investigaciones Biotecnológicas del Ecuador,
ESPOL Polythecnic University, Escuela Superior Politécnica del Litoral,
ESPOL, Facultad de Ciencias de la Vida

Dra. Patricia Manzano works as a researcher at the Escuela Superior Politecnica del Litoral (ESPOL) and as Head Research of Bioproducts and Bioprocess Laboratory at the Centro de Investigaciones Biotecnológicas del Ecuador (CIBE) in ESPOL. She has experience in the area of natural products, and the development of bioproducts and their potential use in agriculture, health, and food industry, especially in the development of biostimulants. She has published 25 articles in indexed journals and four book chapters about phytochemicals.

Maritza Alonzo Macías

Research Professor
Tecnologico de Moterrey, Escuela de Ingeniería y Ciencias.

Dra. Maritza Alonzo has a BS in Biochemical Engineering, a MS in Food Science and a PhD in Process Engineering. Her research work is focused on the area of emerging technologies applied in foods and medicinal plants, extraction of essential oils and biomolecules, and their characterization.

INDEX

β

A

B

C

D

E

F

G

H

I

K

L

M

N

O

P

Q

R

S

T

U

V

W

Z